The
Endometriosis
Health & Diet Program

Get Your Life Back

Dr. Andrew S. Cook, MD, FACOG
Author of *Stop Endometriosis and Pelvic Pain*
Danielle Cook, MS, RD, CDE

Robert
ROSE

Design and Production: Daniella Zanchetta/PageWave Graphics Inc.
Editors: Sue Sumeraj and Bonnie Munday
Copy editor: Linda Pruessen
Recipe editor: Jennifer MacKenzie
Proofreader: Wendy Potter
Indexer: Gillian Watts
Nutrient analysis: Magda Fahmy

Cover photo: Woman holding apple © iStockphoto.com/DragonImages
Back cover photos: Yoga pose © iStockphoto.com/Steex; Healthy salad © iStockphoto.com/Ridofranz

Published by Robert Rose Inc.
120 Eglinton Avenue East, Suite 800, Toronto, Ontario, Canada M4P 1E2
Tel: (416) 322-6552 Fax: (416) 322-6936
www.robertrose.ca

Printed and bound in Canada

2 3 4 5 6 7 8 9 MI 25 24 23 22 21 20 19 18

MIX
Paper from
responsible sources
FSC
www.fsc.org
FSC® C103567

Contents

Part 3: Diet Plan for Endometriosis and Pelvic Pain

Part 4: Recipes for Endometriosis and Pelvic Pain

Introduction

Health is a spectrum and everyone starts somewhere on that spectrum. Movement toward better health along that spectrum is the ultimate goal. Each small change you make is a gift you are giving to yourself, and forward movement in the healing process.

— *Danielle Cook*

As it turns out, there is quite a bit women with endometriosis can do — independent of their doctor or anyone else. Your situation is not hopeless.

Endometriosis is a mysterious disease that is poorly understood by almost everyone, including the vast majority of physicians and health-care providers responsible for treating this condition. Endometriosis can cause unbelievably severe pain, worse than that of surgery or childbirth. Although this is a benign disease, meaning it is not a cancer, its impact can be devastating, effectively robbing a woman of her ability to live a functional life. While there is no known "cure" for endometriosis, there are effective treatments. For example, once treated properly with a surgical procedure known as wide excision, most women will never experience recurrence. While not a cancer, endometriosis is a tumor that needs to be completely removed.

The strict definition of endometriosis is "the presence of lesions in the pelvis similar to the tissue found inside of the uterus," but the reality can be much more far-reaching. One of the authors of this book, Dr. Andrew Cook, has been treating endometriosis — or "endo" — in private practice for 25 years. Over this time, he has seen and learned a lot. Treating endometriosis is not just a job for him; it is a mission in life. The amount of pain, suffering and invalidation a woman experiences as a result of endo is unnecessary, and the lack of care and concern is deplorable; the average "medical care" provided to women with endometriosis is poor and really quite shameful. This has historically resulted in women continuing to live in pain, at the mercy of their treating physician, with no real power to effect a change in their own life.

As it turns out, there is quite a bit women with endometriosis can do — independent of their doctor or anyone else. Your situation is not hopeless. It may be quite difficult, and we are not saying it will be an easy fix, but you do gain a lot of power when you have the correct information. You will need to become educated and actively participate in making healthy choices in your life. This can initially seem overwhelming and confusing, but the information in this book is designed to provide a road map — one you can follow to regain your health and decrease your pain. (If you have significant endometriosis, you may need to combine the work you are doing with excisional surgery to remove the tissue that is causing your pain.) This book will provide you with the most up-to-date, scientifically based, comprehensive information on diet, lifestyle and holistic treatment for endometriosis.

A Call to Action

On behalf of women worldwide and as director of the World Society of Endometriosis Surgeons, Dr. Cook implores and challenges the medical community to once and for all abandon the outdated beliefs surrounding endometriosis and the practices still all too commonly used for women with endometriosis. It is time to turn the page on acceptance of practices that are not supported scientifically and are substandard in the treatment of endometriosis. Patients deserve to be heard, understood and believed. If an OB/GYN chooses to see and treat women with endometriosis as part of their practice, they need to take responsibility for learning the complexity of this disease and how to treat it effectively. Hysterectomy does not cure endometriosis, nor is it alone an effective or appropriate treatment. Coagulation (burning surgery) is substandard and should be relegated to the history books. Wide excision surgery has unequivocally been shown to be the most effective treatment modality for removal of endometriotic tissue with very low recurrence rates.

At Vital Health Institute (VHI), we constantly strive to provide the best treatment strategies, not just for our patients but for all women with endo. That is how this book was born. This is the third book in a series we have published about endometriosis. After reviewing the most up-to-date research, listening to our patients' stories and tapping into the experience gained over 25 years of treating patients with endometriosis, we have devised a comprehensive and integrative program for endo. We wanted to share this program and put the healing power into the hands of women who suffer from this disease, their caregivers and their providers. This book is meant to be a resource, and serves as a starting point for building an individualized program. The plan is meant to be easy to understand yet comprehensive.

Our hope for this book is that it can be a tool in your ever-growing toolbox to help treat and manage endo. Whether you suffer from it, have a loved one who suffers from it or are a practitioner caring for women with this disease, our sincere desire is that the information provided in the following pages can serve as a guide for relief and healing.

We would love to hear your feedback and your stories. Please send these to patientstories@vitalhealth.com.

With love and healing thoughts,

— Danielle and Andrew

> **Whether you suffer from endo, have a loved one who suffers from it or are a practitioner caring for women with this disease, our sincere desire is that the information provided in the following pages can serve as a guide for relief and healing.**

Part 1

Diagnosis, Pathophysiology and Conventional Treatment

Part 1 provides basic information about endometriosis; contributing factors in its development (pathophysiology); and a description of conventional treatment. In this section you will gain a better understanding of the medical side of endo and how various lifestyle factors such as stress may impact the disease. Here you'll find the evidence-based rationale for why various lifestyle changes are being recommended. If you are a person who needs to know the "why," it's a must-read.

Chapter 1
What Is Endometriosis?

What It Really Means to Have Endometriosis

Endometriosis by definition is a disease process whereby tissue somewhat like the endometrium (the lining of the uterus) exists outside the uterus. This "rogue" endometriotic-like tissue most commonly involves the peritoneum, a thin layer of tissue that lines the pelvic structures, the bowel, the bladder and the ovaries. Quite frankly, a lot of this medical stuff can be quite dry and boring and does not convey what it is like for a woman to have this disease or how it truly impacts her family, her career, her sex life and her ability to live her life in very basic ways.

In reality, this disease can be like having tens or hundreds of excruciatingly painful blisters covering the inside of the pelvis. Pelvic pain and infertility are the two most common symptoms of endometriosis. For the lucky ones, the pain lasts just a couple of days during their period; in the worst cases, the pain is 24/7. The fact that women with endometriosis look fine on the outside can cause even well-meaning people to doubt the severity of their pain.

Most women with endo begin to have pain in their teenage years, sometimes even starting in elementary school. While similar in timing, this pain is completely different than normal menstrual cramps. It is not uncommon for these girls to miss several of days of school each month from cyclic pain that can exceed the level of pain patients experience after major surgery.

A lack of awareness of this disease can leave these girls without a correct diagnosis and support from their physicians. This, in turn, can lead to a lack of appropriate treatment for the pain and an invalidation of the patient's situation. Her family may now be led to believe that psychological issues drive the severity of her pain. In this tragic situation, she is effectively held prisoner and tortured by her own body in broad daylight, with no one who fully understands her situation or who can effectively help her.

The symptoms usually progress as she matures into a young woman. Both the severity and duration of the pain typically increase. Initially, most days each month are pain-free, but the number of these pain-free days is slowly replaced by an increasing number of non-functioning pain days. The unpredictability of the increasing number of pain days makes it challenging to maintain a functional life. It becomes increasingly difficult for her to make plans for a future date, as it becomes more likely that it will be a pain day, and she will not be able to follow through on her commitment for any activity.

Endometriosis can take away many additional aspects of a normal life. The days of feeling like a vibrant, desirable woman are long since gone. Acting like the loving, compassionate woman, mother and partner that she truly is becomes more and more difficult. Stress on family relationships is common and real.

Even at this stage, most women fight the disease, refusing to let it completely take over their lives. You would most likely pass right by them in public, having no idea of the devastation with which they are dealing. Most of the time they get up, put on a brave face and do their best to live a normal life.

The medical definition of endometriosis does not even begin to describe the reality of what it means to have the disease. The next time you hear about endometriosis, remember how devastating it can be. If you have a loved one, friend or co-worker who suffers from endometriosis, please remember to treat them with respect and compassion.

There is a lot about endometriosis that we do not understand, including basics such as what causes it, why some women get it and others do not, how it causes infertility and how it causes pain. Medical professionals cannot agree on just what constitutes endometriosis. Is it simply endometriotic implants in the pelvis that can be removed surgically with wide excision to cure the patient of her symptoms? Or is it a more complex systemic (or whole-body), multi-system dysfunction causing underlying health issues, with endometriotic implants in the pelvis as just part of the overall picture? If the first interpretation is correct, then we need to convince surgeons to use wide excision in place of coagulation (burning) to effectively resolve pain. If the latter is true, then a comprehensive holistic approach — in addition to excisional surgery — is required.

In 2005, in a debate hosted by the Endometriosis Association at their 25th annual conference, Dr. David Redwine argued that "endometriosis is a locally-focused disease requiring only good surgery." Dr. Redwine actively promoted the idea of wide excision as the standard of surgery for treatment of endometriosis, which improved treatment for women. However, we now know that a broader definition of the disease is required for successful treatment. Let's look at this topic in a bit more detail.

No, It's Not "All In Your Head"

All too often, it seems that when members of the medical profession do not understand or have good therapies for a medical condition, they question the validity of the physical diagnosis and do not trust the patient. We all have personal issues that may affect how we experience a given situation, and endometriosis patients are not immune from these, but personal issues do not cause the pain. Endometriosis is a real medical condition that causes real pain and health issues for millions of women, affecting their quality of life as well as the quality of life of those in their lives. The pain is real, and not in their heads, as so many women with endometriosis are told. In our experience, women with endometriosis are strong, determined people suffering from a devastating medical illness.

Endometriosis Defined

If symptoms remain after hormonal suppression or surgical treatment, patients are often made to feel that it is all in their head, and that there is no physical basis for their health problems.

The narrowest definition of endometriosis, as we've seen, is the presence of endometriotic-like tissue — tissue very similar to the inside lining of the uterus, called the endometrium — in the pelvis that can result in a variety of symptoms, including progressively painful periods, pelvic pain, pain with intercourse, pain with bowel movements, constant pelvic pain, low back pain, fatigue and infertility.[1] This narrow concept presumes that the root of all of these symptoms is the endometriotic implants. This limited view common in traditional Western medical practices is that symptoms will resolve once the implants are suppressed hormonally or removed surgically. If symptoms remain after hormonal suppression or surgical treatment, patients are often made to feel that it is all in their head, and that there is no physical basis for their health problems.

Over the last couple of decades, this belief has resulted in endo support groups, patients and some health-care providers trying to raise awareness of endometriosis. This campaign has taken shape on two fronts. The first is focused on bringing attention to the fact that the disease exists and is a valid medical condition. The second has been an effort to educate patients and physicians on the importance of using the wide excision surgical treatment option, rather than burning or coagulation, to provide more effective treatment.

Recently, there has been good progress in raising the level of awareness of endometriosis as a disease. There has also been steady progress when it comes to women themselves understanding the importance of wide excision. Unfortunately, there is still work to do with regard to physicians' awareness, not only in believing the true severity of the pain but also on the importance and implementation of wide excision.

It's hard to believe that it has taken so long to bring awareness to a disease that affects so many people. The Internet, available to the public only since August 6, 1991, has been tremendously empowering to women with this disease. Women who previously felt alone, isolated and "crazy" have been able to connect with others going through the same difficult experience. The Internet has also been a vehicle for dissemination of important information about this disease and its treatment.

Many women with endometriosis will have most of their pain resolved with surgical wide excision. But what about those who continue to suffer? The fact that the removal of the implants didn't "cure" these women tells us that there is a missing link in the treatment plan. Scientific research and our clinical experience with endometriosis reveal beyond a shadow of doubt that endometriosis is, at least in a significant number of women, more than just implants in the pelvis.

Evolution of a Definition

Let's review the progression of our understanding of endometriosis over the last couple of decades. Initially, it was thought that endometriosis and its associated pain were a result of abnormal growths of displaced endometrium in the pelvis. The treatment involved coagulation surgery (the burning of the endometriotic implants), a hysterectomy with removal of both ovaries, or GnRH hormonal suppression with increasingly powerful prescription medications, often accompanied by uncomfortable side effects. If a woman continued to have pain after hysterectomy or medically induced menopause, her pain was thought to be psychosomatic (just in her head) and was commonly believed to be secondary to childhood trauma and abuse. Unfortunately, this situation is still all too prevalent today — this is in spite of scientific studies clearly proving endometriotic tissue can continue to grow in the absence of systemic estrogen.[4]

Dr. Cook has surgically removed endometriotic tissue, confirmed as such by surgical pathology specimens, from countless patients without estrogen, including a woman in her late 60s who had gone through a hysterectomy with removal of both ovaries 25 years earlier and who never took estrogen. He recently operated on a transgender male, assigned female at birth but whose gender identity is male, who had transitioned physically and hormonally to male. The patient had a history of pelvic pain and endometriosis and had subsequently undergone a hysterectomy with removal of both ovaries. He was on testosterone treatment; laboratory blood tests confirmed a lack of estrogen and high-normal male values of testosterone. He was a hormonal desert for endometriosis! However, during surgery,

Dr. Cook found endometriotic tissue throughout the pelvis, with confirmation on the surgical pathology specimens. Four days after surgery, the patient looked and felt better than he had the day prior to surgery. This type of unnecessary pain and suffering has been going on for decades.

The overly simplistic definition of endometriosis as nothing more than pelvic implants found in stressed out, over-reactive women that can be easily resolved with the induction of medical menopause, coagulation surgery or even hysterectomy with removal of ovaries is insulting to the women who suffer from this medical condition. The first step is for physicians to recognize and truly believe the plight of women afflicted with this disease and to educate themselves on its complexity and causes. This includes understanding the effectiveness of wide excision surgery as well as the powerful lifestyle changes necessary to correct underlying physiological, immunological and genetic defects. Reaching this milestone as the standard of care would be a huge step in the evolution of treatment of this disease, with a future goal of eliminating unnecessary pain and suffering in a massive number of women.

> The first step is for physicians to recognize and truly believe the plight of women afflicted with this disease and to educate themselves on its complexity and causes.

FAQ

Q. Is endo a disease or a syndrome?

A. A disease is defined as a disorder in a system or organ that affects the body's function — in this case, endometriotic implants in the pelvis that result in pain and infertility. If endo were strictly a disease, the pain would resolve and fertility be fully restored when the implants are completely removed. A syndrome is defined as a collection of signs and symptoms known to frequently appear together but without a known cause. We contend that endometriosis is actually a continuum of health issues, with the simple cases being a disease and the more complex cases a syndrome of health issues. Back in the 1990s, Dr. Cook coined the term MSDS, or multi-system dysfunction syndrome, in an attempt to describe the complexity of the health issues facing many women with endometriosis. This title was the result of years of observation. Dr. Cook consistently noted a combination of malfunctioning systems in the body that negatively influenced one another and that, together, fueled a woman's downward spiral of poor health and discomfort.

What Causes Chronic Pelvic Pain?

The next step in correctly understanding the definition of endometriosis is an appreciation of the large number of other traditionally accepted medical conditions that may be associated with the disease. Chronic pelvic pain is defined as pain located below the belly button that lasts for 6 months or longer. It may or may not be associated with a woman's menstrual cycle. Endometriosis is one of the leading causes of pelvic pain, but it is not the only cause. As we will see in the next chapter, there are many conventional medical conditions that might contribute to a woman's pelvic pain. In order to fully resolve pelvic pain, other forms of medical treatment may be necessary based on which condition or combination of conditions is contributing to the overall pain and symptomology.

These conditions are often contributors to the overall health problems commonly seen in women with pelvic pain, and they are frequently incorrectly attributed to endometriosis itself. Unfortunately, endo can be just one piece of a complex puzzle, and often, other issues such as inflammation, toxins or infections need to be addressed as part of a comprehensive endo treatment plan (we will discuss this further in the next chapter). This is another compelling reason why endometriosis should be considered a medical subspecialty. In the interim, OB/GYNs should be trained in how to screen and diagnose these health problems, and subsequently coordinate care among various medical specialties.

It is our understanding of the complexity of endo that prompted us to write this book. In order to properly and effectively treat endo, the root causes of the condition must be addressed. It is well known that the majority of people in the developed world are not healthy. They may not be sick enough to be diagnosed with a disease, but they are on the road of ill health. Unless changes are made, it is only a matter of time before they cross the line into an official disease state. A significant number of the women with endometriosis that we see are in ill health; perhaps this has contributed to the development of the disease.

To us, it seems that Western medical treatment has reached a point of over-reliance on pharmaceuticals. If you are sick, a pharmaceutical medication is often prescribed. If that medication causes side effects, another pharmaceutical is often prescribed to treat those. The net result is a growing list of pharmaceutical prescriptions that gets us no closer to a healthy body and existence. This is not true health care but rather disease management. Traditional Western medical treatment for endometriosis in the form of hormone manipulation, including medically induced menopause, is crude at best. Women with endometriosis need true health care in order to regain their health, not poor-quality disease management.

The Bottom Line

So what is the definition of endometriosis? Endometriosis has a common thread of implants in the pelvis. In addition, many women have other associated conditions that contribute to their symptoms. Finally, a significant portion of women with endometriosis have underlying issues such as inflammation, altered immune function and insulin resistance. Addressing diet and lifestyle can often help a woman to regain her health and wellness.

In our experience of treating endometriosis and pelvic pain, wide excision surgery, done correctly, is absolutely essential. Without it, it is nearly impossible to heal from endometriosis and the associated pain. If your car was getting really bad gas mileage and you knew something was wrong, you could get new high-efficiency tires and have the engine tuned up, but if the parking brake was stuck on, the tires and tune-up would not make much of a difference. The parking brake would have to be released before a significant improvement in gas mileage would occur. On the other hand, just fixing the parking brake on a car left sitting in a field for years is not going to get that car to start, let alone guarantee good gas mileage. Just like the parking brake, wide excision endo surgery is a critical part of successful treatment, but in many cases it is just the beginning of a complete treatment program.

As a woman with endometriosis, you have tremendous power over regaining your health. The up-to-date scientific information we have provided here can help you change your life for the better. It will augment and potentially improve any treatment — including surgery — that your traditional physician has to offer. In our opinion, the holistic or functional-medicine aspect of treatment, including diet and lifestyle, is just as important as the surgery. Dr. Cook has not found a single treatment that has all of the answers. For this reason, we strongly believe that using a diverse tool kit that includes wide excision surgery, lifestyle changes, and the addressing of underlying causes is the best-known treatment plan for endometriosis.

It may be difficult at first to understand just how important and powerful lifestyle and diet are in regaining your health. The fact that you are still reading suggests you are open-minded about this part of your health-care and healing journey. For women with endometriosis and the associated conditions, obtaining good holistic health advice is probably just as hard as or harder than getting excisional surgery. We hope this book can provide you with a good foundation on which to build your health.

Case Study: Meet Jane

Jane is a 35-year-old real estate agent who came to Vital Health Institute (VHI) as a last resort. She is happily married to a supportive husband and is a mother of two, ages 4 and 2. But when she entered our office, she was exhausted, defeated and desperate for some answers.

Jane began experiencing pelvic pain when she was 25. Around the same time, she started having intestinal problems, including alternating diarrhea and constipation, bloating and stomach pain after eating. In the last 5 years, her sleep had become restless, with several nightly wakeups, which only increased with motherhood. Her fatigue became progressively worse, to the point that she had to take a nap every afternoon in order to make it through evenings with her family.

Before coming to VHI, Jane had been to several medical practitioners, including her general family practitioner, her obstetrician, a gastroenterologist and an acupuncturist. Her obstetrician strongly suspected endometriosis and had recently prescribed birth control pills to manage symptoms. Her gastroenterologist had diagnosed her with irritable bowel syndrome (IBS) and prescribed an antidepressant. Her family practitioner had prescribed Ambien for sleep.

Jane came to us hoping to get off of her medications, stop having pelvic pain and regain her life. She was too tired to play with her children, sex was painful, she couldn't focus and felt like she was always in a mental fog, and she had gained 20 pounds in the 2 years since she started taking an antidepressant. She felt like a failure as a wife and a mother, and just getting out of bed in the morning was a struggle.

From the outside, Jane looked healthy. Although her friends and family tried, they could not comprehend her discomfort. She felt alone and scared.

After extensive consultations at VHI, Jane underwent a successful surgery with Dr. Cook and worked with Danielle to improve her gastrointestinal health, lower her inflammation and address some of her unhealthy lifestyle practices. They worked together on her diet, discussed sleep hygiene and stress reduction, and made a plan to incorporate more daily movement.

Jane felt better immediately after her surgery, and month by month her body, her mental health and her general health improved. She lost 25 pounds, began sleeping 7 to 8 hours a night without medication, eliminated her gastrointestinal distress and had energy from sunrise to bedtime. She felt more connected to her family and friends, felt more confident at work and felt like she had regained her life.

Everything we did with Jane is explained in detail in this book. We hope you have the success Jane did by taking your health and your future into your own hands!

Chapter 2
Symptoms and Associated Conditions

Endometriosis Symptoms

The most common symptom associated with endometriosis is progressively severe pain during the menstrual cycle. When a girl first starts having periods, they are usually not painful at all or perhaps accompanied by mild cramps. These cramps do not prevent her from doing normal activities. Over time, however, the pain slowly becomes more and more severe. In addition, the number of pain days each month typically increases over time. It is not uncommon for the pain to eventually be present all the time. The pain is still usually worse with her period, but it can become constant and severe.

Common endometriosis symptoms include:

- **Severe pelvic pain.** The pain may be cyclical (worsening around menses and ovulation) and/or non-cyclical in nature (constant throughout the cycle). Women describe a burning, throbbing and stabbing pain in different parts of the pelvis. This pain can be even more severe than labor or post-operative pain.

- **Pain during sex.** Endometriosis can cause pain with deep penetration. This is because the area of tissue just beyond the end of the vagina is commonly affected by the disease, making it tender and sore.

- **Pain during urination and bladder pain.** If the disease is present in or near the bladder, this may result in bladder sensitivity and/or pain on emptying the bladder. Another common cause of bladder symptoms is interstitial cystitis, a condition that frequently appears with endometriosis.

- **Pain during bowel movements.** Endometriosis involving the lowest part of the colon (the rectum) may result in pain with bowel movements during menses (or all month long).

- **Pain prior to bowel movements.** Endometriosis involving the colon may result in pain just prior to bowel movements.

- **Cyclical rectal bleeding.** If endometriosis has invaded into the bowel wall, the patient may experience cyclical rectal bleeding.

- **Bloating.** Bloating may result from the inflammatory response to endometriosis involving the pelvis and bowels.

- **Nausea and vomiting.** This may be a symptom of severe pain, of the effect of inflammation on the gastrointestinal tract or, more specifically, a symptom of invasive small bowel disease. Acute vomiting can be a symptom of small bowel obstruction, a rare but serious complication of endometriosis demanding emergency medical intervention.

- **Constipation and diarrhea.** Endometriosis near or involving the bowel may result in IBS-like symptoms.

- **Fatigue.** Severe fatigue is a nonspecific symptom of endometriosis. It is a common symptom experienced by sufferers of chronic illness and pain.

- **Infertility.** It has been estimated that 40% of women with endometriosis struggle with fertility problems. Around 20% of women in a healthy population will experience infertility, meaning that in those with endometriosis the risk of fertility problems is doubled. Infertility may be due to adhesions that result from the disease process or the effect of the disease on the intrauterine environment. In addition, endometriotic tissue releases chemicals that may hinder conception and fertilized egg implantation.

- **Shoulder-tip pain.** If a patient has diaphragmatic endometriosis, she may present with cyclical right-shoulder-tip pain. Diaphragmatic endometriosis is relatively rare.

In those with endometriosis the risk of fertility problems is doubled.

While endometriosis is associated with a range of symptoms, the most common is chronic pelvic pain. You do not have to experience all of these symptoms to have endometriosis. Debilitating pelvic pain is not normal; it is your body's way of communicating that something is wrong. You should seek the help of a doctor who is familiar with treating endometriosis and pelvic pain.

Q. Is endometriosis "just" killer cramps?

A. Endometriosis is not "just" killer cramps. Severe cramping during the menstrual flow can be associated with another gynecological condition called adenomyosis. Adenomyosis occurs when endometriotic tissue is found inside the muscular walls of the uterus, and can cause severe cramping and heavy menstrual bleeding. Adenomyosis can co-occur with endometriosis, which explains why the symptoms of the two conditions are frequently confused with one another. (See page 21 for more on adenomyosis.)

Is My Pelvic Pain Endometriosis Alone?

Even after the correct surgery to completely remove all of the endometriosis, some patients still have pain.

While endometriosis is a leading cause of pelvic pain, it is not the only cause. Imagine a bucket full of fluid. The fluid in the bucket represents the pain you are experiencing. If the fluid is endometriosis alone, it means that 100% of your pain is from endometriosis. The fuller the bucket, the more severe the pain; if it is overflowing, the pain becomes intolerable. If this is your situation, and your bucket is filled only with endometriosis, you will have a complete resolution of pain with surgery. Your bucket is empty, and your pain is gone.

We have talked about the challenges of getting the correct surgery to completely remove all of the endometriosis, but even when that is the result, some patients still have pain. This means that the fluid in their buckets was a mixture of endometriosis and other medical conditions. The 20 medical conditions listed and discussed below are some of the more common co-conditions associated with endometriosis.

Abdominal Wall Neuropathy

The ilioinguinal, iliohypogastric and genital femoral nerves are found in the lower abdominal wall between the belly button and hip bone, down to the groin and upper leg. When these nerves are damaged, a nerve block or trigger-point injection can be helpful; often, a series of nerve blocks can ease the pain. In some cases, a technique called radiofrequency nerve ablation is used to provide longer-lasting relief.

Adenomyosis

Adenomyosis is a close relative of endometriosis. In this condition, endometriotic tissue is found within the muscular walls of the uterus. The two main symptoms of adenomyosis are severe uterine cramping that worsens during menstrual flow and unusually heavy periods. Not all women with adenomyosis have symptoms.

Adhesions

Adhesions are bands of fibrotic tissue (scar tissue) that form between adjacent organs and structures, such as between the ovaries and pelvic sidewall, and between the uterus and bowel. Adhesions can be thin and cobweb-like, or dense and thick like hardened glue. They arise from pelvic disease, infection or injury. Over time, the inflammation associated with endometriosis can cause the formation of scarring and adhesions, and the surgery to remove the disease may result in further adhesions as the body heals.

> **Did You Know?**
>
> **Surgery for Adhesions**
>
> Surgery can be performed to remove painful adhesions. A problem, however, is in preventing the adhesions from reforming during the healing process. The use of adhesion barriers and an early second-look procedure to take down newly forming adhesions before they become established can help provide ongoing relief.

Some patients are more prone to forming adhesions than others. In severe cases, it is almost as if a tube of superglue has been deposited into the pelvic cavity, causing structures to fuse and distorting the pelvic anatomy. If adhesions stretch or constrict a vital structure such as the bowel, this can result in pain and other symptoms, such as bowel obstruction and nausea.

Appendicitis

Appendicitis is a condition in which the appendix becomes inflamed. In the case of acute appendicitis, the onset of inflammation is sudden and is accompanied by severe right-sided pelvic pain that brings the patient to the ER; in this case, the appendix is removed during emergency surgery. Occasionally a patient will present with chronic appendicitis, or her acute pain will be passed off as endometriosis pain, potentially leading to a life-threatening situation if the appendix then ruptures.

Fibroids

Fibroid tumors are accumulations of smooth muscle tissue that form within the muscular walls of the uterus. A woman may develop multiple fibroids, and the tumors can vary in size from smaller than a marble to larger than a grapefruit. If symptomatic, fibroids can cause heavy periods and uterine cramping that worsens with menstruation.

Food Sensitivities and Food Allergies

While technically different, food allergies and food sensitivities can result in similar types of problems. A food allergy, such as to seafood, is mediated by the immune system. The patient may break out in a rash and/or may experience difficulty breathing, and symptoms are immediate. Food allergies can be severe and life-threatening. A food sensitivity, such as to the milk protein casein, is also mediated by the immune system, but symptoms are less severe and can take hours or even days to manifest. Typical reactions include stomach upset, headaches, fatigue and joint pain, and they can contribute to pelvic pain and many of the symptoms associated with endo. Phase 1 of the Endometriosis Diet Plan (see page 137) has a built-in elimination diet to help you discover if you have any food sensitivities.

Foreign Body

Pelvic pain may result from foreign materials left in the body after a previous procedure, such as surgical staples and mesh. A foreign body may result in a chronic inflammatory reaction called a foreign body giant cell reaction. Foreign body reactions can be resolved by removing the source of the reaction. Avoiding the use of foreign non-biodegradable materials in the body can prevent these reactions from occurring in the first place.

Gastrointestinal (GI) Problems

Bowel problems are common in pelvic pain patients. Many patients report bloating, cramping, gassiness and alternating bouts of constipation and diarrhea. Gastrointestinal problems can be caused by food allergies and sensitivities. Other causes may include bowel motility problems or spastic bowel, bowel obstructions due to adhesions, redundant colon (an extra length of colon), diverticulitis (when a small pouch forms in the colon and becomes infected), and anal fissure (a crack in the lining of the anus, often the result of constipation). In addition, infections, a damaged intestinal lining, stress and dysbiosis (an imbalance in the bacteria and yeasts living in the intestines) can cause GI problems.

Generalized Visceral Hypersensitivity

Visceral refers to the internal organs; *hypersensitivity* refers to abnormally increased sensitivity. With generalized visceral hypersensitivity, the entire inside of the body hurts. This is usually because inappropriate signals are being sent by the nervous system, creating neuropathic or centralized pain.

Hernia

Groin hernias include inguinal, obturator and femoral hernias. Inguinal hernias are the most common. Inguinal hernias are actually an uncommon source of pelvic pain and are often over-diagnosed and treated with mesh, which can then become a new source of pelvic pain. For this reason, inguinal hernias should be treated without mesh. Sometimes a patient may develop a painful abdominal wall hernia, including umbilical hernias, incisional hernias and ventral hernias. Surgical correction can resolve the hernia and any associated pain.

Interstitial Cystitis

Interstitial cystitis (IC), or painful bladder syndrome, is a chronic bladder condition that often mimics a bladder infection. The most common symptoms are pelvic pain, pelvic pressure, pain with urination, urinary frequency and urinary urgency. Women with IC typically have smaller bladder capacity, and when the inside of the bladder is inspected via cystoscopy, glomerulations (small capillary bleeding from the bladder wall) and Hunner's ulcers (lesions or sores on the bladder lining) may be observed.

Did You Know?

Treating Interstitial Cystitis

Unlike endometriosis, IC cannot be surgically removed, but there are treatments that can help manage symptoms, including dietary changes, bladder instillations, medications and herbs.

Ovarian Cysts

The most common non-endometriotic ovarian cysts are functional cysts (follicular cysts and corpus luteal cysts). Functional cysts form and resolve as a normal part of the menstrual cycle. Sometimes functional cysts persist longer than normal and cause pain. If the ovary is also involved due to scar tissue or adhesions, the presence of a functional cyst during the cycle can cause a cyclical stretching of the scar tissue, producing a painful pulling sensation. If a cyst ruptures, acute pain may occur. Not all cysts are symptomatic. Sometimes a patient will have large ovarian cysts without any symptoms at all. Non-functional cysts include endometriomas and hemorrhagic corpus luteal and dermoid cysts. Imaging can help differentiate between functional and non-functional cysts. Endometriomas and dermoid cysts do not resolve on their own without surgery.

Ovarian Remnant Syndrome

An ovarian remnant is a small piece of ovarian tissue left behind following the removal of an ovary. This can occur if the ovary is fused by adhesions to the adjacent pelvic sidewall prior to removal. In such cases, the ovary must first be carefully peeled away from the adherent structures without leaving a remnant behind. Ovarian remnant syndrome is when a patient experiences pain as a result of the ovarian remnant. Sometimes a remnant will be identified by the presence of a cyst in the ovarian tissue on ultrasound or by persistently elevated estrogen levels (in the case of removal of both ovaries). Ovarian remnant syndrome can be resolved by surgically removing the remnant of ovarian tissue.

Ovarian Torsion

Ovarian torsion is when an ovary twists on itself. Torsion is associated with acute lower abdominal pain and represents a medical emergency. If the torsion is not resolved quickly, the blood supply to the ovary may be compromised and the ovary may cease to function, resulting in loss of the ovary.

Pelvic Congestion

Pelvic congestion, uterine varicosities and ovarian vein varicosities (varicose veins) are all variations of enlarged pelvic blood vessels and may present as a source of pelvic pain. Pelvic congestion may be manageable conservatively or via radical organ removal (hysterectomy), depending on the site of the varicosities.

Pelvic Floor Muscle Spasm

Pelvic floor muscle spasms are excruciatingly painful and can occur spontaneously or become triggered by activity such as sexual intercourse.

Chronic pelvic pain can result in a tightening of the pelvic floor muscles. When the pelvic floor muscles become overly tight or overly relaxed or loose (such as following childbirth), the patient is said to have pelvic floor dysfunction (PFD). Some patients with endometriosis or other forms of chronic pelvic pain will go on to develop pelvic floor muscle spasms due to a tightening of the pelvic floor muscles in response to ongoing severe pelvic pain. Pelvic floor muscle spasms are excruciatingly painful and can occur spontaneously or become triggered by activity such as sexual intercourse. Pelvic physical therapy can help alleviate the painful and debilitating symptoms of PFD and pelvic floor muscle spasm.

Pudendal Neuropathy and Pudendal Nerve Entrapment (PNE)

The pudendal nerve is located along the side of the vagina. This nerve has three basic branches: an anterior branch to the clitoris; a middle branch to the vaginal and vulvar area; and a posterior branch to the anus. Pain can be present in any portion of the nerve if it becomes damaged or entrapped. The pain is often worse when the patient is sitting. Pudendal neuropathy can be treated with pudendal nerve blocks and pelvic physical therapy. In some cases, radiofrequency ablation of the pudendal nerve may be helpful.

Uterine Prolapse

Uterine prolapse is when the uterus drops down into and sometimes out of the vagina. It is more common in patients who have had vaginal deliveries, as the process of childbirth can loosen the pelvic structures that support the uterus. Prolapse is also more common in women post-menopause, as the drop in estrogen levels can also weaken the support structures in the pelvis. Patients suffering from prolapse may complain of a bearing down sensation and lower back pain. Prolapse may also be associated with stress incontinence (where lifting, coughing, sneezing and/or exercise result in involuntary urination).

> **Patients suffering from prolapse may complain of a bearing down sensation and lower back pain.**

Uterine Retroversion

Normally the uterus is anteverted, which means it is tilted forward slightly, toward the bladder. In approximately one in five women, the uterus is retroverted, meaning it is tilted backward, toward the bowel. While retroversion of the uterus is considered a normal phenomenon, it can be associated with lower back pain, painful sex and painful bowel movements. Retroversion may be more symptomatic in women who have co-occurring uterine pathology such as fibroids and adenomyosis.

Vulvodynia

The vulva is the area surrounding the outside of the vagina. *Vulvodynia* means "pain of the vulva." There are two general types of vulvodynia. Patients with generalized vulvodynia can experience pain anywhere on the vulva; it can involve the entire area or specific, isolated areas, and the pain can be intermittent or constant. Vulvar vestibulitis involves pain of the vestibule — the small area around the opening of the vagina inside the labia minora, or inner lips. Pain is only present with pressure on the area, such as during intercourse or tampon insertion.

Chapter 3
Diagnosis

Technically, the only way to provide an absolute diagnosis of endometriosis is to perform a laparoscopy, take a biopsy and have it confirmed by microscopic analysis. Currently there are no blood tests, urine tests or X-ray images that can absolutely diagnose endometriosis. However, this doesn't mean that a presumptive diagnosis cannot be made without surgery.

Dr. Cook has seen thousands of women with pelvic pain and endometriosis over the last 25 years. Despite new high-tech lab tests and sophisticated equipment, his most important information is gleaned from a careful, detailed patient history. At their initial appointment with Dr. Cook, patients typically spend 1 to 2 hours talking with him, and they undergo a complete physical examination, including a transvaginal sonogram. The patient's story and physical presentation are the most powerful tools we have. The patient knows her body, and many have phenomenal intuition about what may be wrong. If the physician really takes time to listen, and clearly understands what the patient is experiencing, this will provide tremendous insight into her presumptive diagnosis. For example, if a young woman experiences only minimal pain when she first starts her periods, but then experiences progressive and increasingly severe pain over the subsequent years, she has a very high likelihood of endometriosis. In addition, a history of an increasing number of pain days each month is also supportive of the diagnosis of endometriosis.

Did You Know?

Endo Stages

The American Society for Reproductive Medicine (ASRM) staging system for endometriosis ranges from stage I to stage IV. There are basically two types: noninvasive endometriosis and invasive endometriosis. Stages I and II basically correlate with the noninvasive form, while stages III and IV correlate with the invasive form. The peritoneum is a thin layer of tissue that lines the pelvic structures, the bowel, the bladder and the ovaries. In stages I and II, endometriotic implants grow on the surface of the peritoneum — similar to chia seeds on cellophane. In this form, the disease is superficial. In contrast, stage III and IV endometriosis is destructive, invading the tissue and causing scarring and damage to the surrounding organs.

Physical Examination

On physical examination, the patient with noninvasive (stage I or II) endometriosis will have a relatively normal pelvic exam. Although there can be significant pain, the organs, including the uterus and ovaries, and ligaments will all feel normal. The patient with invasive endometriosis (stage III or IV) will have a markedly different exam. In extreme cases, endometriosis can be seen invading the vaginal wall during a pelvic examination. It is not uncommon for a diagnosis of endometriosis to be made on the spot, in the office.

The patient may also have what is called a frozen pelvis. The ligaments of a normal pelvis act like bungee cords, providing support with some flexibility, but returning to a normal position when at rest. A frozen pelvis feels as though somebody has poured concrete into the area. There is no movement with pressure on exam; the pelvis feels like one large, solid mass. Most often, a patient with stage III or IV endometriosis will have a "chocolate cyst" in the ovary, medically known as an endometrioma. This enlarged ovary may be felt during pelvic exam.

In addition, the use of a sonogram (ultrasound) can be very helpful. An endometrioma has a very characteristic appearance on sonogram, and while a diagnosis of endometriosis cannot be made with 100% certainty, a presumptive diagnosis can be made based on this finding. A transvaginal sonogram can also provide other clues. While scar tissue cannot be seen directly, movement with the probe at varying degrees of pressure should result in the uterus and intestines sliding over each other. If there is scar tissue present, they will both move together. Also, the end of the sonogram wand can be used to map out the areas of pain within the pelvis. For example, pressure on the bladder may cause pain, suggesting the possibility of interstitial cystitis, and the uterus can be inspected for changes suggestive of adenomyosis, myometrial hyperplasia and fibroids.

Many of the patients we see experience pain with intercourse. Part of the pelvic examination is mapping out the different areas that are contributing to painful intercourse. Gentle pressure is placed on the vestibule, the area around the opening of the vagina, with a cotton swab. A patient with vestibulitis will experience intense pain with this type of pressure. In addition, we perform a pelvic floor exam, during which the pelvic floor muscles are palpated. These muscles should not be tender or painful; if they are, the patient is suffering from pelvic floor muscle spasm.

Additional exams include examination of the pudendal nerve, bladder, cervix, uterus and ovaries. The pudendal nerve, which is next to the wall of the vagina about halfway up the vagina, is palpated to determine if the patient has a pudendal neuropathy. The bladder is positioned along the anterior wall of the vagina.

Did You Know?

Physical Therapy

After the patient has healed from her endometriosis surgery, she will probably require therapy by a pelvic floor physical therapist, who specializes in the treatment of issues related to pelvic pain.

This is palpated during the exam to determine if pain in the bladder is contributing to the overall pelvic pain. The cervix, posterior cul-de-sac, uterosacral ligaments and pelvic sidewalls are all palpated to locate areas of pain and restriction. The uterus and ovaries are palpated to determine if they are normal in size and/or painful. All of these areas can contribute to pain during sex.

The CA-125 Blood Test

Unfortunately, the percentage of patients with endometriosis who test positive for elevated CA-125 levels is quite low. A patient with a "normal" test result could still have endometriosis.

CA-125 stands for cancer antigen 125. While readings of this antigen can be elevated in patients with ovarian cancer, elevated CA-125 is also found in some patients with endometriosis. In the past, there was hope that this test might act as a diagnostic blood test for endometriosis. Unfortunately, the percentage of patients with endometriosis who test positive for elevated CA-125 levels is quite low. A patient with a "normal" test result could still have endometriosis. If the patient has an elevated CA-125 reading, it is more likely that she has invasive stage III or stage IV endometriosis rather than noninvasive stage I or II. [1]

It seems that some women have endometriosis that produces CA-125 while others do not. This is why it is advisable to check CA-125 on all endometriosis patients preoperatively. If it is elevated, this provides a blood marker through which disease activity can be followed. After the patient is healed, a recheck of her CA-125 can be done to make sure that the level has normalized. This helps confirm removal of the endometriosis (if no adenomyosis is present) and also provides a baseline with which to compare in the future if there is concern about recurrence. [2]

The CA-125 blood level varies throughout the menstrual cycle, with the highest levels during menstruation and a moderate elevation during ovulation. It is therefore important that a patient has subsequent blood tests at the same time in her menstrual cycle.

RESEARCH SPOTLIGHT
Endometrial Biopsy Test

In 2009, a colleague of Dr. Cook's, Dr. Moamar al-Jefout from Jordan, published an interesting paper in the journal *Human Reproduction*, describing a double-blind study looking for the presence of nerve fibers in the functional layer of the endometrium obtained with biopsies from women with endometriosis. His goal was to establish this procedure as a diagnostic test for endometriosis. The conclusion was that an endometrial biopsy, with detection of nerve fibers, provided a reliability of diagnosis of endometriosis close to the accuracy of laparoscopic assessment by experienced gynecological laparoscopists. [3] Unfortunately, this test is not yet commercially available for the diagnosis of endometriosis.

CT and MRI Scan

Use of computed tomography (CT) and magnetic resonance imaging (MRI) scans may be helpful in certain situations. Studies are ongoing to determine the best role of these tests in aiding the correct diagnosis of endometriosis. The results are dependent on both the quality of the CT and MRI machines — better machines provide better resolution, and thus ability to see smaller lesions — and the level of expertise of the radiologist reading the test. At this point in time, CT and MRI studies may aid in clarifying the extent of what is known as deeply infiltrating endometriosis (DIE), which invades beneath the thin layer of tissue lining the pelvic structures. An MRI specifically may also be helpful for the evaluation of adenomyosis, fibroids and endometriomas.[4]

The Bottom Line

A thorough evaluation of a patient with pelvic pain and suspected endometriosis is necessary. Identification of possible coexisting issues with endometriosis is important for a complete and accurate diagnosis. (A more detailed discussion of the diagnosis of these medical conditions can be found in *Stop Endometriosis and Pelvic Pain*, by Dr. Andrew Cook.)

In general, a presumptive diagnosis of endometriosis can be made without surgery. Associated issues that can be treated noninvasively are often addressed first if the pain is not debilitating. Depending on how the patient responds to conservative treatment and the severity of her pain, she may not require surgery or a definitive diagnosis of endometriosis. If she does not improve adequately and/or if her pain is interfering with her ability to function normally, or is severe, then laparoscopic surgery is needed with proper wide excision to treat and remove the endometriosis and associated anatomic conditions effectively.

Chapter 4
Pathophysiology and Contributing Factors

Did You Know?

Recurrence and Worsening

The theory of retrograde menstruation predicts that the disease will recur after surgery and worsen over time with each menstrual flow, yet surgical excision of endometriosis has been found to effectively remove the disease in most patients, with true disease recurrence being rare. Studies examining the extent of disease across different age groups of patients have failed to find an increase in disease with age.

Common Theories of Endometriosis

At this point in time we do not know what causes endometriosis. When considering the origin and manifestation of a disease, we need to consider the factors that determine whether a woman develops the condition or not and, of those women who do develop the disease, the factors that determine how severe her disease ultimately is (how symptomatic, how aggressive, how invasive and how extensive).

Several theories of the origin of endometriosis have been proposed. The aim of a theory of origin is to present an explanation that adequately accommodates all that we know about the disease. Generally, the best-fit theory is adopted and used to guide and predict treatments and outcomes. If new information becomes available over time, the best-fit theory may be surpassed or replaced by a competing theory. Alternatively, it may be adapted in order to accommodate new findings.

Sampson's Theory of Retrograde Menstruation

Perhaps one of the most popular and enduring theories of origin is that of retrograde menstruation, transportation and implantation. This is the belief that endometriosis occurs through a process of endometriotic tissue flowing back along the fallopian tubes during menstruation, entering the pelvic cavity, and implanting and invading the surfaces of the pelvic structures.

Retrograde menstruation, however, is a common phenomenon that occurs in 90% of women, yet only 10% of women develop endometriosis. Furthermore, the refluxed material contains only minimal deposits of endometriotic tissue. While endometriosis consists of tissue that is similar to the native endometrium, it is not identical to the tissue that lines the uterus, suggesting that it is not a mere auto-transplant.

Other phenomena about the disease that cannot be adequately explained by this theory include the presence of endometriosis in stillborn female fetuses, in women without a functional uterus, and in a small number of men undergoing treatment for prostate cancer.

Immune Dysfunction Theory

Research reveals that women with endometriosis are at increased risk for various autoimmune disorders, including allergies, systemic lupus erythematosus, Sjögren's syndrome, rheumatoid arthritis and multiple sclerosis. Based on this finding, a hybrid theory was developed that expands upon Sampson's theory of retrograde menstruation. As mentioned previously, retrograde menstruation occurs in around 90% of women, yet only a minority develops endometriosis. It has been hypothesized that an underlying immune dysfunction interferes with the body's natural ability to clear this refluxed tissue from the pelvis and therefore the tissue is allowed to establish itself and proliferate, resulting in endometriosis.

> **While autoimmune disorders are more common in women with endometriosis, many women with endometriosis do not have any such disorders.**

This line of argument suffers many of the same limitations as the original theory of retrograde menstruation. While autoimmune disorders are more common in women with endometriosis, many women with endometriosis do not have any such disorders. Another important question is whether immune dysfunction truly precedes the onset of endometriosis or rather is a result of the disease process itself. Endometriosis triggers an ongoing immune response, which over time could moderate or disrupt immune function, altering an individual's propensity for developing autoimmune disorders.

Immune dysregulation is discussed in more detail starting on page 42.

Theory of Mülleriosis

The theory of Mülleriosis is the notion that endometriosis is laid down during embryonic development and remains dormant until later in life when hormonal changes (such as during puberty or pregnancy) trigger the disease to become active and symptomatic. During embryonic development, tissue is laid down and differentiated into the various pelvic organs and structures, including the reproductive organs. In women with endometriosis, something goes awry during this process and tissue that would ordinarily be restricted to the inside of the uterus ends up developing in locations outside the uterus.

A helpful analogy is that of a chef who is following a recipe for a full-course dinner. He has all of the right ingredients, but the recipe contains mistakes and some of the ingredients that belong in the appetizer end up in the dessert, and some ingredients intended for the dessert end up in the main course. In the development of the reproductive organs, HOX genes determine which tissue develops where. It is possible that abnormalities in these genes, whether spontaneous or inherited,

The Mülleriosis theory can explain why the disease has been observed in infants and prepubescent girls, as well as the presence of other types of aberrant tissue that may co-occur with endometriosis.

result in coding errors that in turn lead to the presence of aberrant endometriotic tissue outside the uterus.

The Mülleriosis theory can explain why the disease has been observed in infants and prepubescent girls, as well as the presence of other types of aberrant tissue that may co-occur with endometriosis, such as endocervicosis (tissue similar to the cervix found outside the uterus) and endosalpingiosis (tissue similar to the lining of the fallopian tubes present outside the tubes). It could also help explain the unique patterning of the disease — that is, why it occurs more commonly in some locations than others. Interestingly, there is a pattern of abnormalities and anomalies, such as urinary tract and uterine anomalies, adenomyosis, fibroids and peritoneal pockets, that are significantly more common in patients with endometriosis. This syndrome of conditions could be explained by a common underlying pattern of coding errors that manifest during embryonic development.

Embryonic Rest Theory

The embryonic rest theory proposes that cells of Müllerian origin can persist within the peritoneal cavity and under certain circumstances induce the formation of endometriotic tissue. An embryonic rest is a remnant of embryonic tissue that has persisted beyond the embryonic phase of development. Cells of Müllerian origin are the embryonic cells that originally comprised the Müllerian duct, a structure that subsequently differentiated into the female reproductive organs (specifically the fallopian tubes, the uterus and part of the vagina). It is unknown, however, whether these cells really can persist beyond early life.

Stem Cell Theory

A recent theory is that endometriosis arises from endometriotic stem cells located outside the uterus. Stem cells are undifferentiated cells that harbor the potential to regenerate and produce more differentiated "daughter" cells. It is proposed that stem cells located in the pelvis outside the uterus bring about the regeneration and differentiation of endometriotic lesions. These same cells play a role in the monthly regeneration of endometriotic tissue inside the uterus after each menstrual flow.

Theories of Lymphatic and Vascular Spread

In rare cases, a patient will present with endometriosis in faraway places, such as the lung, the brain or even the eye. One explanation for these occurrences is that small amounts of endometriotic tissue can spread throughout the body via the lymphatic and vascular system. It is unclear, however, how this process would occur, and perhaps a more plausible explanation is that the disease presents in these distant sites due to a process of coelomic metaplasia (the transformation of cells or tissue from one type to another).

Coelomic Metaplasia Theory

Coelomic metaplasia rests on the notion that any cell in the body has the potential to become any other cell. All cells have the same basic genetic code but are distinguished by the different ways in which their basic genetic code is expressed. The expression of any given cell's genetic code may be influenced by a number of factors (such as inflammation, exposure to toxins and wound healing).

In the case of endometriosis, the theory of coelomic metaplasia predicts that the genetic material in a cell or group of cells (tissue) becomes expressed differently, causing the tissue to transform into endometriosis. This theory could explain the occurrence of disease in distant sites in the body, scar endometriosis and the presence of disease in men undergoing treatment for prostate cancer.

Other Theories and Contributing Factors
Genetics

We have seen many women in our practice who have mothers, sisters and/or grandmothers who have been diagnosed or have similar "endometriosis symptoms." In fact, it has been estimated that from 5% to 7% of women with a first-degree relative with endometriosis will develop it, and that their symptoms will be more severe than someone lacking this genetic link to the disease.[1] There has been speculation throughout the years that endo may have a genetic component.[2]

A few examples of specific genes that have been studied in relation to endo include CYP1A1, CYP19, GSTM1, NAT2 and COMT. CYP1A1 and CYP19, enzymes in the cytochrome P450 detox system, play an important role in Phase I detoxification in the liver.[3] Mutations in these genes may decrease healthy breakdown of estrogen and environmental toxins.

GSTM1 and NAT2 are Phase II conjugating enzymes, which aid in the detoxification of chemicals, medications, environmental toxins (such as bisphenol A, or BPA), estrogen and oxidative stress. Research has demonstrated an increase in cancer in individuals with these genetic mutations. In addition, GSTM1 is involved in repairing the tissue that lines the ovaries from damage caused by chemicals, medications, environmental toxins and oxidative stress. Mutations in GSTM1 and NAT2 may result in poor estrogen breakdown and tissue damage from toxins.[4]

> There is increasing evidence that endometriosis, like many other chronic health conditions, is an epigenetic disease. All of this evolving research suggests that our genes are not our destiny, and that we have lots of power over our health.

Did You Know?

Epigenetics

Epigenetics is how our genes express themselves depending on their interaction with their surrounding environment.

COMT is an enzyme involved in metabolizing estrogen and catecholamine neurotransmitters such as dopamine, epinephrine and norepinephrine. Alterations in the COMT gene may result in decreased estrogen breakdown and mood alterations. Studies also demonstrate a lowered pain threshold with this genetic mutation.[5]

For some time, we believed genetics determined our health outcomes. In fact, many medical professionals still believe this. While it is true that we are born with a specific genetic code, we are now learning that what we call *epigenetics* may be even more important. Epigenetics, or how our genes express themselves depending on their interaction with their surrounding environment, seems to have a greater impact on our health than the genes that make us who we are.[6] One can think of genes as the books in a library, while epigenetics is the reading assignment telling us which books are to be read. What we expose our genes to can impact whether we develop a chronic health condition, such as endo, and how fast and well we age. Epigenetic instructions are passed down through at least several generations. Thus we are not only talking about the effects of our own environment. What our mothers' and grandmothers' genes were exposed to factors in as well; not only did their environment change their genetic expression, but it can also result in a change in expression in our genes.

An example of an epigenetic switch is the mutation of GATA2 to GATA6, which results in progesterone resistance and endometriosis development.[7] This switch can occur whether or not an individual has a genetic mutation in the gene; what is equally or more important is the environment and exposure to toxins.

RESEARCH SPOTLIGHT
Is Genetic Mutation the Cause?

In addition to simply looking at familial tendencies of the disease, researchers are also working to uncover genetic mutations that explain the etiology (cause) of endo. Research has demonstrated a significant difference in the endometrium of a woman with endo when compared to women without the disease, resulting in more aggressive cell growth and increased aromatase expression (aromatase makes estrogen, which leads to more estrogen production). Women with endo also appear to have endometriotic cells that can attach and turn into a lesion more easily than in women without the disease. In addition, the endometrium of a woman with endo appears to contain more enzymes that facilitate the implantation of endometriotic tissue into tissue outside of the uterus and the formation of lesions.[9] These alterations in physiology may be a result of genetic mutations.

There is increasing evidence that endometriosis, like many other chronic health conditions, is an epigenetic disease.[8] All of this evolving research suggests that our genes are not our destiny, and that we have lots of power over our health. This is great news, and is, in part, why we have written this book. Chapter 6 has suggestions for how to reduce your toxic load and how to gently upregulate your body's natural detoxification processes. In addition, the Endometriosis Diet Plan (see chapter 12) is designed to encourage healthy genetic expression by providing nutrients for optimal enzymatic function, and food chemicals that "talk" to your genes to optimize your health.

Environmental Toxins

Research indicates that incidences of endo are on the rise and it's now occurring at a younger age. An older study conducted in 1998 by the Endometriosis Association discovered that there was a 23% increase between 1980 and 1998 in patient-reported pelvic pain prior to the age of 15. In addition, pelvic pain began at an earlier age and included a greater variety of symptoms.[10]

There is a possibility that endo symptoms are developing at a younger age as a result of an earlier onset of puberty. Nearly 50% of African American girls and 15% of Caucasian girls are developing breasts and pubic hair by the age of 8.[11] The onset of puberty is marked by an increase in hormones such as estrogen. Since endo is an estrogen-driven disease, it's easy to imagine how these additional years of estrogen exposure could alter a woman's health.

A proposed explanation for this earlier onset of puberty and endometriosis is an increased exposure to a variety of environmental pollutants. Experimental studies on animals and epidemiological studies on humans suggest an increased incidence and severity of endo with exposure to chemicals such as organochlorine chemicals, DDT, mirex, toxaphene, poly-chlorinated biphenyl (PCBs), pentachlorophenol and dioxins.[12]

Dioxins and dioxin-like compounds are some of the most toxic chemicals known to exist today and are a serious public health threat (see "Research Spotlight," page 36). They are in a group of highly toxic pollutants known as persistent organic pollutants, or POPs, and are linked to the development of cancer, reproductive and developmental problems, immune system damage and hormone disruption.

Another chemical that has dioxin-like behavior and poses similar threats to our health is polychlorinated biphenyls. PCBs consist of a culmination of several individual chlorinated compounds commonly used between 1929 and 1977 as coolants and lubricants in transformers, capacitors and other electrical equipment. In 1977, these chemicals were banned due to their resistance to breaking down easily in the environment. In fact, they persist in our environment today and have accumulated in our food chain. The most heavily contaminated foods are fish and meats.[19]

Did You Know?

Toxins in Our Food

Our food supply can be a source of toxins. Many times, making more informed choices about where our food comes from and how it is grown can decrease the amount of toxins we ingest. For example, organopesticides (including aromatic fungicides and hexachlorocyclo-hexanes) used on conventionally grown fruits and vegetables have been linked to the pathogenesis of endometriosis.[23] Choosing organically grown produce can reduce our exposure to this toxin. Organopesticides also make their way into other foods we eat, including fish, meat and dairy, when these animals eat feed containing these chemicals. Buying responsibly raised, grass-fed meats and wild fish is another way to limit our exposure to these chemicals.

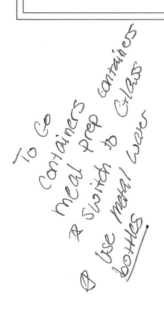

We know that these chemicals are hazardous to our health, but there is also mounting evidence that exposure to dioxins and PCBs may stimulate endo growth as a result of increased chronic inflammation, increased estrogen synthesis, and altered monthly thickening and shedding of the uterine wall, which would normally impede the development of endo.[20]

Another toxin you may have heard about is bisphenol A (BPA). Many of you may have already reduced your use of plastics in an attempt to decrease your exposure to this toxin. BPA and phthalates are used in the manufacture of many plastic water bottles and plastic food containers. Both chemicals have been associated with damage to reproductive and developmental health, and higher rates of endometriosis.[21] BPA has a similar structure to estrogen and can behave like estrogen; however, the body takes much longer to metabolize it. It can attach to estrogen receptors, stimulate the production of estrogen and enhance gonadotrophin secretion — all of which may encourage endo growth and worsen symptoms.[22]

A xenoestrogen is a chemical compound, either natural or synthetic, that has estrogenic activity. BPA, PCBs and phthalates are examples of synthetic xenoestrogens, while phytoestrogens such as soy are an example of naturally occurring xenoestrogens. Mycoestrogens, a type of mycotoxin produced by certain types of mold, are another source of xenoestrogens.

See chapter 6 for ideas for ideas on reducing your toxic load and slowly detoxifying your body. In chapter 11, several herbs and supplements are listed that can be helpful in enhancing the body's natural detoxification processes. Some have stronger scientific evidence to back up their claims than others. Note that supplementation for detoxification will not replace lifestyle and dietary changes. For example, if you continue to use plastic water bottles, lather your body daily with chemicals and ingest foods laden with pesticides, hormones and antibiotics, taking a supplement for detoxification may not be very effective. The diet recommendations in this book (starting in chapter 12) are designed to help your body detoxify daily in a gentle, natural way.

Chronic Inflammation

Scientific studies clearly demonstrate that endo is an inflammatory disease. This contributes to the amount of pain women with endo experience monthly or even on a daily basis. Endo pain is real and supported by current research, which demonstrates that women with endo have elevated levels of several chemical mediators involved in the inflammatory process. For example, concentrations of cytokines, histamine and kinin — all important markers of inflammation — are higher in women with endo than women without the disease.[24] In addition, studies have shown that many women with endo have higher amounts of prostaglandin E2 (PGE2) in their peritoneal fluid than women without endo.[25] PGE2 has been shown to increase inflammation, growth and pain in women with endo.[26]

PGE2 also strongly increases the production of estrogen through an enzyme called aromatase.[27] Aromatase converts testosterone into estrogen. It is found in fat tissue, the brain, the placenta, blood vessels, skin, bone and the ovaries. The fact that it is found in fat tissue is one reason some practitioners suggest fat loss as a strategy to reduce the estrogen load in women with endo. In addition, aromatase can be found in the endometriotic tissue (endo implants), uterine fibroids, breast cancer and endometrial cancer.

You read that right: your endo implants are making their own estrogen, and that estrogen is like fertilizer for more endo growth! (This is why the drug Lupron, hysterectomy with removal of the ovaries, and even menopause do not necessarily cure endo or even relieve the pain of endo.)

One of the main precursors in the formation of PGE2 is arachidonic acid, which is a type of fatty acid made in your body from certain omega-6 fatty acids and consumed directly through the diet in fatty red meats, egg yolks and organ meats. Your body needs some arachidonic acid, but an excess can contribute to increased inflammation. Dietary alterations that balance omega-3 fatty acids, healthy omega-6 fatty acids and healthy saturated fats may help to decrease inflammation, pain and excessive estrogen production. The Endometriosis Diet Plan is designed as an anti-inflammatory diet, with a focus on balanced, healthy fats for reduced PGE2 production.

Caution

There are several herbs and supplements that can be helpful in decreasing inflammation (see chapter 11). Some have stronger scientific evidence to back up their claims than others. It is important to know, however, that supplementation with anti-inflammatories will not replace lifestyle and dietary changes. For example, if you continue to eat a diet high in added sugars and excessive carbohydrates or expose yourself to excessive toxins, taking a supplement to reduce inflammation will probably not be very effective.

Did You Know?

The Oxidation Process

The formation of rust is an example of an oxidation process. Compare the oxidation in your body to a metal hinge left outside in the elements. The hinge becomes rusty, does not open and close as well, and begins to weaken and break apart.

An antioxidant is a molecule that can donate an electron to a free radical and thus has the ability to inhibit the oxidation of other molecules, stopping the chain reaction. Examples of antioxidants include vitamin E, vitamin C, glutathione and negative ions from the core of the earth.

Oxidation

Oxidation occurs when an atom or molecule loses an electron. The process of oxidation results in the formation of free radicals — or atoms that are missing one of their electrons. The loss of the electron makes the atom very unstable, and it will not rest until it can find another stable atom from which it can steal an electron. In a healthy situation, free radicals are formed to help kill off viruses and bacteria. But when free radicals are generated in excess, or are not quickly controlled, they can cause an uncontrolled chain reaction resulting in significant damage to healthy cells and tissue.

One important source of free radicals is the abundant oxygen formed in our bodies by reactive oxygen species (ROS). Our cells use lots of oxygen to make energy, and ROS are generated constantly as part of normal cellular metabolism. Since this type of ROS is a by-product of metabolism in the body, it is known as endogenous ROS. Exogenous ROS come from outside of the body. Examples include hydrogen peroxide, pesticides, xenobiotics (defined as substances that are foreign to the body, such as BPA found in plastics) and tobacco smoke.

Oxygen is especially susceptible to radical formation. An antioxidant is a molecule that can donate an electron to a free radical and thus has the ability to inhibit the oxidation of other molecules, stopping the chain reaction. Examples of antioxidants include vitamin E, vitamin C, glutathione and negative ions from the core of the earth.

Apoptosis is defined as programmed or normal cell death. When a cell is done with its work and is no longer needed it goes through apoptosis. This is in contrast to a cell that dies as a result of damage (sunburn, for example) or infection. Women with endo have been shown to have increased oxidation as a result of apoptotic endometriotic tissue and cell debris from menstrual reflux, all causing elevated inflammation. In addition, women with endo have demonstrated an overproduction of ROS and appear to have lower antioxidant defenses than women without endo.[28]

This research suggests that women with endo may require a particularly robust antioxidant support program. The lifestyle suggestions in this book — such as earthing (a source of healthy negative ions) and exercises to decrease your ROS formation and naturally increase antioxidants — can be incorporated into your daily routine and will help to reduce free radicals in your body. The Endometriosis Diet Plan (starting in chapter 12) is packed with important food sources of antioxidants. In fact, dietary antioxidants may be more beneficial than supplements, as they are typically found in groups, which work synergistically, as opposed to individually. Also, supplementation alone may not be protective against free-radical-producing substances such as toxins and stress.

Blood Sugar Regulation

High blood sugar is a huge contributor to inflammation. There is ongoing, mounting research on how sugar, especially too much sugar, is harmful to our health. In fact, there is an entire website — www.sugarscience.org — that consists of over 8,000 scientific studies on the negative health impacts of sugar in our diet! You may be surprised to learn that sugar consumption can increase your chances of developing Alzheimer's disease and cancer, and even contribute to premature skin aging. Acute inflammation after ingestion or infusion of glucose (sugar) has been shown in numerous studies.

A 2002 study in the scientific journal *Circulation* demonstrated an elevation in inflammatory markers such as interleukin-6 (IL-6) and tumor necrosis factor-alpha (TNF-alpha) after an infusion of glucose.[29] These are strong promoters of inflammation and tend to be higher in women with endo.

This study produced particularly interesting results when the researchers infused both glucose and glutathione (a strong antioxidant) simultaneously. With the antioxidant protection provided by glutathione, they did not see the previous significant rise in inflammatory markers. This suggests that the acute inflammation seen with an increase in blood glucose may be at least partially due to oxidation.

> You may be thinking, "I don't eat candy or sweets." It's important to remember that added sugars don't come only from obvious sources.

What Happens When You Eat Too Much Sugar

- fatigue
- memory loss
- poor circulation
- fatigued and painful muscles
- stiff, painful joints
- wrinkles
- gray hair
- declining eyesight
- headaches
- sensitivity to noise
- depression
- frequent illness/ infection

Earlier, we discovered that women with endo appear to have an increased amount of oxidation (see page 38) as a result of apoptotic endometriotic tissue and cell debris from menstrual reflux and lower antioxidant defenses.[30] This amounts to a more severe and exaggerated inflammatory reaction in women with endo who eat a diet high in sugar.

Every time you eat sugar, you are rusting from the inside! Eating a diet high in sugar will certainly worsen your endo symptoms and most likely contribute to the disease process.

The promotion of inflammation is not the only way sugar is harmful; high glucose levels will also increase insulin secretion.

Did You Know?

Sugar Has Many Names

Sometimes, you really need to be a detective to find out whether sugar is an added ingredient in your foods. Sugar Science lists 61 different names for sugar, including agave nectar, barley malt, beet sugar, cane juice, caramel, corn sweetener, dextrose, evaporated cane juice and fructose.[32] (For a complete list, go to www.sugarscience.org/hidden-in-plain-sight.)

Did You Know?

Sugar Is More Addictive Than Cocaine

Studies on cocaine-addicted rats have demonstrated a stronger preference for sugar consumption than cocaine.[33] We know that both sugar and addictive drugs such as cocaine stimulate dopamine receptors, the pleasure center of the brain. In addition, neuroimaging studies have demonstrated structurally similar changes in the brains of obese individuals and drug abusers.[34]

That, in turn, will lead to a decrease in sex hormone–binding globulin (SHBG). This hormone is responsible for binding up free hormones such as estrogen and testosterone and transporting them around the body. Think of it like a commuter bus for your hormones: if hormones are on this bus, they cannot bind to cell receptors and initiate their action. When SHBG is low, more free hormones, including estrogen, are available to bind to cells. What this means for someone with endo is that more estrogen is available to drive the endo disease process.

You may be thinking, "I don't eat candy or sweets." It's important to remember that added sugars don't come only from obvious sources such as candies, baked goods, sweetened beverages and desserts. Americans consume an average of 66 pounds of "added dietary sugar" each year. You might be surprised to learn that 74% of packaged foods include added sugars in their ingredients.[31]

If you're not eating foods with added sugar, the sources of sugar in your diet may surprise you. All foods that contain carbohydrate break down into sugar. Foods that are innately high sources of carbohydrate include grains and all grain products (yes, this includes quinoa and brown rice!), fruit, milk, starchy vegetables, and legumes/lentils. If you eat a bowl of quinoa, for example, this will break down to glucose (sugar) and raise your blood sugar, creating inflammation. Sure, quinoa has fiber and more protein than other grains; however, it is also carbohydrate-rich. The key is to find out how much carbohydrate you can tolerate without raising your blood sugar too high.

Added Sugar

Even foods that are considered healthy can be laden with sugar. Compare this list of sugar amounts to a typical can of soda, which has 11 teaspoons (46 g) of sugar:

- 8 oz (227 mL) sweetened yogurt: 7 tsp (29 g)
- 1 breakfast bar: 4 tsp (15 g)
- 1 cup (250 mL) bran cereal with raisins: 5 tsp (20 g)
- 8-oz (250 mL) glass of fruit juice: 7 tsp (30 g)

* All figures are averages

One way to do this is to check your blood sugar with a glucometer before eating and again 1 to 1.5 hours after eating. Your blood sugar should not rise more than 30 points; if it does, you have eaten too much carbohydrate. Many people don't want to prick their fingers and check blood sugar if it is not medically necessary (such as with diabetes). Most individuals tolerate approximately 20 grams of carbohydrate in each meal. The Endometriosis Diet Plan is carbohydrate-controlled, and meals

Checklist

How to Remove Added Sugars and Limit Carbs

1. Clean out your cabinets and your refrigerator. This is the most important step. That hidden candy bar in the freezer will get eaten.

2. No sugar-sweetened beverages (soda, juice, energy drinks — anything that tastes sweet). This includes artificially sweetened beverages such as diet sodas and flavored water. Artificial sweeteners have been shown to activate the same pleasure center of the brain — however, because they do not produce complete satiation, they heighten your sugar cravings, resulting in an increased intake of sweets throughout the day.[35]

3. Remove all processed foods from your diet. If you must eat processed foods, make sure to read the labels and look for any added sugars such as those listed on the Sugar Science website (www.sugarscience.org/hidden-in-plain-sight). In addition, look for foods that have 5 ingredients or fewer — ingredients that are actual foods, not chemicals.

4. Limit your fruit to 2 servings daily of lower-sugar fruits such as limes, organic berries, organic green apples and grapefruit.

5. Fill your plate and your belly with more fresh vegetables. Create a rainbow on your plate.

6. Add healthy fats to each meal, such as coconut, olives and olive oil, ghee, avocados, and nuts and seeds. These will keep you feeling full for longer and help to stabilize blood sugar fluctuations.

7. Add to each meal 3 to 5 ounces (the size of the palm of your hand) of protein, such as chicken, fish, grass-fed beef, eggs and turkey.

You may benefit from additional vitamin C in your diet or in a supplement. Examples of foods high in vitamin C include radishes, organic berries, raw broccoli and raw kale.

Follow the Endometriosis Diet Plan, which is low in sugar and carbohydrate-controlled to help balance blood sugar.

are designed to contain 20 grams of carbohydrate or less. Phase 1 of the diet is the lowest-carbohydrate phase. You may tolerate more carbohydrate. After phase 1, you can experiment by eating larger portions of high-carbohydrate foods, such as root vegetables.

Many people are addicted to sugar (see sidebar on page 40). We recommend a complete cold-turkey elimination of added sugars in the diet at least for a few months, as opposed to limiting added sugar consumption based on the addictiveness of sugar. This means no added sugar in the house. If it is in the house, you will eventually eat it, just as an alcoholic will eventually drink alcohol if it's around. The battleground is at the grocery store: Do not bring it home.

Kicking the sugar habit may be a lifelong challenge, just as an alcoholic has a lifelong challenge in avoiding alcohol. In the long run, however, you will be motivated by beginning to feel better and discovering a whole world of new amazing flavors and tastes.

You may have a few rough days or weeks as you are detoxifying from your sugar addiction. Hang in there! Consider planning your schedule to allow extra time for sleeping and resting during this phase. Drink lots of water, take baths with Epsom salts, and set up a support system, such as a good friend you can call when you need a boost.

Immune Dysregulation

Many experts in the medical field consider a dysregulated immune system as a major contributor to the development of endometriosis, and there are numerous studies supporting this theory. It's believed that most women will experience some retrograde menstruation (the backwards flow of blood into the peritoneal cavity) during menses. This blood contains fragments of endometriotic tissue. Normally, a healthy immune system easily scavenges this tissue and destroys it, preventing implantation and growth in tissue outside of the uterus. In order for this endometriotic tissue to translocate onto the tissue outside of the uterus and proliferate, it must first be able to survive the attack of the body's immune system.

There is mounting evidence that impaired immune surveillance, and defects in the innate and adaptive immune cells — specifically macrophages, natural killer (NK) cells and cytotoxic T cells, which normally destroy these tissue fragments — may be involved in the pathogenesis of endo.[36] This can be likened to an army operating without its front-line troops or cavalry scouts. There is no preparation for enemy attacks and, as a result, those attacks are stronger and more effective. This impairment in immune surveillance prevents the immune system in women with endo from being able to adequately destroy and remove these tissue fragments from the peritoneal cavity, leading to uninhibited growth and the development of endo.

For example, NK cells appear to function differently in women with endo.[37] Normally, NK cells destroy target cells such as endometriotic cells by releasing cytoplasmic granules of proteins, which kill the cells. In women with endometriosis, this cytotoxic activity is significantly reduced, allowing endometriotic fragments to develop into lesions on tissues outside of the uterus.

In addition, macrophages, the first-line defense of the innate immune system, are more numerous, but appear to exhibit an inferior ability to destroy endometriotic cells in women with endo.[38] Macrophages also initiate acute inflammation and the production of local cytokines and chemokines, which start and continue the inflammatory cascade. This function of the macrophages appears to continue to work in women with endo, despite the reduced immune function. This combination of increased amounts of endometriotic tissue and inflammation results in greater blood flow, growth factors and tissue inflammation, allowing an optimal environment for the growth and spread of endometriosis lesions.[39] Another difference in the

> **Another difference in the immune system in women with endo appears to be decreased vitamin D3–binding protein.**

Checklist
How to Improve Your Immune System

These 6 components are the foundation to your healing, and to optimizing your health.

1. **Reduce stress.** Daily stress reduction is critical for the immune system (see chapter 7). We highly recommend the incorporation of stress-reduction practices into your daily routine.

2. **Get enough sleep.** A good quantity and quality of zzz's is essential for a strong and well-balanced immune system (see chapter 8).

3. **Get moving.** Safe and effective exercise is important for strengthening your immune system. Exercise helps to build your immune army (see chapter 9).

4. **Detox.** Reduce your exposure to toxins and practice gentle, ongoing detoxification to help prevent damage to your immune cells and genes (see chapter 6).

5. **Charge up.** Charge your body's electrical system to help power up your immune system. We don't often consider the electrical charge of our bodies and how it relates to our health, but this is an important component to healing and staying well (see chapter 10).

6. **Eat well.** Enjoy a diet that aids in gentle detoxification, decreases inflammation and promotes healing. A diet plan, meal plans and recipes start in part 3, which includes a list of endo-busting foods to assist in fueling your body for health and healing.

immune system in women with endo appears to be decreased vitamin D_3–binding protein. A study published in 2011 showed that women with endo have a significantly higher rate of genetic defects in their vitamin D_3–binding protein. This protein is necessary for the activation of macrophages. Mutations in this gene may be one explanation as to why macrophage activity is decreased in women with endo.

Lastly, T cell activity also appears to be decreased in women with endo. Normally, T cells initiate cell death via the Fas/FasL pathway. However, in women with endo, the endometriotic cells appear to be resistant to Fas-mediated cell death, and also have the ability to use this pathway for an attack on the host's own immune system.[40] Again, this leads to uninhibited growth and the destruction of surrounding tissue by endometriotic fragments growing outside of the uterus. The result of all of these alterations in the immune system in women with endo? Pain, discomfort and misery!

Like other bodily processes, the immune system has a checks-and-balances component to regulate and shut off an immune response. This is important for maintaining homeostasis and controlling inflammation. Without it, the immune system can become overactive and begin to attack the body's own tissues, leading to autoimmune disease.

Important players in immune system regulation include regulatory T cells (Tregs) and hormones. Tregs are a subpopulation of T cells important for modulation of the immune system, continued tolerance of self-antigens and prevention of autoimmune disease. Tregs suppress the immune system and help to control immune responses. Normally, the number of Treg cells is high during the follicular phase (first half of cycle) of menstruation and declines during the luteal phase (second half). In women with endo, Treg cell expression continues to be high — and actually continues to increase — during the luteal phase of the menstrual cycle.[41] Because Treg cells are immune suppressive, this alteration allows for endometriotic fragments to survive and easily implant into tissue outside of the uterus.

To enhance and power your immune system further, additional supplements and herbs can be used (see chapter 11), though they cannot replace lifestyle and dietary changes. For example, if you continue to work on your computer late at night, stay indoors all day, and maintain an erratic sleep schedule, taking a supplement to maintain a healthy immune system may not be very effective.

Gut Health and Dysbiosis

Just like all inflammation in the gut, endometriosis-associated intestinal inflammation commonly alters the bacterial balance in the gut. Research on the intestinal flora in female rhesus monkeys with endometriosis demonstrated more severe intestinal inflammation and a reduced amount of aerobic lactobacilli and gram-negative bacteria (beneficial bacteria) than primates without the disease.[42]

Here's why a balanced gut is so important: Dysbiosis (an imbalance in the gut microbiota) can lead to health disturbances such as poor digestion, malabsorption of nutrients, chronic inflammation and an increased prevalence of gastrointestinal infections.[43] The beneficial flora that live in the gut have many important roles, including toxin elimination (heavy metals, et cetera), xenobiotic and drug metabolism, hormone balancing, maintenance of the gut barrier, metabolism of important nutrients such as vitamins K and B, and healthy digestion.[44] Beneficial bacteria that reside in the gut are important for protecting us from infection. They prevent pathogens from binding to the gut and produce their own antibiotics. Without adequate beneficial bacteria in the gut, our defenses are down, and the result is often chronic GI infections and an impaired, dysregulated immune system.

Various dietary, environmental exposures and emotional stressors can impact our gut health. A diet low in fiber and vegetables and high in processed sugars, unhealthy fats and processed meats — the so-called Standard American Diet, or SAD — can negatively alter the gut microbiota, leading to a reduction in important, beneficial bacteria.

> **Antibiotics taken in the first two years of life appear to be especially devastating to healthy microbiota development and increased chronic disease risk.**

The Gut-Estrogen Connection

The gut is an important site for proper estrogen elimination. Remember, estrogen can be like fertilizer for endometriosis growth. Estrogen is metabolized and conjugated (manufactured into a safer, removable form) in the liver and then packaged into bile acids for excretion via the feces. When we eat a meal, especially a meal with fat, we excrete bile acids into the small intestine to aid in fat absorption. Bile then binds to fiber to be excreted in our stools.

Certain bacteria in the gut secrete an enzyme called beta-glucuronidase, which cleaves the glucuronide molecule from estrogen, and converts estrogen into a more toxic form. Basically, this enzyme removes the important packaging done in the liver, and this more toxic form of estrogen is reabsorbed into circulation instead of excreted through the stool. Ultimately, this adds to the total estrogen load. Lactobacillus, a strain of beneficial bacteria that exists in large amounts in our large intestine, decreases the activity of B-glucuronidase.[45] Remember, this type of bacteria was found to be lower in monkeys with endo.

Genetically modified (GM) foods are also problematic. The chemical glyphosate, which is found in GM foods, appears to negatively alter our gut microbiota.[46] Glyphosate is an active ingredient in Roundup, a herbicide sprayed on crops grown from GM seeds. Glyphosate has been shown to negatively impact beneficial bacteria, allowing pathogenic bacteria an opportunity to overgrow and impair health.

Dr. Samsel Seneff, an expert in genetically modified organisms (GMOs), links consumption of foods grown from GMOs with the development of chronic health conditions such as autism, obesity, inflammatory bowel disease, infertility, depression and allergies. For more information on GMOs, visit www.nongmoshoppingguide.com. Buying organic foods or foods labeled non-GMO can greatly reduce your exposure to GM foods.

Antibiotic use is probably one of the most destructive mechanisms for destroying and disrupting our gut microbiota. Even short-term use (7 days) of a broad-spectrum antibiotic has been shown to damage beneficial bacteria, and these microbial changes can last up to two years, if not longer. This can result in a reduction of bacterial diversity, which greatly diminishes one's health and wellness. In addition, the use of antibiotics can induce mutations in healthy gut bacteria, leading to antibiotic resistance.[47]

The majority of women who we see at our practice suffer from gastrointestinal discomfort. The cause of their discomfort varies. However, we have noted an increased incidence of small intestinal bacterial overgrowth (SIBO). SIBO is a syndrome resulting from an elevated number and/or abnormal type of bacteria in the small intestine. Normally, the majority of bacteria reside in the large intestine, with decreasing amounts

Did You Know?

The Most Common GM Foods

- corn and corn products (for example, corn syrup)
- soybean
- cottonseed
- canola oils
- beet sugar

There is strong evidence that psychological stress can have a negative impact on gut microbiota. For example, a reduction in lactobacilli has been observed in humans during school examinations, in rhesus monkeys removed from their mothers, and in mice relocated to a new cage without food and water.[49] We are all exposed to stress throughout our lifetime. Learning how to reduce stress and modify the way our bodies react to stress can help to protect our important GI friends.

as you travel up the small intestine toward the stomach. One study observed an increased occurrence of SIBO in women with endometriosis;[48] in fact, in a study of 50 women with endo (confirmed by laparoscopy), 40 tested positive for SIBO. (For symptoms and risk factors, see "Symptoms and Risk Factors of SIBO," page 47).

The most common test for SIBO is a hydrogen and methane breath test. This simple test can be done in your doctor's office or with a test kit from a specialty lab.

Some individuals will require ongoing and/or targeted probiotic support through diet or a combination of diet and probiotic supplements (see chapter 11). For example, if you have a mutation (polymorphism) in the FUT2 gene, you may require a daily bifidobacteria probiotic.[50] The FUT2 gene regulates the amount of bifidobacteria growing in the gut. A low amount of bifidobacteria increases the risk of developing inflammatory bowel disease, autoimmune disorders and infections such as *Candida* overgrowth. If a person has a mutation in this gene, they may not be able to house a healthy amount of bifidobacteria in the gut without ongoing supplementation.

Other individuals who may require daily, targeted probiotic therapy are those born via a cesarean section, those not breastfed for at least 6 months, and those who were given antibiotics in the first 2 years of life. Passage through the vagina and consumption of breast milk provide critical exposure to beneficial bacteria and immune-enhancing factors, and research has shown an increased rate of chronic disease in children and adults lacking these.[51]

Antibiotics taken in the first two years of life appear to be especially devastating to healthy microbiota development and increased chronic disease risk. Antibiotic use early in life causes imbalances in the gut microbiota, often referred to as dysbiosis. This can lead to immune dysregulation and an increased incidence of chronic health conditions such as obesity, autoimmune disease(s), allergies and atopic disorders, and infectious diseases (for example, viruses and *Candida*).[52]

Increasing the amount of beneficial bacteria in the gut can assist in healthy estrogen elimination, lower intestinal inflammation, improve digestion, strengthen the immune system, improve detoxification and offer protection from intestinal infections. The Endometriosis Diet Plan is designed to balance gut bacteria in a three-step process:

1. Balance gut bacteria and address potential bacterial overgrowth in the small intestine.

2. Recommend specific foods to encourage the growth of beneficial bacteria in a slow, progressive manner to assure tolerance and continued symptom improvement.

3. Add greater amounts of prebiotic foods to further grow and strengthen your army of beneficial bacteria.

Symptoms and Risk Factors of SIBO

Typical symptoms of small intestinal bacterial overgrowth, or SIBO, may include:

- bloating
- flatulence
- abdominal pain
- diarrhea
- constipation
- weight loss
- weight gain
- fatigue
- pelvic pain

- steatorrhoea (fat in stools)
- malabsorption
- excessive burping after meals
- skin problems such as rosacea
- iron deficiency
- B$_{12}$ deficiency
- vitamin D deficiency
- leaky gut

Risk factors for developing SIBO include:

- constipation
- poor intestinal motility
- neurological damage to the gut
- frequent use of antibiotics
- low beneficial bacteria
- adhesions or blockages in the intestines
- low stomach acid (this includes individuals on proton pump inhibitors)
- heavy alcohol consumption

- smoking
- hypothyroidism
- chronic stress
- frequent use of opiates (pain medication)
- chronically elevated cortisol
- ileocecal valve dysfunction (the valve between the small intestine and large intestine)
- birth control pill use (possibly)

A very important but often neglected component to gut health and proper digestion is mindful eating. Eating with awareness is critical to the digestive process. Just thinking about food initiates digestion by increasing salivation and the production of digestive juices. Observing and smelling the foods we are about to consume further enhances this process. (For more on mindful eating, see "Checklist," page 48.)

Mitochondrial Dysfunction

Mitochondria are the cell's energy powerhouse. Interestingly, mitochondria started off as bacteria, but they evolved acting as the host's energy supplier. The most important function of the mitochondria is cellular respiration, which is the cell's system for producing adenosine triphosphate (or ATP — our body's energy currency). Energy is obtained by the oxidation (breakdown) of proteins, carbohydrates and fats into ATP. In addition to energy production, the mitochondria also assist in building hormones

> A diet low in fiber and vegetables and high in processed sugars, unhealthy fats and processed meats — the so-called Standard American Diet, or SAD — can negatively alter the gut microbiota, leading to a reduction in important, beneficial bacteria.

Checklist
How to Eat with Awareness to Improve Digestion

1. **Make sure you are relaxed before eating.** Eating when you are stressed will impair digestion. Deep belly breathing is a great way to relax; it also activates the vagus nerve, which coordinates the nervous system with the digestive process. We often recommend four rounds of 4-7-8 breathing before meals. For directions on how to perform this technique, see chapter 7.

2. **Chew your food thoroughly.** This is an important first step in healthy digestion. We recommend chewing each bite 30 to 60 times, or until it is a liquid. This makes it easier for digestive enzymes to interact with food and break apart large complexes (for example, protein) into easily absorbable molecules such as single amino acids. By simply chewing, we can sometimes alleviate digestive discomfort. One of the biggest causes of heartburn is not chewing our foods enough.

3. **Eat with awareness.** Refrain from eating while working, answering emails, watching TV or driving.

4. **Be adventurous.** Try new flavors by using herbs and spices.

5. **Stop eating as soon as you feel full.** There is no need to clean your plate. Overeating can cause digestive discomfort and overwhelm your body.

6. **Eat a variety of foods.** Eating the same things every day can contribute to the development of food sensitivities if you have a damaged intestine. We recommend rotating your protein sources every 4 to 5 days and eating a variety of vegetables.

such as testosterone and estrogen, the production of enzymes for detoxification, pyrimidine and lipid biosynthesis, metal metabolism, calcium homeostasis and flux, neurotransmitter synthesis, heat production and proper insulin secretion. This important cell organelle plays a critical role in apoptosis, or programmed cell death. If the mitochondria becomes damaged, this can impair organ function and lead to irregular cell growth. In fact, it is speculated that several health conditions could be a result of mitochondrial damage or dysfunction, including cancer, diabetes, fibromyalgia, bipolar disease, accelerated aging, anxiety and chronic fatigue syndrome.[53]

The mitochondria play a key role in activating the immune system and controlling the inflammatory response.[56] The mitochondria become activated by cellular damage due to trauma, toxins (for example, pesticides, heavy metals, BPA), drugs (for example, statins, antidepressants, metformin, antibiotics), free radicals, stress, lack of sleep and infection. Once this activation occurs, the mitochondria send out a signal to turn on the immune system, which includes the initiation of the inflammatory cascade.

Not only is inflammation painful, but it also creates a vicious cycle: inflammation damages the mitochondria, impairing mitochondrial function, which leads to symptoms such as fatigue, a weakened immune system and accelerated aging. This strengthens the argument that adequate sleep, daily stress reduction, proper diet, reduction of toxic load and the ruling out of chronic infections are imperative for endo management. The program presented in this book provides information on how to reduce toxic exposure, improve sleep, eat to fuel your mitochondria and increase antioxidants, and reduce your daily stress.

Even if you have genetic mutations in your mitochondrial DNA or damage to your mitochondria, you can repair and optimize mitochondrial function and stimulate mitochondria production. For example, there are proven dietary strategies, such as a ketogenic diet (see "FAQ," page 50), fasting or intermittent fasting, that accomplish these goals.

Fasting is another strategy. It typically takes a few days on a water fast to switch from burning glucose to burning ketones. You would then need to follow your fast with a ketogenic diet. Although there is great evidence that fasting can improve mitochondrial function, we typically do not recommend fasting if you are not healthy or are nutritionally depleted. Many endo patients already suffer from severe fatigue, and malnutrition is common. An extended fast may exacerbate these conditions. For these patients, intermittent fasting may be more beneficial.

RESEARCH SPOTLIGHT

The Role of DNA in Endo

Mitochondria have a small amount of their own DNA (mtDNA), which is essential for their normal function. There can, however, be genetic mutations in this DNA, and, in addition, it is highly susceptible to free-radical damage. We have discussed the role of oxidation and free radicals as they relate to inflammation and the pathophysiology of endometriosis (see page 38). Antioxidants can greatly reduce free radicals, thereby protecting all cells and the DNA within them.

Genetic polymorphisms (mutations) in mitochondrial DNA have been discovered in research, and these may increase a person's risk for developing endo. For example, the mitochondrial DNA 16189 variant appears to be higher in patients with endo.[54] This could make a woman with this genetic mutation more susceptible to developing endo. Mitochondrial proteins have also been found to be different in women with endo than in healthy controls, and quality of oocyte — an immature egg that is rich in mitochondria and important for fertilization — is decreased in women with endometriosis.[55] These differences may impact both the disease process and fertility.

Even if you have genetic mutations in your mitochondrial DNA or damage to your mitochondria, you can repair and optimize mitochondrial function.

There are several ways to manage intermittent fasting. Our favorite is to limit eating to only 4 to 10 hours of each day. This can easily be achieved by eating your first meal in the late morning and your last meal in the early evening, allowing for a 12- to 20-hour fast each night. Others prefer to do 1 to 2 days of 24-hour fasting each week in order to achieve health benefits. The easiest way to do this is to eat your last meal sometime between 3 p.m. and 5 p.m. and then fast until the same time the following day, allowing much of the fast to happen while you are sleeping. You may be thinking, "I cannot go even a few hours without eating or I get dizzy and cranky and have low energy." This is most likely because you are on a blood sugar rollercoaster. When in ketosis, you will be less hungry and your energy will be more stable.

These strategies are not for everyone. However, a ketogenic diet and some form of fasting can be highly therapeutic, especially if you have a lot of inflammation, estrogen dominance and neurological damage. We do not recommend ketogenic diets or fasting if you have low thyroid function, adrenal dysfunction, are pregnant or breastfeeding, are very active (especially if you do frequent, high-intensity workouts), are malnourished, have a history of kidney stones or have gallbladder disease.

FAQ

Q. What is a ketogenic diet?

A. It's a very low-carbohydrate, very high-fat diet that allows the body to use fats, rather than sugar, as fuel. A brief period on this diet (1 to 2 months), or cycling on and off, can be very healing to our bodies when appropriate and if done correctly. With the ingestion of ample carbohydrates, our body uses glucose for fuel. Carbohydrates are oxidized for energy and free radicals are produced. In addition, glucose in the blood can be glycosylated (a sugar and a protein attach, creating a substance much like caramel), creating inflammation and causing damage to arterial walls. When carbohydrates are limited, the body switches to using ketones, a cleaner fuel. A healthy state of ketosis has been demonstrated to starve cancer cells, induce mitochondrial production, reduce the number of free radicals produced, increase production of GABA (a calming neurochemical often referred to as "natural valium"), increase tolerance to emotional stress and reduce inflammation.[57]

In addition to the positive health impacts of running on ketones, ample fat in the diet is also essential for building functional mitochondrial membranes. Ketogenic diets can also help with small intestinal bacterial overgrowth, which is common in women with endometriosis (see pages 45–47 for more information about SIBO).

In addition to diet, exercise can be an important component in improving mitochondrial function, decreasing inflammation and slowing the aging process. Exercise is a form of stress on the body, which increases the number and function of mitochondria. Like calorie restriction (achieved by fasting and intermittent fasting) and ketosis, exercise stimulates amp-activated protein kinase (AMPK), which triggers the production of new mitochondria.[58] Overeating and inactivity appear to decrease AMPK activity. As mentioned, according to research, regular exercise appears to stimulate AMPK activity.[59] AMPK can also greatly reduce inflammation. We have included an entire chapter on exercise (see chapter 9) and have provided a few examples of exercise programs to get you started.

There are some essential nutrients that can be helpful in supporting mitochondrial function and protecting the mitochondria, although it's important to note that supplementation for mitochondria support will not replace lifestyle and dietary changes. Find a complete list of some of our favorite supplements and herbs to aid in mitochondrial health and function in chapter 11.

Caution

If you are following a ketogenic diet, fasting or doing intermittent fasting, you most likely need more carbohydrates if you have the following symptoms:

- difficulty recovering from your workouts
- cessation of menstruation or irregular cycles
- trouble sleeping
- worsening fatigue

Hormone Imbalance

When discussing endo, it's important to have a basic understanding of hormones. An entire book could be written about the role of hormones in endo's pathophysiology and disease; however, this section is meant to provide a brief overview of hormones and some examples of how your disease may be impacted by hormone imbalances.

Balance among hormones is vital: sex hormones (estrogen, progesterone and testosterone), adrenal hormones (cortisol and DHEA) and thyroid hormones all work in harmony. Think of each hormone as an instrument in a beautiful orchestra. If one instrument is out of tune, or is playing considerably louder than the others, the tune will be negatively altered. This is why it's not advantageous to focus on one specific hormone, even estrogen. It makes better sense to concentrate on balancing these hormones. This normally involves enhancing detoxification, dietary strategies, stress reduction, exercise and movement, herbs and nutrients, and, occasionally, hormone replacement.

A basic understanding of estrogen metabolism is important for the treatment and management of endometriosis. Endo is known to be an estrogen-related disease; therefore, modulation of production and enhanced elimination of estrogen may aid in slowing the progression of the disease or recurrence of endo following a surgical intervention. As stated earlier, estrogen can be thought of as a fertilizer for endo, and decreasing a woman's estrogen load may help to control the disease. Estrogen is produced by converting testosterone and androstenedione into estrone through a process called aromatization, which is

Estrogen's 28-Day Cycle

In premenopausal women, the ovaries are responsible for the majority of estrogen production, which is produced at varying amounts based on a woman's menstrual cycle. The ovaries and the pituitary gland (located in the brain) work together to prepare a woman's body for pregnancy each month. If there is no fertilization, the result is menstruation, which occurs on average every 28 days.

- Day 1 of the menstrual cycle is the first day of full bleeding (not spotting). On the first day of the cycle, estrogen is at its lowest.

- Ovarian estrogen levels gradually increase and peak around day 12 to 14, during ovulation, when the unfertilized egg is released from the follicle (the fluid-filled sac in the ovary that houses the egg).

- The corpus luteum (ruptured follicle) releases decreasing amounts of estrogen until about day 24, and if the egg is not fertilized, estrogen levels rapidly drop, which results in menstruation.

facilitated by an enzyme called aromatase. The ovaries, placenta, adipose tissue, skin, brain, and other human tissues contain aromatase.[60] In the peripheral tissues, estrone is converted into the most active form of estrogen, estradiol.

The presence of estrogen is a signal for the uterine lining to thicken. (We will come back to this when we discuss estrogen's relationship to progesterone in uterine-lining thickness.) Estrogen is toxic in large amounts, and therefore the body has a sophisticated system for metabolizing and detoxifying it for elimination. Through the work of a series of enzymes in the liver, estrogen undergoes a four-step process that results in a variety of estrogen metabolites. These metabolites are then packaged into bile and excreted into the small intestine when a meal is consumed. Estrogen metabolites bind to fiber in the intestines and are eliminated in the stool.

In women with endometriosis, there is some evidence of altered estrogen production and, many times, decreased elimination. First, an increase in aromatase expression has been observed in women with endo.[61] Second, endometriotic implants and endometriomas have elevated levels of aromatase messenger RNA, and are capable of producing their own estrogen. These two factors alone can result in a lot of endo fertilizer: estrogen.

To further complicate matters, aromatase can be stimulated by prostaglandin E2, which is released mainly by macrophages during an inflammatory response. Remember, macrophages are found in greater amounts in women with endo. And here's more bad news: estrogen induces PGE2 formation, creating a vicious cycle.[62] If you are overweight, there will also be estrogen produced in fat tissue, which will further increase your estrogen load.

If you are overweight, there will also be estrogen produced in fat tissue, which will further increase your estrogen load.

If your estrogen production is increased, the metabolism and detoxification of estrogen becomes a critical function to reduce your total estrogen load. Genetically, differences in important genes for estrogen metabolism have been observed in women with endo, which can result in increased amounts of estrogen. For example, mutations in the CYP2C19 and HSD17B1 — genes associated with estrogen metabolism — appear to exist more frequently in women with endo.[63] CYP2C19 encodes cytochrome P450 detox system enzymes (enzymes involved in the first phase of estrogen metabolism in the liver). A reduced function of this enzyme would result in elevated circulating estrogen. Another example is COMT,[64] which detoxifies estrogen by hydroxylation in the second phase of estrogen metabolism in the liver. Note that both of these examples involve detoxification of estrogen in the liver. The liver is our main site for detoxification of hormones, toxins, ammonia, most drugs (including pharmaceuticals) and alcohol. This is where supporting your body's detoxification and limiting your toxic exposure play a huge role in estrogen metabolism.

> **If your estrogen production is increased, the metabolism and detoxification of estrogen becomes a critical function to reduce your total estrogen load.**

How Your Liver Handles Toxins

The liver has only a certain amount of the enzymes and key nutrients needed for detoxification. Think of your liver as a bucket with a hole at the bottom — into which a very viscous solution of toxins (including estrogen) is being poured. The bucket contains enzymes to break down the thick liquid into a watery liquid, allowing it to easily flow out through the hole. As long as the amount of thick liquid being poured into the bucket does not exceed the rate of its breakdown into water, the bucket does not overflow. If, however, the liquid is poured too quickly into the bucket, or there are not enough enzymes to transform it into a thin liquid, the solution will overflow. This is also how it works in your body. If you are exposed to more toxins than your liver can detoxify, toxins such as estrogen will accumulate in your body and cause damage and poor health.

An elevated estrogen load can certainly cause a lot of problems and contribute to endo disease progression. However, many times it is not simply a surplus of estrogen alone that contributes to disease progression, but rather an imbalance of estrogen with other hormones. You could say the estrogen is drowning out the other "instruments" in your hormonal orchestra.

Progesterone is an example of a hormone that, when in balance with estrogen, maintains harmony. It prevents the estrogen-driven growth of the endometrium by preventing continued thickening of the uterine lining during the luteal phase — or second half — of the menstrual cycle. If estrogen levels continue to dominate in the luteal phase, the uterine lining will be thicker, which will most likely result in heavier, more painful menses. Many women with endo appear to be progesterone-resistant, which contributes to endometriotic tissue survival and proliferation outside of the uterus.

In addition, progesterone activates an enzyme called 17b-HSD type 2, which converts estradiol (the most active form of estrogen) into estrone (a significantly less active form).[65] The result is an increase in active estrogen, which may contribute to an increased concentration of estradiol and enhanced growth of endometriotic lesions.

Estrogen also has an intimate relationship with adrenal stress hormones such as cortisol. Cortisol is critical for our survival. However, as is the case with other hormones, we want just the right amount — not too much, and not too little. Cortisol is important for reducing inflammation, and levels of production are increased when the body is injured or fighting infection, as well as when we are psychologically or physically stressed. When cortisol levels remain elevated, or over time become depleted, hormonal balance is affected. For example, progesterone is converted to cortisol. If cortisol needs are continuously high, progesterone levels become depleted. This, aside from the ramifications of low progesterone, creates estrogen dominance.

Another example of cortisol's impact on hormones can be found in its relationship to thyroid hormones. Both high and low levels of cortisol affect thyroid hormone levels and reduce thyroid receptor site sensitivity. In addition, prolonged cortisol elevation reduces the liver's ability to detoxify estrogen, which results in increased amounts of thyroid-binding globulin (TBG). This hormone transports thyroid through the body, but when thyroid is attached to this hormone, it cannot attach to cells. Therefore, if levels of TBG are excessive, someone may experience symptoms of a low thyroid.

You may be wondering how to synchronize all of these hormones. Working with an experienced, qualified practitioner for fine-tuning may be necessary, but you can begin the process on your own by following the Endometriosis Diet Plan, practicing daily stress reduction techniques, moving your body, getting adequate sleep, and supporting your body's natural detoxification processes. In addition, we have provided suggestions as to herbs and nutrients that may gently assist in balancing hormones (see chapter 11).

> **Cortisol is critical for our survival. However, as is the case with other hormones, we want just the right amount — not too much, and not too little.**

Stress

It is well known that stress weakens our immune defenses,[66] increases the inflammatory process,[67] alters blood sugar regulation,[68] contributes to infertility and menstrual cycle irregularities,[69] impairs gastrointestinal function[70] and alters the delicate microbial balance in the gut.[71] When discussing stress, it is imperative to distinguish between different types of stress. Stress can be classified as acute stress, episodic acute stress, and chronic stress.

> **People who are known as Type A personalities and worrywarts tend to experience high levels of episodic stress.**

- **Acute stress.** A specific event or situation in which our safety or ego is threatened typically causes an acute stress response. The event is brief and the body quickly returns to a relaxed state. Examples of acute stress are nearly hitting another car, giving a speech and even an intense bout of exercise. Because acute stress is short-lived, it doesn't have enough time to do the extensive damage associated with other, ongoing types of stress.

- **Episodic acute stress.** This refers to frequent episodes of acute stress. Common causes are having too many obligations, poor time management, lateness and an overall slew of self-inflicted demands and pressures competing for your attention. People who are known as Type A personalities and worrywarts tend to experience high levels of episodic stress. Physiological symptoms common with this type of stress include frequent tension headaches, migraines, high blood pressure, anxiety, depression, sleep abnormalities, high blood sugar, gastrointestinal discomfort, anger and heart disease.

- **Chronic stress.** This is the relentless stress that wears people down from day to day. It's the type that accompanies poverty, a dysfunctional home life, an unhappy marriage and job dissatisfaction. Chronic stress is never-ending, and typically the person views their situation as hopeless. Those who suffer from it tend to become mentally accustomed and numb to it; however, this type of stress is very harmful to your health. It can result in death from suicide, violence, heart attack, stroke and other chronic diseases.

After learning a little more about the changes that occur in your body in response to stress, you may better understand how stress can worsen your endo symptoms. For example, endo has many physiological abnormalities, such as a dysfunctional immune system, chronic inflammation, hormonal imbalances and dysbiosis. Stress — specifically, episodic and chronic stress — negatively influences these physiological changes. Everyone experiences stress at some point in their life. You may be

The 6 Steps of Stress Response

When we experience psychological or physiological stress, the hormones of the hypothalamus-pituitary-adrenal (HPA) axis control the response. Here is a step-by-step description of the stress response:

1. A stressful event occurs. Examples include a life-threatening situation (almost being hit by a car), giving a speech, too much caffeine and a chronic infection.

2. The hypothalamus — which is located in the brain and serves as the command center of the stress response — is activated. It communicates with the entire body through the autonomic nervous system (ANS), which controls functions such as breathing, heart rate and the dilation and constriction of blood vessels. The ANS consists of two subsystems: the sympathetic nervous system (SNS) and the parasympathetic nervous system (PNS). The SNS, often referred to as the "fight or flight" nervous system, prepares the body to respond quickly to danger. It can be likened to a gas pedal in a car. The PNS is also known as the "rest and digest" nervous system, as it's active when you are sleeping and eating. It serves to calm the body down after the initial danger has passed. It can be thought of as the car's brakes.

3. The hypothalamus activates the SNS by way of the autonomic nerves to the adrenal glands. These glands sit on top of the kidneys. The adrenal glands respond by releasing the hormones epinephrine (also called adrenaline) and norepinephrine into the bloodstream. Epinephrine triggers several physiological changes, such as an increase in the heart rate to circulate more nutrients to muscles, a dilation of the small blood vessels in the lungs to increase oxygen consumption, and an increase in the release of glucose (blood sugar) from the liver and fats from adipose tissue to supply fuel to the muscles.

4. Following the initial surge of epinephrine, the hypothalamus then activates the HPA axis. The HPA axis holds the gas pedal down to the floor, and will continue to do so until the brain perceives that the body is once again safe. The hypothalamus releases corticotropin-releasing hormone (CRH), which stimulates the pituitary gland to release adrenocorticotropic hormone (ACTH).

5. ACTH stimulates the adrenal glands to release glucocorticoids such as cortisol. Cortisol stays elevated until the threat passes. Cortisol has several physiological roles, such as increasing blood sugar, increasing potassium excretion, dampening the immune response and causing damage to the hippocampus (the memory center of the brain). Long-term elevated levels of cortisol and epinephrine can contribute to a weakened immune system, anxiety, poor sleep, weight gain (especially in the abdominal region), thyroid disorders and high blood sugar.

6. Once the brain believes the danger has passed, the PNS is activated, which essentially shuts down the stress response. The main neurotransmitter released is acetylcholine. It acts to slow the heart rate, dilate blood vessels in the GI tract, stimulate the salivary glands, increase peristalsis, fill male and female genitals with blood, and constrict the bronchioles in the lungs. In addition, serotonin and GABA are released. These two neurotransmitters are responsible for calming the nervous system and achieving restful sleep and healthy digestion. Unfortunately, when we are chronically stressed, these feel-good neurotransmitters can be depleted, leading to depression, insomnia, digestive issues, sexual and menstrual dysfunction and poor sleep.

experiencing one or all of these types of stress right now. In fact, living with a chronic illness such as endo is a cause of episodic and chronic stress.

There is also strong evidence that living with stress, either current or from past trauma, can make your endo symptoms worse.[72] Practicing a daily stress reduction program and resolving past trauma can be essential for optimizing your general health and controlling your endo symptoms. Chapter 7 can assist you with stress reduction and give you ideas to help you heal from adverse childhood experiences.

> **Living with stress, either current or from past trauma, can make your endo symptoms worse.**

RESEARCH SPOTLIGHT
When Your Childhood Affects Your Health

Past experiences and traumas that conjure up negative emotions can cause a stress response in your body each time you think about them. There is an ongoing area of research referred to as the Adverse Childhood Experiences (ACEs) study. Conducted by the Centers for Disease Control and Prevention (CDC) and Kaiser Permanente, the study aims to assess how negative childhood experiences such as abuse and neglect can predict your risk for developing major chronic diseases.[73]

There are 10 types of ACEs, including separation or divorce of parents; physical, sexual or emotional abuse; physical and emotional neglect; domestic violence; mental illness in the family; substance abuse in the household; and incarceration of a family member. Each type of experience prior to the 18th birthday counts as one ACE.

According to research, 60% of women who suffered sexual abuse develop fibromyalgia; two or more ACEs increase the risk of developing autoimmune conditions by up to 80%; and a person with six or more ACEs has a reduced lifespan of 20 years. For more information on ACEs and to determine your ACE score, go to www.acestoohigh.com.

The Types of Sleep

Once you fall asleep, you experience different types and phases of sleep:

Quiet Sleep (or Non-REM Sleep)

Stage N1

- This is the time between wakefulness and light sleep.
- You are no longer aware of your surroundings; however, you can easily be awakened.
- This is the period when you are dropping into sleep.
- During this phase, the predominant brain waves are theta waves.
- Your body temperature begins to drop, your muscles relax, and there is a usual side-to-side eye movement.

Stage N2

- Your eyes slow to stillness and your heart and breathing rates slow.
- Brain-wave activity is irregular, with slow waves mixed with short bursts of faster waves.
- About half of the night is spent in this phase.
- In this stage, there may be periods of muscle twitching alternating with muscle relaxation.

Stages N3 and N4

- These are also referred to as deep sleep or slow-wave sleep.
- Delta waves become the primary brain waves in this stage.
- Heart rate and blood pressure continue to drop until reaching a 20% to 30% reduction from waking rates.

Sleep Deprivation and Poor-Quality Sleep

Everyone sleeps. In fact, we spend one-third of our lives sleeping! We need sleep just as we need water and food to survive. It is critical to maintain moods, memory, cognitive performance, and to assure normal function of the endocrine and immune systems. A lack of sleep or poor-quality sleep can be linked to a wide variety of chronic health conditions including obesity, diabetes, hypertension, Alzheimer's disease and mood disorders such as depression. The problem is that most of us don't get enough. According to a sleep survey conducted by the National Center for Health Statistics (NCHS) in 2013-2014, approximately one-third of U.S. adults do not meet the minimal recommendation of 7 hours of sleep each night.[74]

Did You Know?

How Much Sleep Is Ideal?

- Age 18–25: 7–9 hours
- Age 26–64: 7–9 hours
- Age 65-plus: 7–8 hours

- This is the stage of sleep when much of your bodily repair occurs.
- Slowed heart rate and blood pressure give the heart a much-needed rest.
- Blood flow is diverted toward the brain, cooling the temperature.
- Large amounts of human growth hormone are released from the pituitary gland, stimulating tissue growth and repair.
- The greatest amount of growth hormone is released between 10 p.m. and 2 a.m.
- The immune system is strengthened during this phase, aiding your body in protecting you from infection and illness.
- Approximately 20% of your sleep time is spent in this stage when you are young; however, this decreases as we age, and after age 65, deep sleep is nearly absent.

Dreaming Sleep (or Rapid Eye Movement [REM] Sleep)

- Your brain is very active thinking and dreaming.
- REM sleep gets its name because your eyes move rapidly back and forth behind closed eyelids.
- During REM sleep your body temperature, heart rate, blood pressure and breathing increase back to daytime levels.
- Your sympathetic ("fight or flight") nervous system is very active during this period.
- REM sleep is important for brain restoration; it is believed to help clear unnecessary information from your brain and help to process new information. It is like an efficient filing system, constantly removing irrelevant files and replacing them with new.
- REM sleep occurs three to five times a night, approximately every 90 minutes, increasing in duration with each REM cycle.

To better understand how much sleep we actually need, 18 leading scientists from the National Sleep Foundation formed an expert panel to review more than 300 scientific publications on sleep.[75] According to these experts, sleep needs vary depending on a person's age. Young adults (ages 18–25) and adults (ages 26–64) require 7 to 9 hours, and older adults (over 65) do best with 7 to 8 hours. In addition to not getting enough sleep, 35% of Americans reported that their sleep was only poor to fair quality, and 25% of women wake feeling unrested.[76]

Unfortunately, patients with endo and pelvic pain often have a difficult time sleeping. Chronic, severe pain can certainly hinder a good night's rest. Women with endo have been shown to have significantly worse sleep quality than women without the disease.[77] And here's where the double-edged sword comes in: lack of sleep and poor-quality sleep can worsen pain![78]

FAQ

Q. How are hormones affected by poor sleep?

A. Here are a few examples:

1. Cortisol is increased, resulting in elevated blood sugar, weakened immunity, an increase in central fat deposition (belly fat) and, over time, an increase in inflammation.
2. Follicle-stimulating hormone (FSH) and luteinizing hormone (LH), which are both tightly tied to reproduction and menstrual cycles, are released during sleep. Sleep irregularities could lead to hormonal imbalance.
3. Growth hormone production and secretion is also increased during sleep. This important hormone delegates the body's proportions of fat and muscle during adulthood and aids in nightly bodily repair.
4. Inadequate sleep may reduce levels of leptin, which regulates appetite and carbohydrate cravings.

These are just a few examples of how sleep deprivation can negatively impact your health. In regards to your endo pain, changes in the above hormones may contribute to your disease by altering healthy blood sugar regulation, hormone balance and immune regulation.

Why does a lack of sleep contribute to pain? When we sleep we are not merely closing our eyes and resting. Sleep is a time when our bodies are making important changes, recharging and healing. During sleep, many cells demonstrate an increased production of proteins needed for cell growth and repair. Sleep is also a time when the body secretes several important hormones that impact growth and energy production, and control metabolic and endocrine functions.[79]

In order to better understand how to improve your sleep, it's important to have a basic understanding of how sleep patterns are regulated and what normally occurs while you are asleep. This gives you an underpinning for why specific activities are recommended or discouraged to improve your sleep.

> **Our sleep and wake cycles rely on specific brain activity and chemicals produced by our bodies, controlled by sleep homeostasis and circadian rhythms.**

Our sleep and wake cycles rely on specific brain activity and chemicals produced by our bodies, controlled by sleep homeostasis and circadian rhythms. In humans, the 24-hour sleep/wake cycle consists of approximately 8 hours of nocturnal sleep and 16 hours of daytime wakefulness. Sleep homeostasis is not fully understood, but it is believed that a chemical called adenosine has a lot to do with it. During the day, this chemical builds up, inducing our need to sleep. As we sleep, this chemical decreases, and we are able to wake refreshed.

When and what chemicals get released is determined by the body's internal clock, known as the circadian rhythms. A person's circadian rhythms are established within the first few months of life, but can be altered by travel (change in time zones), night-shift work, pregnancy, certain medications, changes in sleep routines (staying up late or sleeping in), various medical problems such as Alzheimer's or Parkinson's disease, stress and mental health problems.

The type of light and the time of day you are exposed to this light plays a central role in establishing your circadian clock. The shorter-wavelength blue light that is emitted from the sun and digital screens (such as those found on smartphones, computers, tablets and television screens) signals our brains to stay awake. This type of light suppresses melatonin, a hormone released by the pineal gland in the brain, which tells the body to sleep. Melatonin also triggers the release of other hormones such as testosterone, estrogen and human growth hormone.

The release of melatonin at sundown made perfect sense in the world of our ancestors. When the sun went down, it was time to go to sleep. They did not have artificial light, and were in perfect sync with the earth's natural lighting flow. Exposure to this light during the day is important for production of serotonin, which is converted into melatonin after dark. This is why exposure to sunlight in the beginning part of the day, without wearing sunglasses, is important for sleep.

However, watching TV, reading on a tablet or a smartphone or working on your computer at night can lower melatonin production and contribute to sleeping problems. One way to block the blue light is by wearing amber/yellow-colored glasses after dark. In addition to your exposure to light, the time you go to bed and rise also impacts your circadian rhythms, and research suggests that the time you rise may be more important.[80] Sleeping in on the weekends may throw off your circadian rhythms more than the time you go to bed, which will make waking on Monday morning more difficult. Turning in earlier, awaking at sunrise each morning and getting some morning sunlight each day are the best ways to set a healthy internal sleep-and-wake clock.

Typically, a person with a healthy sleep pattern moves predictably through each stage of sleep (see "The Types of Sleep," pages 58–59), alternating between non-REM and REM sleep. In adults aged 18 to 25, four to six non-REM and REM cycles occur throughout the night, with the majority of deep sleep occurring in the first half of the night. An adult requires, on average, 7 to 9 hours to complete these cycles; teenagers require approximately 9.5 hours. As we age, less N3 sleep and more N1 sleep takes place, resulting in more waking during the night.

> **Exposure to sunlight in the beginning part of the day, without wearing sunglasses, is important for sleep.**

Did You Know?

How to Get a Good Sleep

- Turn in earlier
- Awaken at sunrise
- Get some morning sunlight each day

As you can see, sleep is an important factor in your overall health and your healing journey with endo. See chapter 8 for information on how to improve your sleep quality and quantity, including lifestyle and diet tips.

Diet and Food

There is evidence that specific dietary patterns and foods can reduce or increase inflammatory markers, which are often high in women with endo.

Although there are several purported "endometriosis diets," no specific diet has been studied for its use and success with treatment or management of the disease. A few studies on diet and its relationship to endo have been carried out; however, all of them were observational and not experimental. What this means is that populations or groups who had higher rates of endo were isolated and then their dietary patterns were studied. This does not show a causative effect of how their diets contributed to their disease progression, but rather shows one possible factor that may have encouraged the disease process.

Also, these types of studies analyze only a select part of a diet, such as red meat intake, versus a specific test diet with controlled components such as macronutrient (carbohydrates, fats and proteins) ratios, types of fats, et cetera. In addition, other important influences on health such as caloric intake, BMI, genetics, toxic exposure and lifestyle are not considered. As a result, looking to the scientific literature for the perfect endo diet is difficult, if not impossible.

There is evidence that specific dietary patterns and foods can reduce or increase inflammatory markers, which are often high in women with endo.[81] Dietary recommendations in this book are based on optimizing hormone balance, controlling inflammation, strengthening the immune system, balancing the gut microbiota, fueling the mitochondria and balancing blood sugar.

With this said, it is still important to discuss the available studies on this topic. No studies have yet been done to observe the relationship between macronutrient intakes and endo. However, a few studies on fat intake and endometriosis exist. Unfortunately, the results are inconsistent.[82]

Here's what is clear in the literature:

- Trans fatty acids and an imbalance in the ratio of omega-6 to omega-3 fatty acids enhance the production of inflammatory cytokines (increase inflammation).[83] Therefore, avoiding trans fatty acids (hydrogenated oils, partially hydrogenated oils, fried foods, margarine, shortening and all products containing these ingredients) and balancing the ratio of omega-3 to omega-6 fatty acid consumption is most likely a helpful dietary strategy for endo.

- Over-consumption of carbohydrates most likely worsens endo symptoms. Literature supports the idea that high consumption of added sugars and carbohydrates increases estrogen levels and contributes to inflammation and pain.[84]

- Excessive circulating insulin signals the ovaries to increase testosterone production and lowers SHBG levels, increasing free estrogen.[85] Elevated insulin levels also stimulate inflammation, resulting in increased pain, an upregulation of aromatase activity (whereby more estrogen is made) and immune suppression.[86]

A lower carbohydrate diet may be helpful in controlling endo symptoms and disease progression. Following the Endometriosis Diet Plan, starting in chapter 12, can help you to achieve this goal, as it is carbohydrate-controlled.

FAQ

Q. Is avoiding meat a good thing?

A. There are some "endo diets" that recommend complete avoidance of meat or abstinence from red meat. There is one study in the literature supporting this notion. The researchers found an increased incidence of endo in women who ate more red meat (7 or more times a week versus 3 or fewer times a week) and ham (3 or more times a week versus less than 3 servings a week).[87] Unfortunately, the study failed to include a few very important details about the quality of the meat consumed.

First, if the women in this study consumed conventionally raised grain-fed cattle, they may have increased their total estrogen load. Conventionally raised cattle in the United States are routinely supplemented with estrogen to increase milk productivity and improve the taste and consistency of the meat.[88] This is also true for chickens raised in the United States.[89]

Second, how the animal was raised and slaughtered contributes to the health aspects of the meat. If animals are raised and slaughtered under stressful conditions, the stress hormones are increased, which leads to the production of pro-inflammatory cytokines.[90] When we consume the meat, these stress hormones and inflammatory cytokines are ingested and negatively impact our health.

Lastly, the diet of conventionally raised animals consists predominantly, if not solely, of grains, which contain large amounts of omega-6 fatty acids, pesticides and chemicals. Ingestion of these meats increases our omega-6 fatty acid load, altering our omega-6 to omega-3 fatty acid ratio, resulting in increased inflammation. Purchasing and consuming meats from animals that have been humanely raised and slaughtered and raised in the absence of hormones and antibiotics, and have spent their lives grazing ("free range") may reduce or ameliorate the observed association of meat consumption and a higher incidence of endometriosis.

The scientific literature is also unclear about the association between dairy and endometriosis. One study demonstrated a reduced risk of endo with higher dairy consumption.[91] The researchers attributed this to the positive impact of vitamin D and calcium on the immune system. On the flip side of the argument, there are those who recommend avoidance of dairy to women with endo. This makes sense for milk from conventionally raised cows, as these cows are given estrogen to increase their milk production, and much of this estrogen ends up in the milk.[92]

Another argument for avoidance of dairy — as well as beef, fish and poultry — is that they are a large source of dioxins, regardless of how they are raised. In addition, many individuals react negatively to dairy (whether due to a sensitivity, intolerance or allergy). Eating dairy may increase inflammation in dairy-sensitive individuals.

We recommend eating meats in moderation (a palm-sized portion one to three times daily) and consuming only meats that are grass-fed, organic, antibiotic-free, hormone-free and humanely raised. Consumption of small amounts of dairy by dairy-tolerant individuals — especially fermented dairy in the later phases of the Endometriosis Diet Plan — is also permitted.

Choose Smaller Fish

Fish are a fantastic source of omega-3 fatty acids. But some fish, especially larger varieties, are also a source of dioxins and other toxins such as heavy metals. Eating smaller fish (such as sardines) and avoiding large fish (such as tuna) can greatly reduce your exposure to toxins. In addition, we recommend eating only wild-caught fish, as farm-raised fish are lower in omega-3 fatty acids (due to their feed) and contain higher amounts of certain toxins.

A healthy omega-6 to omega-3 fatty acid ratio can be helpful in controlling inflammation. Unfortunately, the Standard American Diet has a 15:1–17:1.75 omega-6 to omega-3 fatty acid ratio. A 2:1 to 3:1 omega-6 to omega-3 fatty acid ratio has been recommended in order to decrease inflammation. In rabbits, ingestion of omega-3 fatty acids reduced endometriotic implant size, and in cells in petri dishes (in vitro), the addition of omega-3 fatty acids significantly slowed the growth of endometriotic cells.[100]

We often recommend increasing the amount of omega-3 fatty acids in your diet to decrease the synthesis of highly inflammatory cytokines and prostaglandins (increase inflammation and pain). In addition to fish, other fantastic sources of omega-3 fatty acids include flaxseed, grass-fed beef, dark green vegetables, chia seeds and hemp seeds.

FAQ

Q. Is it okay to eat soy?

A. Probably. A recommendation to avoid eating soy is common for those with endometriosis. There has been only one human study done on this topic, and it took place in Japan. The researchers observed a correlation between higher soy intakes and lowered endo occurrence.[94] It's important to note that the soy consumed in Japan is often fermented, unlike the majority of the soy consumed in North America, which is highly processed. Soy is very hard to digest, and fermenting it "predigests" the soy and also provides beneficial bacteria.

In addition, the Japanese eat only small amounts of soy in comparison to North Americans. And the soy consumed in Japan, unlike the soy we have in North America, has not been genetically modified.

Many believe that soy may contribute to endo disease progression because it is rich in phytoestrogens, which are believed to contribute to the total estrogen load. However, phytoestrogens have a weak estrogen effect, and may help with symptom management in small doses. In fact, in animal studies, consumption of soy reduced the weight and surface area of endometriotic lesions. Soy appears to inhibit aromatase and estrogen receptor expression, resulting in a reduction of total estrogen concentration.[95] Based on this research, small amounts (a few servings per week) of organic or non-GMO fermented soy appear to be safe for women with endo.

A common recommendation made by many endometriosis specialists is to avoid gluten. We typically recommend that our patients try it for at least 6 months, especially if they have gastrointestinal discomfort and/or other autoimmune diseases (such as thyroid disease). Following a gluten-free diet for 12 months was shown to significantly reduce endo-associated pain in 75% of 207 subjects.[93]

The duration of this study suggests that it may take some time to see benefits from the elimination of gluten from the diet. We have several patients who report that they avoided gluten for a month or two and failed to see any improvement. It may take longer. This might have something to do with the contribution of gastrointestinal inflammation to systemic pain. Gluten is very hard to digest and can cause a great deal of inflammation, especially in someone with an inflamed gut (see the box on page 66 for more information about gluten-containing grains and your health). Also, endometriosis is a condition of immune dysregulation, and GI inflammation can greatly alter the immune system.

How Wheat and Other Gluten-Containing Grains May Be Contributing to Your Health Problems

Gluten is a protein found in wheat, as well as barley, bulgur, Mir (a cross between wheat and rye), rye, seitan and triticale. Oats don't contain gluten but are often processed in plants that produce gluten-containing grain products and may be contaminated with gluten. Gluten is also used in many processed foods.

We used to believe that individuals with celiac disease, an autoimmune reaction provoked by the ingestion of gluten, were the only people who needed to avoid gluten. But a growing number of individuals now appear to be gluten-sensitive, a condition that has come to be known as non-celiac gluten sensitivity (NCGS). People with NCGS should also avoid consumption of gluten-containing foods.

Wheat also contains other proteins that can pose health problems, such as wheat germ agglutinin and amylase trypsin inhibitors (ATIs).

Eating wheat and other gluten-containing foods may contribute to your disease in the following ways:

- **Gut inflammation:** If you are sensitive to gluten, your body will react by mounting an immune response, leading to gut inflammation. Wheat germ agglutinin also stimulates inflammation in the gut's cells. In addition, ATIs can set off an immune response in the GI tract by stimulating immune cells. Both gluten and ATIs may also contribute to overall inflammation and pain in the body.

- **Intestinal permeability ("leaky gut"):** Your intestinal lining forms an important barrier that protects your body from viruses, bacteria, yeasts and fungi, toxins and undigested proteins. When your gut is inflamed, cells that are normally wedged close together become separated, turning your protective shield into a sieve. Moreover, when you eat gluten, your gut releases a protein called zonulin, which stimulates the tight junctions between cells to loosen. Together, inflammation and zonulin contribute to a leaky gut, which is a key contributor to the development of autoimmune diseases.

- **Increased risk for developing autoimmune diseases:** When your gut is permeable, pathogens and undigested proteins leak through into your general circulation, stimulating an immune response. The immune system forms antibodies to these pathogens and undigested proteins. The trouble is, some of these proteins look similar to cells in the human body, and the body starts attacking itself! In addition, because 80% or more of your immune system is in your gut, chronic gut inflammation can weaken and unbalance your immune function.

- **Brain inflammation:** There is a strong connection between the gut and the brain, and if your gut is inflamed, your brain likely is too. Brain inflammation may lead to depression, dementia or Alzheimer's disease.

In addition to gluten, other foods such as eggs, dairy and soy may be poorly tolerated and induce inflammation in sensitive individuals. An effective tool for eliciting food sensitivities and intolerances is an elimination diet. Phase 1 of the Endometriosis Diet Plan utilizes an elimination diet.

Knowing what foods to consume is as important as knowing what foods to avoid. There are a handful of studies on foods that may potentially help with endo. For example, a higher intake of fruits and vegetables may be useful.[96] This is most likely due to several protective health qualities of fruits and vegetables:

- Vegetables contain high amounts of folate, methionine and vitamin B_6, which are critical for DNA methylation (important in estrogen detoxification). Scientific literature has demonstrated an association between DNA methylation abnormalities and women with endometriosis.[97]

- Fruits and vegetables are rich sources of phytonutrients (chemicals found in plants that protect them and keep them healthy) and antioxidants, which have been shown to reduce oxidation and inflammation in women with endometriosis.[98]

- Fruits and vegetables are abundant in fiber, aiding in regular bowel movements, which is essential for estrogen elimination. We recommend eating 7 to 10 servings of fruits and vegetables daily (1 to 2 of which are fruit), and striving to consume every color of the rainbow at each meal or at least daily.

- Pesticide exposure has been strongly associated with endometriosis; therefore, we recommend eating organic produce whenever possible.[99]

See part 3 of this book for a diet created specifically for those with endo, including meal plans. In part 4, you'll find 100 recipes that are suitable for the Endometriosis Diet Plan.

Pesticide exposure has been strongly associated with endometriosis; therefore, we recommend eating organic produce whenever possible.

Chapter 5
Conventional Treatment of Endometriosis

If you are seeing a traditional OB/GYN, you will usually be offered one of two basic types of treatment for endometriosis. The first option is medical treatment in the form of some kind of hormone manipulation. The second is surgery, usually laparoscopic burning or coagulation of the endometriosis implants, although a much better option is wide excision surgery.

Medical treatment can be especially helpful if the limitations of this approach are appreciated. The typical medical treatment for endometriosis provided by most OB/GYNs is the manipulation of hormones, primarily estrogen and/or progesterone levels. The concept behind this approach is that estrogen tends to stimulate the growth of endometriosis and progesterone balances or stabilizes the effect of estrogen. In a very simple example, one can think of estrogen as fertilizer for the lawn and progesterone as the lawn mower. The goal of medical treatment of endometriosis is to increase the ratio of progesterone to estrogen (progesterone-only treatment), decrease the amount of both estrogen and progesterone (birth control pills) or eliminate estrogen from the body (gonadotropin-releasing hormone, or GnRH, treatments such as Lupron, which induce a temporary menopause).

Natural menopause occurs with the depletion of eggs and the associated hormone-producing cells in the ovaries, resulting in plummeting levels of estrogen and progesterone. Menopause can also occur following removal of the ovaries or medical suppression. The common side effects of the hormone drop that comes with menopause — whether natural, surgical or medically induced — include hot flashes, trouble sleeping, weight gain, bone loss and irritability.

The medical profession used to think that elimination of estrogen — via either surgical menopause (hysterectomy with removal of the tubes and ovaries) or use of GnRH agonists such as Lupron to induce medical menopause — would eliminate endometriosis. Unfortunately, endometriosis can continue to grow despite hormonal manipulation or lowered or even absent estrogen levels. Dr. Cook has observed uninhibited endometriosis growth in both post-menopausal women and women on birth

> The typical medical treatment for endometriosis provided by most OB/GYNs is the manipulation of hormones, primarily estrogen and/or progesterone levels.

control. It turns out that it is possible for endometriosis to produce aromatase enzyme activity, which is the enzyme needed to produce estrogen. A recent study of 42,079 women with endometriosis showed 17.09% of those with endometriosis were perimenopausal (45 to 54 years old) and 2.55% were postmenopausal (55 to 95 years old).[1]

As you can see, the medical treatment options for endometriosis are fairly crude, and commonly come with unacceptable side effects. They do not provide a cure for the disease, and work only for a portion of endometriosis patients. Even when the treatment option is effective, the results are only temporary. And the use of a GnRH agonist such as Lupron to cause a temporary medical menopause may not be effective in treating endometriosis, as the endometriosis lesions can produce their own estrogen and remain active, and potentially invasive, despite ovarian suppression.

This chapter explores the medical treatment options for endometriosis in detail.

> **Unfortunately, endometriosis can continue to grow despite hormonal manipulation or lowered or even absent estrogen levels.**

Progesterone-Only Treatment

All endometriosis treatment options using bioidentical progesterone or a progestin (a synthetic hormone that has progesterone-like effects on the body) are trying to suppress the effect of estrogen on the endometriosis. This option can be effective in some women, especially if the patient's pain is primarily around the time of her period and she does not tolerate estrogens (for example, due to nausea).

The different kinds of progesterone treatments used to treat endometriosis include bioidentical compounded progesterone creams, a pharmaceutical bioidentical oral micronized progesterone, oral synthetic progestins, progestin-only birth control pills, Depo-Provera and the Mirena IUD.

Topical

Progesterone cream is the most common form of topical progesterone. Non-prescription progesterone creams usually do not have enough progesterone to alter the menstrual cycle. However, some women find this low dose of hormone to be effective. Prescription progesterone cream is usually made in a compounding pharmacy at the strength requested by the ordering physician. It can be difficult to get consistent and adequate absorption of progesterone using this delivery method.

Oral

Oral progesterone can include compounded bioidentical progesterone pills; oral micronized progesterone in oil pill (Prometrium); synthetic progestin Aygestin (norethindrone acetate) or Provera (medroxyprogesterone); or the progestin-only birth control pill. The latter do not have any estrogen, and the amount of progestin is about one-third the dose of progestin (thus the term "mini-pill") found in the average combination estrogen/progestin pill.

Injectable

Depo-Provera is a long-acting form of progestin that is given as a shot and lasts for months. The most common side effects include weight gain, breakthrough bleeding and depression.

Mirena IUD

The Mirena IUD as a treatment option for endometriosis delivers a daily dose of about 20 micrograms (mcg) of the progestin levonorgestrel. Birth control pills with levonorgestrel contain a daily dose of 90 mcg to 150 mcg. This is 4.5 to 7.5 times the dose of the Mirena IUD. On average, women using the Mirena IUD have about a 50% to 90% reduction in their menstrual flow, and 20% stop having a period within one year. This is only temporary, and periods start again shortly after removal of the Mirena IUD.

Combined Estrogen and Progesterone Treatment

Combination birth control pills are commonly the first step in treating patients who have endometriosis, pelvic pain and painful periods. If most of the pain a woman is experiencing is around the time of her period, then reducing the intensity of pain and/or the frequency of periods with the use of birth control pills may be an effective endometriosis treatment. With cyclic use of birth controls pills for treatment of menstrual cramps associated with endo, the period is often lighter and less painful. Some women can take the pill continuously (skipping the sugar pills each month and taking hormone pills every day without a break), either completely avoiding periods or significantly reducing the number of periods over time (for example, four periods a year instead of 12).

Even though this endometriosis treatment involves taking estrogen and progestin, women taking a combination birth control pill every day actually experience a significant reduction in the amount of estrogen and progesterone in their body. At first this may not make sense, but the ovaries make a lot more estrogen than that found in the pill. The small, consistent dose of estrogen and progesterone in the pill is enough to signal the ovaries not to make estrogen, temporarily turning the ovaries off and eliminating their relatively large release of estrogen. Less estrogen in the body as a result of the pill can result in less stimulation and activity of the endometriosis. Periods are usually shorter and lighter on the pill because there is less stimulation and growth of the endometrium (the inside lining of the uterus that sloughs off during menstruation).

The most common treatment option in this category is the standard combination estrogen/progestin birth control pill. Other forms of combination estrogen/progestin treatment include the NuvaRing and the Ortho Evra patch. The patch, however, delivers about 50% more estrogen than a standard 35 mcg birth control pill, and thus is not the best for endometriosis treatment.

If your doctor prescribes a particular birth control pill as treatment to help with your endometriosis symptoms, it may work well without any side effects. If this is the case, you have found a good treatment option for your endometriosis, despite the fact that the treatment manages your symptoms without eradicating the disease.

Unfortunately, the pill does not always work well. Also, patients may have significant side effects, such as weight gain, migraines, moodiness, acne, nausea, low libido and sleep disturbances. Breakthrough bleeding is another possible side effect (see "Breakthrough Bleeding and the Pill," page 72). In these cases, a different birth control pill may work better, but there are so many on the market that it can be confusing trying to decide which option is right for you. Not all birth control pills are the same. Understanding the differences will help you and your doctor choose the best pill option to treat your endometriosis symptoms while minimizing side effects.

The difference in the various pills comes down to:

- the amount of estrogen;
- the type and amount of progestin; and
- the balance or relative amount (ratio) of estrogen and progestin.

> The small consistent dose of estrogen and progesterone in the pill is enough to signal the ovaries not to make estrogen, temporarily turning the ovaries off and eliminating their relatively large release of estrogen.

Did You Know?

Alternative Options

If you have significant side effects with your current pill — such as nausea, decreased sex drive and not feeling well — consider one with a different type of progestin, a different estrogen dose, or a different ratio of estrogen and progestin. It may be a better option for managing your pelvic pain.

Breakthrough Bleeding and the Pill

One of the more common side effects patients experience is breakthrough bleeding (BTB), which is bleeding in between their normal period time. This is often associated with cramping and pain. Birth control pills in part provide an effective option for endometriosis treatment by eliminating or reducing the number of bleeding and pain days. There are many causes of BTB on the pill and your OB/GYN should be able to help resolve this for you. It's often a result of either the wrong overall estrogen level or an inappropriate ratio of estrogen and progestin for your body. There are more than 100 different brands of combination birth control pills.

One of the many possible contributing factors to your BTB can be a dominance of either estrogen or progestin. When your doctor performs a transvaginal ultrasound, he or she will be able to measure the thickness of the endometrium. BTB can result from the lining of the uterus being either too thick or too thin. If you are on the pill, changing the balance of the estrogen and progestin in the pill may help.

If the endometrium is thin on sonogram (<5 mm), one option is to switch to a higher estrogen pill (or less progestin), and/or a pill with a higher estrogen-to-progestin ratio. If the endometrium is thick on sonogram (>5 mm), one option is to switch to a lower amount of estrogen in the pill, and/or a pill with a lower estrogen-to-progestin ratio, or a progestin-only pill.

The type of estrogen is the same in virtually all of the combination birth control pills (ethinyl estradiol); it's a synthetic form of estrogen. The amount of this estrogen in the pill can vary from 10 to 35 mcg. The combination pill has one of eight types of progestin. The types of progestin in the pill include norgestimate, desogestrel, norethindrone, norethindrone acetate, ethynodiol diacetate, drospirenone, levonogestrel and norgestrel. NuvaRing has a different progestin than found in any other pill; it's called etonogestrel.

Danazol Treatment

Danazol (brand name Danocrine) was approved in 1976 by the Food and Drug Administration (FDA) as the first medication specifically for treatment of endometriosis. It is a synthetic hormone — there is nothing natural about this treatment option — and is a cross between progesterone and testosterone. If a woman with endometriosis has severe pain around the time of her period and only minimal pain during the rest of the month, then stopping her period can be a very effective treatment option. Unfortunately, a significant percentage of women will continue to have a period even when taking the birth control pill continuously (meaning they skip the "sugar pills" and take the hormones pills without a break). Danocrine can be an effective treatment option, as the medication will usually stop a woman's period while she is taking it.

But it also has potential, significant drawbacks, including the possibility of acne, oily skin, extra hair growth and a deepening voice. These are uncommon, and the medication can be stopped immediately if any are noticed. The medication has to be taken two to three times a day, which can be an advantage: if there are significant side effects, danazol is rapidly excreted from the body, enabling rapid alleviation of the side effects. But it can also be a disadvantage; consistently taking any medication three times a day is certainly challenging.

GnRH Treatment

Lupron is one medication in a class of drugs known as GnRH agonists. GnRH stands for gonadotropin-releasing hormone. *Agonist* means the medication activates the same cellular receptors as the natural hormone. Gonadotropin-releasing hormone is normally released by a part of the brain called the hypothalamus. It is released in little doses at specific intervals. This, in turn, stimulates the pituitary gland at the base of the brain to release FSH (follicle-stimulating hormone) into the bloodstream, which stimulates the ovaries to both mature an egg and produce estrogen. A GnRH agonist temporarily shuts down the ovaries' production of estrogen.

At first, it might seem counterintuitive that giving a medication that does the same thing as the natural hormone can have the very opposite effect. The GnRH agonist, however, is released continuously, not episodically like the natural hormone. Continuous stimulation of the hypothalamus by the GnRH agonist shuts down the release of FSH and thus the ovaries. As soon as the Lupron wears off, the episodic release of gonadotropin-releasing hormone resumes, as do ovulation and the ovarian production of estrogen.

Estrogen stimulates the growth of endometriosis. Since Lupron stops the ovaries from producing estrogen, this medical therapy results in a temporary medical menopause, creating a low-estrogen environment in the body. The idea is that without estrogen from the ovaries, endometriosis would be inactivated. Even under the best circumstances, though, the pain relief provided by this treatment is temporary. In addition, there are several significant problems with the use of GnRH agonists for endometriosis treatment. First, they may not work. Endometriosis can produce its own estrogen, and in these cases Lupron will not suppress the endometriosis activity or pain. In more advanced cases of endometriosis, even if the Lupron suppresses the endometriotic implant activity, it does nothing for the pain caused by scarring and the fibrosis resulting from the invasive endometriosis.

Did You Know?

How Does a GnRH Work?

The GnRH agonist is released continuously, not episodically like a natural hormone. Continuous stimulation of the hypothalamus by the GnRH agonist shuts down the release of follicle-stimulating hormone (or FSH, which stimulates the ovaries to both mature an egg and produce estrogen) and thus shuts down the ovaries.

The side effects of GnRH treatment can be severe. Some of the more common side effects include hot flashes, night sweats, moodiness and irritability, nausea, insomnia and possibly mental fog. One also has to be concerned about the risk of bone loss, which is why this drug is approved only for 6 months of use. There may be indications for prolonged use, but in these cases, nutrients and/or medications to encourage bone growth are incorporated, as is bone density surveillance.

The standard approach by the vast majority of doctors is to start a patient on this treatment with a long-acting form of GnRH agonist such as Lupron Depot, which lasts from 1 to 3 months, depending on the dose given.

It does not make sense to start a long-acting form of a treatment that offers no chance of a cure, but rather just helps to relieve symptoms temporarily. In addition, this drug has a fairly high chance of severe and unacceptable side effects. Why not start out with a short-acting GnRH agonist such as Synarel? This is a nose spray that is given twice a day. If a patient finds this to be a good option for endometriosis treatment with minimal side effects, she can then switch over to a long-acting form such as the 1- or 3-month Lupron Depot shot. If, on the other hand, she experiences significant side effects, the nose spray can be stopped and the effects of the drug will wear off fairly quickly.

We have found that part of the frustration with many patients who have had a bad experience with Lupron is related to the prolonged time it takes for the side effects to wear off. Another common complaint is from patients who feel misled by their doctors, who either did not adequately inform of them of the prolonged side effects, or the possibility that the treatment would not work.

Aromatase Enzyme Inhibitors Treatment

Aromatase enzyme converts a precursor hormone (testosterone) to estrogen. Blocking aromatase enzyme prevents estrogen production anywhere in the body, potentially including the endometriosis implant itself. Examples of aromatase enzyme inhibitors include letrazole (Femara) and anastrozole (Arimidex). Unfortunately, this group of medications does not provide a cure for endometriosis. It's effective temporarily, and it can have the same severe side effects as GnRH agonists (Lupron), including significant bone loss. Finally, it does not successfully treat all endometriosis-related pain.

Surgical Treatment

Unfortunately, most surgeons treating endometriosis are still using coagulation, cautery or fulguration — basically burning — to treat endometriosis implants. This results in a very non-specific surgical burning of tissue. In addition, this approach usually leaves a significant amount of endometriosis behind, resulting in continuing progression of the disease and a relatively rapid return of symptoms and pain. A recent study demonstrated that in the vast majority of cases, surgical burning of the disease leaves endo behind. Tissue analysis of samples treated by monopolar cautery revealed residual endometriosis 81% of the time; for treatment with bipolar cautery, it was a whopping 90% of the time.[3]

> **In the vast majority of cases, surgical burning of the disease leaves endo behind.**

How could any surgeon in good consciousness subject their patient to surgery when there is only a 10% to 19% chance of eradicating the disease? It is no wonder coagulation surgery has a reputation for being marginally effective with high recurrence.

There seems to be a significant disparity in endometriosis treatment outcome between specialized endometriosis physicians with an expertise in the excision of endometriosis and general OB/GYN physicians who cauterize or burn the endometriosis. Outcomes are more successful with specialized endo physicians (see "Research Spotlight," page 76).

The burning type of surgery is crude and outdated. While it is technically much easier and quicker than excisional surgery, we believe it is time to relegate this procedure to the history books. Excisional surgery completely eliminates endometriosis in the vast majority of cases, with high treatment success rates and low recurrence rates. Our own data shows that excisional surgery performed on our patients (who on average have had three to four surgeries elsewhere) results in an average reduction in pain of 75%, with over half experiencing complete resolution of pain. The re-operation rate in this group of difficult patients is only about 15%. In only about half of these repeat surgeries is endometriosis revealed to be present.

Wide Excision Surgery

Wide excision surgery for endometriosis is very effective at removing endometriosis implants and improving quality of life in a large number of patients.

As an increasing number of patients appreciate the importance of excision surgery verses the ineffective burning surgery, there is a growing push for physicians to provide this treatment. The problem we are now starting to see is that some surgeons are cutting a small piece of endo out, either alone or in combination with burning surgery, and calling it excision surgery. Wide excision requires the ability to recognize and remove *all* of the endometriosis. Removing a small portion by excision alone or in combination with burning is not wide excision surgery, and to claim so is deceptive and ineffective.

The key concept in surgical endometriosis treatment is that of wide excision. In other words, the surgeon needs to cut around and under the outer edges of the entire area affected by endometriosis. It may sound simple, but in reality it can be very difficult, as the tough fibrous endometriosis is in essence "glued" to normal delicate tissue such as the bowel, bladder, blood vessels and ureter (the tube that runs from the kidney to bladder). These vital structures can be easily damaged during the removal of endometriosis. Successful, safe excision of endometriosis takes highly specialized surgical skills that are not part of the 8 years of training that OB/GYN doctors receive.

The top three requirements in correct surgical endometriosis treatment are:

1. Complete excision of the endometriosis
2. Complete excision of the endometriosis
3. Complete excision of the endometriosis

Please note that "hysterectomy" is not on this list. In certain cases, it may be appropriate to remove the uterus and/or ovaries in addition to complete excision of the endometriosis, but that complete excision should never be comprised or abbreviated. Situations in which a hysterectomy may be considered are:

- significant adenomyosis
- significant pelvic congestion
- a history of "killer periods" since they first started, in spite of complete excision of endometriosis
- symptomatic fibroids
- women who have finished having children

The decision to have a hysterectomy is very significant and personal. The woman should always be well informed, with correct information provided about the pros and cons for her individual situation, needs and beliefs. A hysterectomy

FAQ

Q. Is robotic surgery better than traditional laparascopy?

A. Surgical endometriosis treatment is almost always done laparoscopically. There has been a recent trend toward use of robotically assisted laparoscopy by general OB/GYNs, but this surgical tool, despite certain claims, does not provide a better approach to the treatment of endometriosis. For an advanced laparoscopic surgeon, it offers no benefit; only limitations. Many OB/GYNs experience severe disorientation while trying to perform traditional laparoscopic surgery, which limits the types of surgery they can perform. The robot primarily helps make the surgery less confusing for the surgeon, as it helps with spatial orientation.

Endometriosis and pelvic pain are known for having poor surgical treatment outcomes and a high recurrence rate. Unfortunately, much if not most of the surgery currently performed for endometriosis is done poorly and improperly, whether using a traditional laparoscopic or a robot-assisted approach. The current surgical treatment for endometriosis and pelvic pain is not perfect, but if done properly, is effective and does provide good results.

> The decision to have a hysterectomy is very significant and personal. The woman should always be well informed, with correct information provided about the pros and cons for her individual situation, needs and beliefs.

can remove the body of the uterus (the part where bleeding and cramps originate) but leave the cervix. This is called a laparoscopic supracervical hysterectomy. Or, a hysterectomy can remove both the body of the uterus and the cervix; this is a total laparoscopic hysterectomy. Neither of these involves removal of the ovaries, and thus they do not affect hormone production. A hysterectomy does not cause the patient to go into menopause.

Removal of one ovary or both ovaries is also an option. If both ovaries are removed, the patient will go into surgical menopause. Removal of an ovary may be considered (but not necessarily required) if there's a history of recurrent endometrioma ("chocolate cysts") or recurrent extensive scar tissue involving the ovary and resulting in pain.

Successful, complete removal of stage III or stage IV endometriosis requires very specialized training, surgical skills and experience. This type of endometriosis can invade just about any organ in the pelvis, including the bowel, ureter, vagina and bladder. Removal of endometriosis from these vital structures is the preferred and most common approach. In cases where an organ has been partially replaced with endometriosis, removal of part of that organ may be required, followed by reconstruction.

Wide excision surgery for endometriosis is very effective at removing endometriosis implants and improving quality of life in a large number of patients. Unfortunately, it is not the complete answer in all cases. It seems the majority of endometriosis specialty centers and patient support groups push the idea that if correct wide excision surgery is performed, then endo will be completely resolved. If the pain still persists, patients are often told that it is not related to endometriosis and are left to find help on their own. In addition, many patients believe that if any persistence or recurrence of symptoms is present, their endometriosis has recurred. As we discussed earlier, however, there could be several other causes of their pelvic pain.

Further Information

For a more detailed discussion of surgery, consider reading *Stop Endometriosis and Pelvic Pain: What Every Woman and Her Doctor Need to Know* or *The Endo Patient's Survival Guide: A Patient's Guide to Endometriosis & Chronic Pelvic Pain*, by Andrew S. Cook et al.

Holistic Treatment

Holistic health care is a culmination of several different modalities and frameworks with the goal of addressing health versus focusing on an illness or symptoms. The underpinnings of a holistic approach involve the patient and the practitioner(s) working as a team to encourage the body's innate healing capabilities using a variety of health-care practices. Possible treatment modalities include nutrition and diet changes, stress management, sleep hygiene, epigenetic medicine, immunotherapy, herbs and supplements, energy medicine and conventional treatments.

Some integrative health practitioners may have a poor understanding of endometriosis and pelvic pain. Holistic treatments and therapy are part of the answer, but they can also be quite complex and poorly understood, even by many of the physicians specializing in this type of medicine. Unfortunately, the message all too often sent to those learning about integrative or holistic health care is that endometriosis is easily treated with supplements and some hormonal manipulation. Many integrative health-care practitioners do not believe surgery helps.

How wrong they are. This is just another example of why it is so difficult for women with this condition to find good, balanced treatment. The holistic aspect is a very important part of an overall treatment plan to improve a person's health — and we feel very strongly about the importance of this type of treatment for women with endometriosis. Diet and lifestyle are hugely important in effective treatment of endometriosis. Using a combination of conventional treatments such as surgery and a variety of holistic and more "alternative" treatments seems to be most effective in the treatment of this complex disease. That's why this book includes chapters on diet and lifestyle.

A Personal Note from Dr. Cook about the Holistic Approach

I do not have endometriosis, but I do have insulin resistance. Over the years, I had gained some weight and required an increasing number of prescription medications to control symptoms that included high cholesterol, high blood pressure and asthma. I am a medical doctor, have seen physicians over the years, and have undergone the traditional medical approach to disease management. I knew I should follow the recommendations that I was providing to my own patients about lifestyle and diet. Yet, I had fallen into the same health-care trap that so many of us experience.

When I decided to implement a healthier lifestyle, I was quite frankly scared and did not know if I could make the necessary changes. I was a sugar addict. (Watch the movie *Fed Up* and it will help you to understand.) Danielle Cook, currently the director of integrative health at Vital Health Institute and the co-author of this book, started working at VHI in 2012. After joining us, she had some concerns about her job security. She wasn't concerned about getting fired — rather, she saw my poor health as a ticking time bomb. She gently prodded me to start making some dietary changes, got me started in a yoga class and pushed me to start making some time for myself and not work myself to death. Basically, she gave me the same advice and information you will find in this book. Over the next year, I lost 35 pounds and eventually got off all of my meds. My lab tests are now normal.

I was speechless. I had been a big proponent of holistic health care for years, but it took Danielle's encouragement for me to finally take my own advice. I was eating a plant-based diet and working out most days. Despite my medical knowledge, I began to finally understand how powerful these lifestyle and dietary changes really are. This approach to health actually fixed the problem and provided much better results than the pharmaceutical approach of Western medicine.

Honestly, part of me was upset. I loved the taste of my sugar and my processed foods. I really did not want to give them up permanently, but I had reached the point of no return. I refused to go back to my previous ill health. It has now been nearly three and a half years since I made these changes and I continue with my new approach to life. It is a new lifestyle, not a fad. Yet, just like an alcoholic, I am tempted every day, and I am not perfect. But I have found a sustainable approach to healthy living.

I am so excited about making this book available to you. Danielle and I have organized and written down the essential information needed for you to take control of your health. So many of you have asked me for a guide to get out of the living hell of the non-functional life resulting from your endometriosis. I hear again and again, "Please help me, I will do anything to get better." This book can be the roadmap you have been looking for to regain your health. As you turn the page and start on part 2, you are taking the next step. I want you to enjoy the same benefits that I experienced, and probably even bigger changes. It may not be easy; it could even be the most challenging thing you ever do. It was for me. I challenge you to dig deep and find the determination I see so often in women with endometriosis. I have confidence. I know you can do it. Here's to your future health and happiness.

Case Study: Norma's Story

Norma, a 25-year-old lawyer, came to Vital Health Institute with painful and irregular periods, insomnia, joint pain, headaches, severe fatigue, bloating, constipation, abdominal pain, burping after meals and acne. She and her husband were discussing having children before she turned 30.

Like many Americans, Norma typically made food choices that were high in processed carbohydrates (such as breads, crackers and pastas), high in unhealthy fats, high in sugar and low in fruits, vegetables, healthy fats and fiber. She ate fast foods a few times a week, avoided most vegetables and other high-fiber foods, as they made her bloat more, and struggled with what she described as "an unrelenting sweet tooth." She typically worked 60 hours a week.

We did several lab tests on Norma to investigate her gastrointestinal health, nutrient deficiencies and hormone levels. Norma tested positive for small intestinal bacterial overgrowth, with excessive methane-producing bacteria; she had a very low amount of beneficial bacteria and an mild overgrowth of yeast in her large intestine; she was low in magnesium, B vitamins, iron, vitamin D and zinc; she was estrogen-dominant; and she had elevated cortisol levels in the evenings.

We advised Norma to follow the phase 1 diet, discussed sleep hygiene and routine stress reduction, encouraged daily movement and getting outside, and suggested the following supplements: betaine hydrochloride with meals, omega-3 fatty acids, Atrantil, zinc carnosine, magnesium, phosphatidylserine, a multivitamin with vitamin D and 2 tablespoons (30 mL) of ghee per day.

At Norma's 1-month follow-up, she reported having more energy, no bloating or burping after meals, regular bowel movements, improved sleep, clearer skin and less joint pain. But her last period had still been painful. We had her continue with the diet and lifestyle changes, encouraged her to use more turmeric when cooking and added a curcumin/boswellia supplement and a soil-based probiotic to her regimen.

At Norma's 2-month follow-up, she reported that she continued to feel better and that her last period had been on time and less painful. We recommended advancing to phase 2 of the diet and continuing to take a multivitamin with vitamin D, omega-3 fatty acids, Atrantil, daily ghee and betaine hydrochloride with meals. We changed her probiotic to one specific for the strains she lacked and added some fermented vegetables to her diet. We suggested that she use the curcumin/boswellia and magnesium supplements the week before her period and during her period only.

At Norma's 3-month follow-up, she was feeling great. Her periods continued to be regular and less painful. We encouraged her to add in foods from phase 3 of the diet and increase her portion sizes, while continuing her lifestyle changes and supplements. We also discussed some more aggressive detoxification options to reduce her toxic load.

At Norma's 6-month follow-up, her skin was glowing and she had more pep in her step. She continued to feel better and better as she kept up the changes she had made. We discussed preparing her body for pregnancy.

Part 2

An Integrative Lifestyle Plan for Managing Pelvic Pain

Part 2 consists of an integrative lifestyle plan that will get to the core of many underlying health problems contributing to endometriosis and its related symptoms. Here, you will learn how to strengthen your body and optimize your health. Topics include detoxification, stress reduction, optimizing sleep, electrically charging your body, smart, effective exercise, and helpful supplements and herbs. Chapter 6 teaches you how to optimize your body's natural detoxification processes using foods and various activities such as exercise and saunas. Chapter 7 gives you information on how to start practicing stress reduction, and provides a small sample of available methods. Chapter 8 is full of great resources for improving your quality of sleep. In chapter 9, you will learn how different types of exercise can impact your health and well-being. (Included is an example of an exercise program that is an effective and safe way to start.) Chapter 10, on electrically charging your body, includes groundbreaking information on the importance of being electrically charged, and a few simple energy-charging practices to incorporate into your healing program. And chapter 11 is all about supplements. It's split into categories based on symptoms. For example, there are lists of herbs and supplements that enhance sleep, reduce inflammation and support mitochondrial function. (A sample general supplement program for endo is also included.)

At first glance, this section may seem a bit overwhelming. We suggest you start by skimming the entire section with an open mind. Then, sit down in a quiet space and write down something you believe would help your health and something you feel confident that you can do. For example, maybe you are very stressed; you may decide to start doing 4-7-8 breathing twice daily for a week or two. After mastering this skill, and making it a habit, you may decide to add another lifestyle change. Just remember: health is a spectrum and everyone starts somewhere on that spectrum. Movement toward better health along that spectrum is the ultimate goal. Each small change you make is a gift you are giving to yourself, and forward movement in the healing process.

Chapter 6
Lightening Your Toxic Load

There is no question that today's world is laden with chemicals, many of which are toxic to human health. Although some of these chemicals have positive benefits and have made many aspects of our lives easier, there is collateral damage. We have already covered the impact of toxins on your general health, on endo and on pelvic pain disorders (see chapter 4). Now that you have a better understanding of where these toxins are found and how they negatively affect your health, we want to offer some solutions for how to reduce your overall toxic load and increase the elimination of toxins from your body with diet and lifestyle strategies.

The Detoxification Systems

There are six main organs/organ systems that are important for detoxification: the liver, skin, kidneys, gastrointestinal tract, lymphatic system and lungs. These six organs/organ systems work together to gather toxins in the body, convert them into less toxic forms and rid your body of them. Urination, defecation, sweating and respiration are the main ways in which the body excretes toxic compounds. In addition, the lymphatic system is important for optimal detoxification.

The Kidneys and Urination

The kidneys are the main organs responsible for detoxification through urination. They process approximately 200 quarts of blood daily, from which they filter out roughly 2 quarts of waste products and toxins. These waste products and toxins are combined with excess water and are safely eliminated from the body through urination. This important detoxification system can function well only if there is an adequate volume of water flowing through the kidneys to carry away waste.

The GI Tract and Defecation

This is perhaps the body's most important method of toxin excretion. The gastrointestinal tract is often given credit only for digestion, absorption and elimination of undigested fragments of food. We need to give this overachiever more credit. The gastrointestinal tract is a dumping ground for unwanted toxins. Sources include toxins and metabolic waste from the liver

Did You Know?

The Endometriosis Diet Plan

The diet presented in part 3 of this book is designed to assist your body's natural detoxification processes and help you to establish and maintain a healthy balance of bacteria in your gut.

(the body's main detoxification organ), metabolic waste from intestinal bacteria, toxins and chemicals in our foods and beverages, and toxins produced by bacteria, fungi and parasites. All of this toxic waste must be bound and eliminated from the intestines through defecation.

The Skin and Sweating

The skin is the largest organ in the body. It has many functions, including:

- regulating body temperature
- preventing loss of body fluids
- serving as a barrier against penetration of toxic substances into the body
- protection against sun and radiation
- serving as a sensory organ for touch, heat, cold, and sexual and emotional sensations
- synthesizing vitamin D
- providing the body structure
- excreting toxic substances through sweating

RESEARCH SPOTLIGHT
Sweating and Detoxification

In a 2011 study published in the *Archives of Environmental and Contamination Toxicology*, researchers concluded that "induced sweating appears to be a potential method for elimination of many toxic elements from the human body."[1] Several toxic elements appear to be preferentially excreted through sweat. Studies have found sweating helpful in the elimination of phthalates[2] and heavy metals.[3] Since toxins may potentially encourage the development of hormone-related conditions such as endo, increased detoxification may help to manage symptoms, slow disease progression and decrease chances of recurrence after surgery.

The Lungs and Respiration

Oxygen is vital to human life. Even a few minutes without oxygen can result in tissue damage, and longer deprivation can lead to death. All cells in the body require continuous oxygen in order to function. This includes cells and tissue involved in detoxification. This may seem like a moot point, since we all breathe automatically. However, how we breathe is important. Many of us have become accustomed to shallow breathing and even holding our breath. This may occur when we are under stress, have poor lung function, poor posture or stiff muscles

Deep breathing allows for oxygen-rich air to reach the depths of your lungs and expel toxins.

or are sedentary. An exchange of fresh oxygen for waste products occurs with each breath. Shallow breathing allows stagnant air and pollutants to accumulate in the lower portion of your lungs. The lungs are a muscle, and just like other muscles in your body, they require conditioning. Deep breathing allows for oxygen-rich air to reach the depths of your lungs and expel toxins. In addition, routine deep breathing will strengthen your lungs to bring in more highly oxygenated air and optimize detoxification.

The Lymphatic System and Drainage

The lymphatic system consists of fluid-filled nodes, blood vessels, glands and organs; its network touches almost every area of the body. This system has two main functions: to cleanse toxins and to protect against infection. Within the lymphatic system, toxins and waste are carried away from tissues and deposited into the bloodstream. The waste is then transported to the spleen, where blood is purified. The spleen contains a reserve of red and white blood cells, making it an optimal organ for fighting infection. In addition to the spleen's immune defense, a robust number of immune cells also travel throughout the lymphatic network. Since endometriosis is often thought to involve immune dysregulation[4] and poor detoxification,[5] optimal function of the lymphatic system may be important for management of the condition.

Proper function of the lymphatic system requires some work on your part. Unlike the blood circulatory system, the lymphatic system does not have a pump. Therefore, it can become sluggish and stagnant, resulting in a buildup of toxic debris. This may be experienced as poor immunity (chronic infections), cellulite, edema (fluid retention), chronic pain and fatty deposits. Here's the good news: you can optimize your lymphatic function by doing various activities, staying hydrated and consuming specific herbs.

Supporting the Detoxification Systems

Urination

Drinking adequate water is critical for proper elimination of toxins through the kidneys. On average, we recommend drinking half of your body weight (in pounds) of fluid in ounces daily. For example, if you weigh 110 pounds (50 kg), you would drink at least 55 ounces (1.6 L) of fluid daily. If you are sweating or have diarrhea, you will need to increase your fluid intake to accommodate for increased loss. We generally recommend water, but any non-caffeinated beverage such as lemon water, herbal tea or coconut water (in moderation) will help hydrate your body. There are also several foods, herbs and nutrients that can support the kidneys to improve this route of detoxification. Some examples include parsley, fruits and vegetables, horsetail (herb), marshmallow root, cranberry, beet juice, lemon juice and organic raw apple cider vinegar.

Defecation

In order to explain how to support elimination through defecation, it's important to understand the key players and functions of this process:

Bacterial Balance

There are 100 trillion bacteria (approximately 3 pounds, or 1.36 kilograms) residing in your gastrointestinal tract. This complex living system has several important jobs in the body; however, right now we are going to focus only on its role in detoxification. There are several different strains of bacteria in the gut — some that benefit our health and some that harm it. Keeping the beneficial bacteria numbers higher helps this army of troops outnumber and suppress the overgrowth of pathogenic bacteria.

At our clinic we often use what is commonly referred to as the 5R program to repair and rebalance the gut. This program was designed to treat gastrointestinal infections, restore a healthy microbial balance, repair the intestinal barrier, rebalance important hormones involved in proper digestion, and optimize digestion by replacing inadequate digestive enzymes and/ or stomach acid. The 5 steps in the 5R Program are: Remove, Replace, Reinoculate, Repair and Rebalance. These steps may occur simultaneously or in a step-by-step progression, depending on your needs.

1. **Remove.** The goal here is to remove any gastrointestinal stressors. These include food sensitivities, parasites, viruses and pathogenic bacteria and yeasts. Phase 1 of the Endometriosis Diet Plan has been designed to help "starve" bad bugs such as pathogenic bacteria and yeasts. An addition of various drugs or herbs may be helpful in eradicating a particular pathogen.

2. **Replace.** The goal of this step is to replace essential digestive secretions necessary for proper digestion. These secretions may be reduced by diet, medications, medical conditions, stress, aging and other factors. Examples of digestive secretions that we often replace include digestive enzymes, hydrochloric acid and bile acids. For example, adequate stomach acid is needed to begin the process of

digesting proteins. If stomach acid is too low, proteins from your foods are not fully digested. This results in the fermentation of protein by bacteria in your gut (which may cause bloating and gas), development of food sensitivities, a damaged intestinal barrier and other digestive complaints such as constipation. We may recommend a trial of betaine hydrochloride (HCl) with meals to increase stomach acid and improve digestion.

3. **Reinoculate.** The goal of this step is to rebalance the gut bacteria. Phase 2 of the Endometriosis Diet Plan is designed to help replace beneficial bacteria such as bifidobacteria and *Lactobacillus* species. This is accomplished by eating a diet high in prebiotic foods (which feed beneficial bacteria) and probiotic foods (which add healthy bacteria to your gut). Some examples of prebiotic foods include onions, jicama, artichoke and asparagus. Examples of probiotic foods include fermented foods such as kefir, sauerkraut and yogurt. We also recommend specific probiotic supplements when necessary.

4. **Repair.** The goal of this step is to repair the lining of the GI tract. Various foods and nutrients are helpful for accomplishing this step. All phases of the Endometriosis Diet Plan include foods that contain these key nutrients. Targeted supplementation may be helpful for expediting repair. Common supplements include zinc carnosine, fish oil, glutamine, and vitamins A, C and E.

5. **Rebalance.** This last step of the 5R program is often overlooked. The goal is to rebalance the nervous system and hormones, which play an integral role in GI health. For example, chronic stress can raise cortisol levels, which can lead to a leaky, damaged GI lining. This step involves practicing daily stress reduction, sleeping 7 to 9 hours nightly, engaging in regular exercise and making healthy lifestyle choices.

Motility

Poor motility is a cause of constipation, which is one of the most common complaints we hear in our clinic. This can happen for several reasons, including: inadequate fluid; nerve damage to the gastrointestinal tract; neurotransmitter deficiency; parasympathetic overdrive (chronic stress); too little or too much fiber; structural blockages such as blind loops in the bowel and strictures; intestinal inflammation; and an imbalance and/or overgrowth of bacteria in the gut. Investigating the root cause of your constipation is important. However, you can try to make changes for some relief (see "Checklist," page 89).

Checklist
How to Relieve Constipation

Try making one change at a time:

1. Drink lots of water. Aim to drink half of your body weight (pounds) of fluid in ounces daily. For example, if you weigh 110 pounds (50 kg), you would drink at least 55 ounces (1.6 L) of fluid daily.

2. Aim for 25 to 50 grams of fiber daily. You can achieve this by increasing fruits, vegetables and non-gluten whole grains (food choices will vary depending on what phase of the Endometriosis Diet Plan you are in). *Always* increase fiber slowly and make sure you are increasing your fluid intake as you increase fiber intake. If not, too much fiber and not enough fluid can make you more constipated. Envision a sponge sopping up water. The sponge is the fiber. You want the sponge to become soft and pliable, not remain hard and inflexible. If adding fiber to your diet makes you more gassy and constipated, it may indicate small intestinal bacterial overgrowth, and adding fiber to your diet at this time may not be the answer; it may need to wait until phase 2 or 3 of the diet.

3. Do some deep breathing before eating. Take 2 to 5 minutes to do this before a meal. It relaxes your tight muscles, activates the parasympathetic branch of your nervous system (the "rest and digest" part) and activates your vagus nerve (important for proper digestion). The 4-7-8 breathing exercise is extremely effective. To do this, sit in a comfortable position and close your eyes. Inhale for 4 seconds through your nose, hold for 7 seconds and exhale through your mouth for 8 seconds. This is 1 round. Do 4 rounds to start. You can increase the number of rounds you perform as you get more comfortable.

4. Gently rub your belly. Do so in a clockwise motion for a few minutes before and after eating. This encourages the downward movement of food through your digestive tract.

5. Take magnesium citrate. Have it before going to bed. We generally recommend starting with 400 mg and increasing by 100 to 200 mg every few nights until you have a soft, well-formed bowel movement the following morning.

6. Try a probiotic. Start with our favorite, MegaSporeBiotic. Begin with one daily with a meal and see how you feel. If it worsens your symptoms, stop this supplement and try it again in phase 2 of the Endometriosis Diet Plan. Another helpful probiotic is Align. It contains *Bifidobacterium infantis*, which can be helpful with improving constipation. There is some evidence that *Bifidobacterium infantis* has some prokinetic effects — in other words, that it helps with motility.[6]

Sweating

Your skin in your largest detoxification organ. Sweating is a great way to detoxify the body and, luckily, there are several methods for raising your body temperature to increase detoxification through sweating. Some of our favorite methods include the following:

Far-Infrared Saunas

Infrared saunas are a great option for detoxification of heavy metals and chemicals.[7] Infrared bulbs heat your tissues to a depth of several inches, which raises body temperature to encourage sweating. In addition, circulation is enhanced, which helps to clear toxins and oxygenate tissues. Heating the body can also help to kill off viruses and other microbes. General recommendations for infrared saunas are as follows: 120°F to 180°F (49°C to 82°C) for 15 to 30 minutes. If you have never taken a sauna before, start with only a few minutes. For each subsequent sauna, add a minute and work up to 15 to 30 minutes. It is also important to shower immediately after a sauna. If you do not wash off the released toxins, they will be reabsorbed.

You can start by taking a sauna a few days a week and work up to daily. In addition to the chemicals and heavy metals released in sweat, good minerals are also released. It is important to replace these minerals. Seaweed, alfalfa, nettle and trace element salt (such as Real Salt) are all rich in minerals.

Biomat

The Richway Biomat uses a combination of far-infrared rays, negative ions and the conductive properties of amethyst crystals. It is an FDA-approved device for the relaxation of muscles and increase of local circulation where it is applied. It can be used for temporary pain relief and it supports the immune system, improves sleep (if associated with pain relief), reduces inflammation and increases tissue oxygenation. In addition, the professional-sized Biomat can be used for detoxification if used on a high-heat (red) setting to induce sweating.

Further Information

For more information on the Richway Biomat, see www.vitalhealth.com and click on the "Store" link. We have also included some studies on using the Biomat for pelvic pain.

Biomat Pain Relief

The Biomat can relieve:

- minor muscle pain
- minor joint pain and stiffness
- joint pain associated with arthritis
- muscle spasms
- minor sprains
- minor strains
- minor muscular back pain
- stress and fatigue
- tight muscles

Exercise

Exercise has so many positive health benefits, and detoxification is one. Exercise increases your body's ability to detoxify in multiple ways. First, if you are exercising vigorously or in a warm climate, you will eliminate toxins through your skin by sweating. Second, moving your muscles pumps your lymphatic system. Lastly, exercise increases your body's production of important antioxidants and protective proteins. For example, when you exercise — especially in short, intense bouts — you produce more glutathione.[8] Glutathione is the body's main antioxidant and also plays a critical role in detoxification. Research has found that endometriotic cells have increased oxidative stress (free radicals) and have alterations in their detoxification pathways.[9]

Hot Bath

There is no scientific literature specifically on the use of baths for detoxification. However, there is some evidence supporting various aspects of this popular recommendation. In the second edition of his book *Beating Lyme Disease*, Dr. David Jernigan highly recommends using an Epsom salt detox bath to aid in detoxification. He has a wonderful blog (http://beatinglymedisease.blogspot.com/2011/06/epsom-salt-detox-bath.html) on this topic, with a detailed explanation for each ingredient, and easy-to-follow directions for preparing this bath.

Lymphatic Drainage

There are several ways to increase lymphatic circulation and improve detoxification. Here are some of our favorites:

Dry Skin Brushing

This is a common Ayurvedic technique to improve lymphatic flow and boost circulation. Dry skin brushing stimulates the sweat glands, opens pores and sloughs off dead skin cells. This technique stimulates lymphatic circulation. It may help with certain skin conditions and reducing cellulite. Dry skin brushing is easy to do; we recommend doing it before showering each day. Using a dry brush with coarse bristles, brush the skin in short strokes toward the heart. Start at the fingers and toes and work your way in toward your trunk.

Rebounder Trampoline

Rebounding is not only fun, but is also one of the easiest ways to pump the lymphatic system. Jumping up and down on a trampoline moves the lymphatic system by stimulating blood flow. Studies have shown that doing 10 to 30 minutes of rebounding daily can be highly effective.

> **Further Information**
> To learn how to do dry skin brushing, you can find several excellent video demonstrations online.

Yoga

There are several ways that yoga improves lymphatic flow. First, inversions — such as placing your legs up a wall, or a headstand — help to drain lymph (fluid containing white blood cells) toward the heart, which increases the rate in which it is circulated and filtered. Second, twists squeeze the muscles and organs, forcing lymph to exit tissues. Lastly, the movement through yoga poses contracts and relaxes muscles, which is how lymph is circulated through the body.

Exercise

As mentioned above, exercise is a way to pump the lymphatic system and encourage detoxification. In addition, if you are sweating, you are also releasing toxins through the skin. Last, exercise helps to raise glutathione levels, which protects the cells from damage and plays a critical role in detoxification.

Water

As mentioned earlier, water plays a huge role in detoxification. Sweat, urine and feces contain water — these three waste products are the body's greatest forms of elimination. If you are sweating or have diarrhea, you will need to increase your fluid intake to accommodate for increased loss. Each day, aim to drink, on average, half of your body weight (in pounds) of any non-caffeinated beverage (preferably water) in ounces. For example, if you weigh 110 pounds (50 kg), you should drink at least 55 ounces (1.6 L) of fluid daily.

Did You Know?

Deep-Breathing Detox

In a study of heroin addicts who were in withdrawal, participants' urine was measured for heroin metabolites. The researchers found that the participants in the deep-breathing test group cleared heroin from their systems significantly faster than other test groups.[10]

Deep Breathing

When we breathe deeply we bring more oxygen into our bodies. Oxygen is essential for the absorption of vitamins and nutrients, which are used in enzymatic detoxification reactions. Oxygen also increases the production of white blood cells and improves lymphatic flow. The expansion and contraction of the diaphragm stimulates your lymphatic system much like exercise does.

Methylation

Methylation is an important biochemical process involved in virtually every system in your body. It occurs billions of times each second. This process turns genes on and off, repairs your DNA, plays an integral role in detoxification, recycles important molecules involved in detoxification, balances neurotransmitters critical for mood stabilization, strengthens the immune system and modulates inflammation. Poor methylation increases your risk for a variety of diseases (see "Risks of Poor Methylation," below).

Poor methylation increases your risk for a variety of diseases.

Factors that impact your methylation process include genetics, diet, smoking, malabsorption, low stomach acid, certain medications (for example, oral contraceptives and proton-pump inhibitors), hypothyroidism, kidney disease, pregnancy and high toxin exposure. There are ways to gain insight into your methylation status, such as red blood cell size, homocysteine levels, B_{12} levels and urinary amino acid levels. In addition, genetic testing can determine your genetic polymorphisms, or defects.

There are several ways you can enhance your methylation. Dietary strategies are built into the Endometriosis Diet Plan, starting in chapter 12. In addition to diet, we suggest you:

- avoid caffeine (excess consumption depletes B vitamins)
- limit alcohol to 3 drinks or less per week (alcohol depletes B vitamins)
- don't smoke (smoking inactivates B_6)
- avoid medications that interfere with methylation
- achieve a healthy gut microbial balance
- increase stomach acid (if necessary)
- try methylation supplements (see page 117)

Risks of Poor Methylation

- osteoporosis
- diabetes
- cervical dysplasia
- cancer
- depression
- dementia
- heart disease
- stroke
- chronic infections
- irritable bowel syndrome
- chronic fatigue syndrome
- hormone imbalances

Chapter 7
Taming the Stress Monster

Stress reduction should be an integral part of any treatment plan for chronic disease, including endometriosis. After learning a little more about the stress response and the changes that occur in your body, you may better understand how stress can worsen your endo symptoms. Practicing a daily stress-reduction program and resolving past trauma can be essential for optimizing your general health and controlling your endo symptoms.

Some people envision stress reduction as hours of sitting in deep meditation. For many, the very thought of this may be unappealing and uncomfortable. Luckily, meditation is only one of many forms of stress reduction that exist. In addition, you can mix and match stress-reduction techniques depending on your needs at various times. For example, if you are stressed and feeling nervous, anxious energy, you may want to engage in an active type of stress reduction, such as dancing, playing music, shaking or the emotional freedom technique (see page 98), rather than practicing a seated meditation. However, if you are feeling run down and stressed, you may benefit from seated meditation, gentle yoga or guided visualization.

This book is not a guide to stress reduction. There are several wonderful resources available for this purpose. However, we wanted to include some basic stress-reduction techniques and ideas for you to consider adding to your toolbox for controlling your endo. This is not an exhaustive list, but simply a starting point that includes a few of our favorites. In addition, we have listed some supplements and herbs that have been shown to support the body when under ongoing stress.

> **Practicing a daily stress-reduction program and resolving past trauma can be essential for optimizing your general health and controlling your endo symptoms.**

Stress Supplements and Herbs

There are many supplements available on the market for stress reduction. Some have stronger scientific evidence to back up their claims than others. Note that supplementation for stress will not replace lifestyle changes. For example, if you continue to overbook your schedule, sleep only 5 hours a night and eat an unhealthy diet, then taking a supplement to support your body under stress will not be very effective. In addition, these supplements are generally for chronic stress as opposed to acute bouts of stress. For a complete list of supplements and herbs that can help support the stress response for women with endometriosis and pelvic pain, see page 128. Note that the dosages listed are for general guidance. Before using any of these herbs or supplements, discuss it with a qualified practitioner.

Starting a Stress-Reduction Program

Starting a stress-reduction regimen can sometimes feel daunting, and can be viewed as yet another commitment or task. We have provided a few tips and recommendations to help you prepare for this important healing journey.

- Make the decision and a commitment to practice stress reduction. This is a wonderful gift you can give to yourself. Consider viewing this as an opportunity to take care of yourself and practice self-love.

- Commit to practicing every day. If possible, set aside a specific time (or few times) to practice each day. Put it in your schedule as a priority. Some find it is easiest to do it first thing in the morning, before other tasks and responsibilities demand your time.

- Consider a 2-week trial of each of the stress-reduction techniques in this chapter. You may find techniques that work better for you. This is just another opportunity to get to know your body in a positive manner.

- Be gentle, nonjudgmental and patient with yourself. You may miss a day here or there, or even a few weeks at a time. You may feel like you are not doing the technique correctly. Remember, this is a *practice*. As with any new skill you are trying to develop, it will take time to feel comfortable doing it, and repetition to transform it into a routine. The great thing about stress reduction is that it is an incredibly forgiving practice, and there is no right or wrong way to do it.

- If your schedule is very busy, add stress reduction into your daily life. For example, you can meditate while commuting on the bus or train or while waiting for an appointment. Practice deep breathing while doing housework, mowing the lawn or walking your dog. If you exercise, focus your attention on your body and coordinate your breathing to your movements with weight training.

- Consider keeping a journal. Write down what type of stress-reduction technique you performed, how you felt before and after, and how long you practiced.

- Turn off the sound on your phone.

- If you live with others, request that you have some privacy during your stress-reduction practice. If needed, explain to them why you are doing this; let them know that by practicing stress-reduction techniques, you will be more relaxed and happy — and more pleasant to be around!

> The great thing about stress reduction is that it is an incredibly forgiving practice, and there is no right or wrong way to do it.

- Dress appropriately. Loose clothing is great for breathing, seated meditation, guided imagery, prayer and the emotional freedom technique. Make sure you are warm enough, but not too hot.

Deep Belly Breathing

Most people take very shallow breaths and use very little of their lung capacity. Breathing deeply from the abdomen brings more oxygen into your body than very shallow breaths from your upper chest. The more oxygen you offer your body, the better you will feel. Oxygen is essential for your cells to make adequate energy.

When you do what is referred to as "deep belly breathing," you instantly activate your parasympathetic nervous system (the part of your nervous system that's active during sleep and digestion). You will quickly feel less tense, more relaxed and more focused. Here are a few steps to master the basics of deep belly breathing:

1. Sit in a comfortable position with your back straight. Place one hand on your chest and one on your belly. (You may want to practice this lying on your back to learn how to belly breathe and then perform this exercise in a seated position.)

2. Inhale through your nose. The hand on your stomach should rise and the hand on your chest should barely move.

3. Now exhale through your mouth and push out as much air as possible while pulling your belly button to your spine. The hand on your stomach should move toward your spine as you exhale, and the hand on your chest should move very little, if at all.

4-7-8 Breathing

Once you've mastered deep belly breathing, try our 4-7-8 technique. It takes very little time to be effective, and you can do it virtually anywhere. Here's how:

1. Sit comfortably with your back straight. You can also do this lying down, especially if you want to fall asleep. This breathing exercise can be very effective for falling asleep, and getting back to sleep if you awaken during the night.

2. Place the tip of your tongue behind your front teeth on the small ridge (this is the area behind your teeth — the part that gets burned when you bite into a hot piece of pizza). Your tongue will remain in this position throughout the exercise.

3. Exhale through your mouth, creating a whooshing sound.

4. Close your mouth and slowly inhale through your nose for a count of 4.

5. Hold your breath for a count of 7.

6. Exhale completely through your mouth making the same whooshing sound for a count of 8. This completes one round.

We recommend starting with four rounds of 4-7-8 breathing two or more times daily. After a month, you can increase to eight rounds in one session. One option is to do the exercise first thing in the morning when you wake and again before bed. If you have digestive issues, it can be done before each meal.

Guided Imagery

Guided imagery utilizes directed thoughts and suggestions to guide your imagination in order to achieve relaxation and focus. An instructor, audio recordings or scripts are often used for this process. Guided imagery is based upon the concept that the mind and body are interconnected.

Guided imagery is based upon the concept that the mind and body are interconnected.

Let's try this simple exercise to demonstrate this point. Imagine a shiny, juicy apple. Imagine the shape of the apple, the texture, smell and taste. Is it cold when you touch your tongue to it or is it freshly plucked from a tree and warmed from the sun? Breathe deeply and inhale its smell. Imagine sinking your teeth into the apple. Imagine the sound when your teeth break the crisp skin. Imagine the juice squirting into your mouth and dripping down your chin. Imagine slowly chewing that luscious bite of apple, savoring the sweetness. Many people salivate when they perform this exercise. This is an example of how your body responds to your thoughts.

Guided imagery can be a powerful tool to relaxing your stressed body, strengthening your immune system, reducing pain and inflammation and sharpening your mind. Many athletes use this technique to improve their performance.

There are several terrific guided imagery tools available for purchase or for free. One of our favorite resources is the University of California – Los Angeles Mindful Awareness Research Center, which has several free downloadable guided meditations (in English and Spanish) to get you started. There are also several free podcasts.

The Emotional Freedom Technique

The emotional freedom technique (EFT), also called "psychological acupressure," consists of tapping specific acupuncture points on the body while verbalizing negative emotional experiences. The goal of EFT is to restore energy flow throughout the body. EFT is based on the belief that negative emotions may block energy flow. It is believed that when we experience a negative emotion or event, the body's natural energy system is disrupted. This can lead to poor health habits, anxiety, depression, pain and chronic disease. EFT can help resolve past traumas. By combining acupressure with the verbalization and acknowledgment of negative emotions, energy blockages are opened and healthy energy flow is restored.

Stress elevates levels of cortisol, which may contribute to endometriosis and pelvic pain. A study published in *Journal of Nervous and Mental Disease* in 2012 found a significant decrease in cortisol levels after 1 hour of EFT treatments.[1] In addition, self-reported anxiety, depression and overall severity of symptoms were decreased after EFT treatments.

EFT is easy to learn; search YouTube for demonstrations. Many patients who do EFT combined with acupuncture have found this to be helpful with pain and other areas of stress in their lives.

Meditation

> **As a result of this external focus, we tend to attribute our pleasure, pain, happiness, et cetera, to what is going on around us, and not to what is occurring inside of us.**

There are hundreds of scientific studies on the benefits of meditation. Meditation involves turning your conscious awareness inward and focusing on the present moment. In day-to-day life, we are typically focused on external stimuli such as the smell of dinner, what someone is wearing or what we have to do that day. As a result of this external focus, we tend to attribute our pleasure, pain, happiness, et cetera to what is going on around us, and not to what is occurring inside of us.

In addition, meditation involves concentration. It is very common for a person's mind to wander from one thing to the next. Often, negative thoughts take hold. Through meditation, the awareness is refocused to a single, specific thought, such as your breathing, the flame of a candle or a picture of a deity. There are many benefits to practicing meditation and honing these skills, including improved focus, a stronger immune system, a healthier emotional well-being, a reduction in pain and much more. An excellent summary of the benefits of meditation and a compilation of scientific studies on meditation can be found at http://liveanddare.com/benefits-of-meditation.

There are several books and websites that walk you step-by-step through starting a meditation program. In many areas, there are also local meditation centers where you can practice for free or at a very low donation cost. There are several types of meditation, including Zen — or Zazen — meditation (see "How to Meditate," page 99), transcendental meditation, Qigong, Kundalini yoga and mantra meditation.

How to Meditate

These are the steps to doing a Zen meditation, also known as seated meditation.

1. Set a timer. Start by doing 5 minutes, and slowly increase your sitting time as you become more proficient at this practice.
2. Sit in a comfortable position with your back straight. You can be cross-legged, seated on a pillow or seated on a chair.
3. Close your mouth and lower your gaze to about 2 to 3 feet in front of you on the floor, or close your eyes. Rest your hands on your knees, relax your shoulders and begin breathing.
4. Pay attention to your breath; observe it rather than trying to control it.
5. Now it's time to focus your mind. There are several techniques for doing this, but counting your breath is typically recommended for beginners. Count one breath in and one breath out. Continue this for 10 breaths and then return to one again. If your mind wanders, start again at one.

   You are now meditating!

Dance

Dance is a well-known therapy used for healing. In fact, there is a field called dance movement therapy (DMT), and you can become a registered dance therapist (DTR). The American Dance Therapy Association defines DMT as "the use of movement as a process which furthers physical and emotional integration of an individual."[2] DMT has been shown to be an effective treatment for oncology patients (reduction of depression and anxiety) and fibromyalgia sufferers (reduction of pain and increased energy), as well as in stress reduction and an overall improved quality of life.[3]

Have you ever turned up the music and danced around your house? Or do you look forward to dancing socially? How does it make you feel? People often say they feel "elated," "free," "light," "happy" and "invigorated." This is a very effective — and free — therapy you can give yourself if you are feeling stressed, anxious, depressed or trapped in your body. A little movement and expression can soothe your mind and help you feel comfortable in your body. Turn your favorite music up and start moving!

Laughter

"Laughter is the tonic, the relief, the surcease for pain."

— Charlie Chaplin

Just as with dancing, laughter is something we were born to do. It's free, and you can do it anywhere. A good laugh can melt away stress and make us feel happy. Its health benefits have been lauded since biblical times ("A merry heart doeth good like a medicine: but a broken spirit drieth the bones." – Proverbs 17:22). More recently, laughter therapy, also called humor therapy, has utilized humor to promote overall healing and wellness; it's growing in popularity.

There are now laughter clubs and even laughter yoga. We commonly hear patients tell us that they feel down and the sweetness of life is gone. Laughter may be a tool to improve your mood, tone your abdominal muscles and help you on your healing journey. Watch a funny movie or a comedian, join a laughter club or spend time with a friend who makes you laugh.

Other Helpful Therapies

These therapies are also helpful for healing past traumas and Adverse Childhood Experiences (ACEs):

- NLP stop technique
- the Gupta Programme (GuptaProgramme.com)
- somatic experiencing
- hypnosis
- eye movement desensitization and reprocessing (EMDR)

Chapter 8
Optimizing Your Sleep

In chapter 4 we covered how a lack of sleep or poor-quality sleep can negatively impact your pain, weaken your immune system and alter hormones. Now that you have a better understanding of sleep biology and some of the important physiological activities that occur during sleep, let's delve into how to improve your sleep quality and quantity.

Just as eating healthily takes some planning and effort, sleep also requires a good plan. You can experiment with the following suggestions to improve your sleep; they include lifestyle and dietary strategies. In addition, herbs and supplements to support sleep can be found in chapter 11, although they can't replace lifestyle and dietary changes. For example, if you continue to work on your computer late at night, stay indoors all day, and maintain an erratic sleep schedule, taking a supplement to help you sleep may not be very effective. We typically recommend first improving lifestyle to enhance sleep and then trying one herb at a time at its lowest dosage.

Lifestyle Tips

Here are some ideas you can try that could help you sleep better. Some of them may take a little planning and effort, but the potential payoff makes it all worthwhile.

- **Prepare your body for sleep.** Avoid cleaning, working, paying bills, having upsetting conversations and watching the news or disturbing shows before bed. One hour before bedtime, start preparing your body for sleep. Make a list of anything on your mind or tasks you need to complete. If there are a few things you can quickly accomplish that night, such as packing your lunch for the following day, cross them off your list. Complete your hygiene routine (teeth-brushing, washing your face, et cetera). During the 10 to 20 minutes before you go to bed, prepare your brain for sleep. Your brain needs time to power down at night. It does not have an on/off switch! Do meditation or HeartMath (www.heartmath.com), read scripture or practice any other relaxation exercise.

- **Avoid napping.** This can alter your natural sleep/wake cycles.

The right snack a few hours before bedtime could help stabilize blood sugar, leading to better sleep. Some to try:

- one of the smoothies in this book (pages 170, 177 and 182)
- ½ cup (125 mL) of homemade yogurt and berries
- a small handful of nuts and ½ cup (125 mL) of berries
- a cup of bone broth
- a spoonful of almond butter
- half a banana and a handful of shelled sunflower seeds

- **Avoid coffee, smoking and alcohol.** All of these impact sleep. Coffee may be well tolerated if you have it at the beginning of the day. If you have sleeping problems, however, you may want to avoid coffee and caffeine completely.

- **Get daily movement and exercise.** Vigorous forms of exercise should be done early in the day, no closer than 4 hours before bedtime. Gentle, restorative forms of exercise, such as yin yoga, may be done in the evenings to calm the nervous system.

- **Avoid eating large meals late in the evening.** Try to eat at least 2 hours before going to bed, and 4 hours if the meal is large and/or heavy. A light snack a few hours before bed can be helpful if your blood sugar is dropping during the night and causing a cortisol surge. One indicator that this may be occurring is if you are waking at the same hour on a regular basis. For example, you may wake at 3 a.m. every morning. If so, make sure you are eating a breakfast with adequate protein and having well-rounded meals every 3 to 5 hours throughout the day to support your adrenal function and stabilize blood sugar. If these diet changes do not improve sleep, you can experiment with a light snack a few hours before bed, including complex carbohydrates, healthy fat and protein. See the sidebar for a few snack examples.

- **Avoid blue light after dark.** Blue light is emitted from your TV screen, computers, tablets, smartphones and florescent lights. Exposure before bed can disrupt your sleep cycle. If you must use one of these devices or have florescent lights in your home, wear amber or yellow-colored glasses after dark. Also, consider putting orange light bulbs into lights you routinely have on at night. There are also some great apps for your phone and computer that adjust the lighting of your screen at night (for example, Twilight app and F.lux).

- **Get some sun early in the day.** Exposure to natural light helps to set your sleep cycles. Try to get some sunlight (without wearing sunglasses) for 10 to 15 minutes at the beginning of the day.

- **Stick to your sleep schedule.** Have the same bedtime and wake-up time daily. This helps to set natural sleep/wake cycles. Go to bed by 10 p.m. and rise at the same time each morning (preferably 8 to 9 hours later). This includes the weekends; try hard to stick to a regular wake time.

- **Use your bedroom for sleeping and sex only.** Avoid watching TV, studying or listening to the radio in bed — although some people are okay to read non-stimulating literature before bed, to fatigue their eyes.

- **Create an optimal sleeping environment.** Make sure your room is cool; an optimal sleeping temperature is between 60°F and 67°F (15.5°C and 20°C). Use blackout shades to ensure the room is completely dark. Place your alarm clock at the other end of the room, away from your head. Purchase a comfortable bed (a latex mattress or non-toxic mattress is best). Most mattresses have a life expectancy of 9 to 10 years. Use earplugs or white noise to block out sounds that may wake you during the night.

- **Turn off and unplug.** Electromagnetic fields (EMFs) may disrupt sleep. Some examples of EMF sources in your bedroom include cell phones, cordless phones, electric blankets, TVs, Wi-Fi and stereos. Unplugging your Wi-Fi in your home and all electronic devices in your room can significantly reduce your exposure to EMFs while you sleep.

- **Move when you can't sleep.** If you cannot fall asleep after 20 minutes, consider leaving your bed and doing a stress-reduction activity such as guided imagery (see page 97) in another room until you are tired.

- **Talk to your partner.** If your partner snores or keeps you awake at night, you may need to have a serious talk about the importance of sleep for your recovery and find some solutions. And consider leaving pets outside of your bedroom.

Foods That Help You Sleep

The power of food shouldn't be underestimated; making the right choices can actually help you get more sleep.

- **Complex carbohydrates.** Eating some complex carbohydrates as part of your dinner may help with sleep. Examples include roasted root vegetables such as squash, yams and beets. Avoid simple carbohydrates such as breads, pasta and sweets.

- **Proteins with high tryptophan.** Tryptophan is an amino acid that is used as a building block for serotonin. Having food that's high in tryptophan, either with dinner or as a light snack before bed, may help with sleep. Examples are chicken, turkey, fish, goat's milk kefir and avocado.

- **Vegetables with calcium and magnesium.** Dark-green leafy vegetables are high in both calcium and magnesium, which help you to relax and fall asleep. Add foods like kale and collards to your evening meals.

- **Foods high in B$_6$.** Vitamin B$_6$ is necessary to form melatonin, which helps you sleep. Bananas, chickpeas and sunflower seeds are examples of foods that are high in B$_6$.

- **Bone broth and gelatin.** Both are high in glycine, an amino acid that improves sleep and reduces daytime sleepiness. A cup of bone broth for an evening snack or with dinner may be a great sleep aid.

Did You Know?

Alarm Clocks

Alarm clocks emit electromagnetic fields (EMFs) and light, which may impair sleep.

Did You Know?

Chamomile Tea

Chamomile helps to soothe the nerves. A cup of this tea after dinner may help your body start to unwind after a stressful day.

Chapter 9
Exercising the Smart Way

Sleeping well, eating right and drinking enough water are all essential to good health. So, too, is moving your body. Physical inactivity is the fourth-leading cause of death in the world, and its impact on health has been compared to smoking tobacco.[1] Exercise and diet are our most powerful medications — and are much more effective than pharmaceuticals. The good news is that both are within your control, and you don't need a prescription!

How Physical Activity and Exercise Help Endo Symptoms

Most of us know that physical activity is good for us, but you may not realize that moving your body is important for managing endometriosis symptoms and pelvic pain. We have covered how blood sugar dysregulation, toxins, too much body fat, hormone imbalances, stress, inflammation and the immune system are involved with endometriosis and chronic pelvic pain. Physical activity has an impact on each of these components. Like anything else, the right type(s) and the right "dosage" of exercise are important for symptom management. Exercise should not be uncomfortable or make your symptoms worse. You may want to talk to a pelvic floor physical therapist about pelvic floor exercises for relaxation and/or strengthening. He or she most likely will be able to offer guidance on what types of exercise are best for you. (For more, see "Pelvic Floor Physical Therapy," page 105.)

It is important to distinguish between exercise and physical activity. Physical activity includes all body movements that use muscle contractions and result in energy expenditure. Examples include cleaning your house, taking the stairs instead of the elevator, parking your car farther away from your destination or walking your child to school. Exercise, or physical fitness, is a subset of physical activity; it's planned, structured and repetitive, with the purpose of improving physical fitness. Health-related components of physical fitness include cardiorespiratory endurance, muscular endurance, muscular strength, body composition and flexibility.

Exercise comes in many forms, and finding the best fit for you may take some experimentation. Both exercise and frequent physical activity are beneficial to your health, and a combination of both is important. If you do only the recommended 30 minutes of moderate to intense exercise daily, and then sit the rest of the day, your health outcomes may still be poor. In addition, a temporary bout of exercise (for example, a 30-minute jog) does not appear to be protective against being sedentary for the remainder of the day.[2] Based on this, and on mounting evidence, we recommend staying active throughout the day by doing frequent physical activity (such as taking breaks from your computer every 30 minutes and walking up and down the stairs a few times) and engaging in exercise 3 to 6 days a week. (See the sample exercise plan on page 112 for more details.)

Pelvic Floor Physical Therapy

Endometriosis can cause pelvic floor dysfunction (PFD). The pelvic floor includes the muscles, connective tissue and ligaments that form a sling from the pubic bone to the tailbone. This sling supports the abdominal and pelvic organs and is involved in sphincter and sexual functions. When these muscles become weak or are in spasm, it is referred to as PFD. PFD can result in pain, urinary problems and difficulty having bowel movements. Physical therapists educated about PFD may be able to provide exercises to help relax and strengthen the pelvic floor muscles. For a list of pelvic floor physical therapists in your area, speak to your medical practitioner, or check these websites:

- www.hermanwallace.com
- www.womenshealthapta.org

Exercise Helps Decrease Blood Sugar

Exercise and, more specifically, frequent bouts of physical activity can help to decrease blood glucose (sugar).[4] When we perform physical activity and exercise, our bodies use glucose and free fatty acids (fat) as the energy currency to fuel bodily movement. The glucose comes from our blood, liver and muscles. When we first start moving, the majority of the glucose is derived directly from the blood — therefore, if blood glucose is high, it gets used by our cells, which lowers the amount of glucose in our blood.

After approximately 15 minutes, glycogen (a storage form of glucose) is broken down to provide additional glucose for another 30 minutes (more or less, depending on intensity and diet) of movement. After about 30 minutes, fatty acids become the primary fuel source.

Another way physical activity helps to decrease blood glucose is by helping the cells to become more sensitive to insulin. You can think of insulin as a key that opens the doors of your cells and allows glucose to enter. When we are physically inactive, our cells can become desensitized to insulin, and the insulin does not work as well — it's like trying to open a door with the wrong key. After we eat a meal, blood glucose rises, which stimulates the pancreas to release insulin into the bloodstream. If the cells are sensitive to insulin — all the keys are fitting into the locks — blood glucose levels will quickly return to normal.

When we do regular physical activity, insulin works better, more doors open, and more glucose is taken up at rest. You can see how exercise is a powerful tool for keeping blood glucose at healthy levels. It helps to lower glucose in the short-term when you exercise, but it also has a beneficial long-term impact on helping glucose get into the cells.

Another way physical activity helps to decrease blood glucose is by helping the cells to become more sensitive to insulin.

Exercise Helps Detoxify

Exercise has an important role in detoxifying your body. There are a multitude of mechanisms in which exercise increases the body's ability to detoxify. First, if you are exercising vigorously or are in a warm climate, you will eliminate toxins through your skin by sweating. Second, moving your muscles is a way to pump your lymphatic system, which tends to be stagnant in sedentary individuals. Toxins can build up in the lymphatic system and weaken the immune system. Lastly, exercise increases your body's production of important protective proteins and antioxidants, such as glutathione. When you exercise, you deplete your glutathione, a powerful antioxidant important for detoxification; however, routine exercise conditions the body to adapt and then increase its production of glutathione.[5] Short bouts of intense exercise, such as interval training, are especially helpful in increasing glutathione production.[6]

Exercise Metabolizes Estrogen

Exercise also appears to help with estrogen metabolism. We have covered the impact of exercise on glutathione production. Besides its ability to generally detoxify, glutathione is also important in estrogen detoxification. High amounts of glutathione are contained in the liver. The liver has two main detoxification pathways, and glutathione is involved in both. Glutathione behaves as an anti-oxidant and protects cells from oxidation. (Research has found that endometriotic cells have increased oxidative stress, or free radicals.[7])

Glutathione is involved in conjugation, whereby it is combined with estrogen for easy elimination. In addition, glutathione aids in the detoxification of alcohol, and studies have demonstrated that even small amounts of alcohol can increase estrogen levels in the blood.

Exercise appears to improve estrogen metabolism by significantly increasing the 2-hydroxyestrone (healthy estrogen metabolite) ratio.[8] Higher levels of 4- and 16-hydroxyestrone increase the risk of estrogen-related cancers such as breast and ovarian. There is some evidence that rates of those cancers may be higher in women with endometriosis; however, the pathophysiology is unknown.[9]

Finally, exercise appears to lower circulating concentrations of total and free estradiol — the most potent of estrogens — and increase sex hormone–binding globulin , which acts to bind up estrogen in the blood, making it unavailable to cells.[10]

Exercise Boosts Mood

Physical activity, especially certain types of exercise such as gentle yoga, can help to relieve stress, improve mood and aid in sleeping well. We have all heard the term "runner's high." Exercise helps to improve your overall mood by increasing the brain's production of feel-good neurotransmitters called endorphins. Endorphins may also help to decrease your pain. Research has shown a decrease in dysmenorrhea (painful periods) with both stretching and aerobic exercise.[11]

The repetitive movement of many exercises is a form of moving meditation, especially if we focus on our breathing and our bodies. For example, if you are doing push-ups, inhaling as you lower yourself and exhaling as you push up, while also concentrating on correct body movement, your mind is able to rest from the ongoing stress of the day. Focusing on form and how your body is feeling with each movement is a way to turn your attention inward. Also, regular physical activity is a great way to improve your self-confidence and body image. Just taking the time to do something good for your body and focusing on *you* can reinforce your self-worth. Lastly, staying active improves sleep, which will have the ripple effect of lowering anxiety and depression.

> **The repetitive movement of many exercises is a form of moving meditation, especially if we focus on our breathing and our bodies.**

Recommended Types of Exercise

There are many different ways to increase your physical activity and add exercise to your lifestyle. As covered earlier in this chapter, both planned exercise and staying physically active throughout the day are important to good health and managing your endo symptoms. Choosing what type of planned exercise you should do, how often and for how long and determining how much rest you require is a process unique to each individual. The following recommendations are general, and are based on recent scientific literature and experience with patients. A consultation

The Latest Thinking on Exercise

Many people exercise to lose weight or body fat. Have you ever noticed the heart rate training zones displayed on your favorite piece of cardio equipment at the gym? Usually, they have a "fat burning" zone. This is typically somewhere around 60% to 70% of your maximum heart rate. This level of intensity requires moderate effort, a level in which you could carry on a conversation, but with some effort. The recommendations that encouraged performing 30 to 60 minutes of moderate-intensity exercise on most days of the week for weight loss, cardiovascular health and overall health are outdated. More recent research has found that this type of exercise is not as effective as other forms of training programs, and that long-duration endurance exercise (such as triathlons and long-distance running) is actually damaging to your health.[12]

with your doctor and/or physical therapist is always a good idea before starting any exercise program.

The type of exercise you choose depends on your health and fitness goals, how much time you have in your schedule, your current health condition, any physical limitations, your energy level and what type of exercise you enjoy. Here are some recommendations.

Further Information

Here are a few examples of HITT-style programs:

- http://www. metaboliceffect. com/about-us/

- http://fitness. mercola.com/sites/ fitness/archive/ 2012/04/06/high- intensity-training- benefits.aspx

- http://draxe.com/ benefits-high- intensity-interval- training/

High-Intensity Interval Training (HITT)

High-intensity interval training, or HIIT, has become increasingly popular. There are several variations on this type of training, but in general, it involves alternating between high- and low-intensity exercise(s), or between high-intensity exercise and a short period of recovery (rest). For example, a short sprint for 30 seconds and then walking for 60 to 90 seconds, or a set of burpees followed by push-ups on a bench, with this combination repeated 4 to 10 times.

In general, HITT workouts are intended to be short — less than a total of 30 minutes. They have a different hormonal effect than moderate-intensity workouts. While both involve an increase in stress hormones such as cortisol and epinephrine (also called adrenaline), in HITT workouts both testosterone and human growth hormone (HGH) are significantly increased, which mitigates the catabolic, or muscle-breakdown, effect of cortisol. In addition, the calorie burn after workouts is much longer with HITT. Lastly, HITT workouts create a short-term stress response in the body, which conditions the body to adapt to stress. HITT workouts can be adapted to meet the needs of the individual, making them suitable for everyone, regardless of fitness level.

Although exercise has several positive effects on our bodies, there is always the risk of overtraining, injury and hormonal imbalance if the correct amount of rest between workouts is not taken. HITT, as its name implies, is intense and hard on the body, especially without proper rest, sleep and nutrition. Overtraining has been shown to lower blood levels of glutamine, dopamine and 5-HTP, which can result in depression and feeling chronically fatigued. In addition, chronically elevated cortisol levels with overtraining can result in increased fat storage (especially around the abdomen), leaky gut, insomnia, immune suppression, elevated blood sugar and hypothyroid symptoms.

Does this mean you should not exercise? Absolutely not! You just need to be smart, pay attention to the symptoms of overtraining, nourish your body properly, get adequate sleep and allow recovery time between workouts. For more details about frequency and duration of workouts, see page 111. And for a sample workout plan, see page 112.

Did You Know?

The Benefits of Weight Training
- more muscle strength
- improved body composition (more muscle, less fat)
- pain management
- improved mobility
- better balance
- increased bone density and strength
- better posture
- improved insulin sensitivity

Resistance Training

Resistance training, or weight training, can benefit your body in many ways (see sidebar). Since many women with endometriosis have been on Lupron or medications to suppress estrogen — which deplete bone density — resistance training may be a critical part of any endo program. When you lift weights, the muscle pulls on your bones, causing tension. The bones adapt to this stimulus by increasing strength and density. It may be a good idea to talk with a physical therapist who specializes in pelvic floor dysfunction before beginning a resistance training program. This is especially true if you plan to do exercises involving the core and hips. If you have very tight muscles in those areas, or have been diagnosed with pelvic floor dysfunction, you want to make sure you are not making symptoms worse by increasing tension.

Walking and Hiking

Walking and gentle hiking are a great way to get outside and move your body. They are also fantastic activities for active rest days between more intense workout days. Taking the time to get sunlight and enjoy nature is healing for your body and soul. If you can, take your shoes off and put your feet in the dirt or in the sand at the beach for 20 minutes or more to ground yourself. Grounding, or earthing, can benefit your health in many ways, including balancing your sympathetic and parasympathetic nervous systems, reducing inflammation, increasing energy and strengthening your immune system.[13]

Why "Earthing" Is So Good for You

Until recently, humans had always been in direct contact with the earth. Now, however, we wear shoes and don't go outside nearly as often as we used to. Why does this matter?

The earth has a negative charge at its surface, which includes soil, the ocean and sand. The human body requires a negative charge to function optimally. When we are in direct contact with the earth — walking barefoot, swimming in the ocean or lying on the ground — the earth's negative charge is conducted to our bodies, literally flooding them with electrons that we use to counteract free radicals and inflammation and to charge ourselves with electrical energy. This positively impacts things such as hormonal cycles, circadian rhythms and emotional health.

In addition to our lack of direct contact with the earth, we are also constantly bombarded with electro-pollution — or "dirty energy" — from cell phones, cell phone towers, wireless routers, electrical cardio equipment at the gym and other electromagnetic frequency (EMF)–emitting devices. This energy weakens the body.

A great resource on earthing and available earthing products can be found at www.grounded.com.

Yoga

Yoga is a great gift you can give your body. There are many different types of yoga, so choosing the right form for you is important. In general, yoga is fantastic for balancing the sympathetic and parasympathetic nervous systems, strengthening bones and muscles, and getting all of the other great benefits of exercise. Here are just a few of the different yoga styles and how each affects your body.

Ashtanga

Ashtanga yoga is a rigorous style that includes specific poses done in the exact same order each time. It is typically a hot, sweaty and physically demanding practice. This type of yoga is harder than others on the body, and daily practice may be too much, especially if you have any adrenal dysfunction or chronic fatigue. It may be best to build up to this type of practice when you are feeling strong, and alternate it with more gentle forms of exercise such as walking or a restorative style of yoga.

Bikram

Bikram classes are similar to Ashtanga as they also follow a specific sequence (but a different one than Ashtanga). The 90-minute practice is done in a heated room, typically around 104°F (40°C), and consists of 26 postures done in the same order each time. This style of yoga is physically demanding on your body due to the high heat as well as some challenging poses held for what can sometimes feel like forever. In addition, Bikram and other types of hot yoga can activate your stress response and, over time, cause adrenal dysfunction. Just as with Ashtanga, Bikram yoga may be best practiced a few days a week, with special attention to proper hydration and electrolyte replacement.

Hatha

Hatha yoga is a general term for any type of yoga practice that teaches physical postures. Most yoga classes in the West are in the Hatha style, and they are often gentle and for beginners. Hatha yoga may be a better choice for less conditioned individuals and those looking for a more restorative type of practice. Hatha yoga, especially beginner classes, are great for active rest days between more rigorous exercise days.

> **Hatha yoga may be a better choice for less conditioned individuals and those looking for a more restorative type of practice.**

Yin or Restorative Yoga

Yin yoga, the opposite of heat-producing yang, is a great way to relax and soothe your nervous system. Most classes use props such as bolsters, blankets and blocks to help you achieve passive poses, held for longer periods of time in order for the body to experience the benefits of the pose with very little effort. This is a great style to do daily, especially if your energy is very low or you are anxious, and it's fantastic for active rest days between more strenuous workout days.

Vinyasa

Vinyasa classes are fluid, movement-intensive practices. These classes move from one movement to the next in a choreographed style. Many teachers play music in their classes. The intensity can be low to very rigorous, depending on the level and the teacher. On yoga studio schedules, these classes are often labeled based on skill and intensity level. Depending on the intensity, vinyasa classes can be used for active rest or as a more physically demanding workout.

Guidelines to Exercise Frequency and Duration

The right frequency and duration of exercise greatly depend on what type of activity you are performing and its intensity. What is important is that you are giving your body adequate rest time to receive the benefits of exercise. Just as with so many other healthy things, such as vitamins and nutrients, the proper "dose" is essential: remember, too much of a good thing can become unhealthy.

As a general rule, you should feel energized and physically better after your workouts and for the remainder of the day. You should sleep better, be in less pain and feel less anxious. However, here are some signs that you probably need a restorative type of exercise in order to heal:

- You need to take a nap after exercise.
- You drag through the rest of your day.
- You find each successive workout feels harder than the last.
- You notice that your sleep is less restful.
- You start gaining weight.
- You feel more anxious.

You may feel great doing some interval training for a few months, and then start noticing some of the above-mentioned symptoms. If you do, you may be overtraining and need some rest.

Sample Weekly Exercise Plan

This is a general plan to help you avoid overtraining while optimizing your health. It is meant for individuals who are generally healthy and are not chronically fatigued. If you suffer from severe fatigue, we recommend you start with only restorative types of exercise, such as walking and gentle styles of yoga. It is important to check with your local health-care provider and/or pelvic floor physical therapist before starting any exercise program.

Day	Exercise Option 1	Exercise Option 2
Monday	Interval training with resistance (see page 113)	Vigorous yoga class
Tuesday	Walk for 30 to 45 minutes	Restorative yoga class
Wednesday	Interval training with resistance	Vigorous yoga class
Thursday	Enjoy a rest day	Restorative yoga class
Friday	Interval training with resistance	Vigorous yoga class
Saturday	Walk for 45 to 60 minutes	Restorative yoga class
Sunday	Walk for 45 to 60 minutes	Restorative yoga class

Every 3 months, take a full week off. Rest! Some walking and gentle yoga are okay to do.

Interval Training with Resistance

Start with 1 set of each exercise and slowly work up to 6 sets of each. Do not exceed 30 minutes. YouTube has some great examples of how to do many of these exercises.

1. **Warm-up: Slow jog or brisk walk (5 minutes).**

2. **Chair squats (1 minute).** Stand in front of a chair, its seat just behind you. Squat as if you are going to sit in the chair, but do not touch the seat of the chair with your behind; then stand again. Repeat for 1 minute.

3. **Push-ups (1 minute).** Depending on your strength, you can do either the easier version of push-ups (with your knees on the floor) or a regular push-up (with your toes on the floor). You can also do these against the wall or the side of a counter. Repeat for 1 minute.

4. **Wall run (1 minute).** Place your hands against the wall. Then run in place while trying to push the wall over. If you need to take breaks to catch your breath, that's okay. Just start running again when you can. Repeat for 1 minute.

5. **Row with resistance band (1 minute).** Resistance bands come in several different tensions; pick the one you're comfortable with. Tie the middle of the band to a doorknob, leaving equal lengths on each end. Facing the door, with an end in each hand, pull hands back, stopping just under your chest. Do this for 1 minute.

6. **Plank (30 seconds).** Get down into a regular push-up position with toes on the floor, but balance on your forearms instead of your hands. Your elbows should be directly below your shoulders, and your body should be in a straight line from head to toes. Tighten up your glutes (butt muscles) and pull in your belly button — imagine you have a flame under your belly and you don't want to get burned. Stay in this position for 30 seconds. *Caution:* During a plank, if your butt begins to lower and your back sways (with your belly button moving toward the floor), lower your knees to the floor and hold this position. A swayed back puts lots of pressure on your back and may do more damage than good.

7. **Burpees (1 minute).** Burpees are a full-body exercise. They are a more advanced movement, so if you are just getting started, you may want to either skip them or do them slowly, step by step.
   - Stand with your feet hip-width apart and your arms at your sides.
   - Lower into a squat position and place your hands on the floor in front of you.
   - Kick your legs backward, jumping into a push-up position.
   - Push your chest up and jump back into a squat.
   - Jump straight up and raise your arms above your head as if you are trying to block a ball at the net in volleyball.
   - Repeat for 1 minute.

8. **Cool down: Walk (5 minutes).**

Chapter 10
Charging Your Body

Additional Resources

- *Earthing* by Clinton Ober and Dr. Stephen T. Sinatra

- *The Fourth Phase of Water: Beyond Solid, Liquid, and Vapor* by Gerald H. Pollack

- Biomat: www. painreduction. thebiomatcompany. com

Most of us think about food and calories as the fuel that enables our bodies to function. We have devoted a large portion of this book to diet. Although the macronutrients fat, protein, carbohydrates and water are all important building blocks for our cells to produce energy — called adenosine triphosphate (ATP) — there is another type of energy produced in the cells that charges our bodies. This is electrical energy, much like the energy that powers a lightbulb or your computer. Our bodies are controlled and charged by electrical signals.

We all learned about atoms in high school. Atoms consist of protons, neutrons and electrons. Protons are positively charged, neutrons have a neutral charge and electrons are negatively charged. When the charges are not balanced, the atom can become either negatively or positively charged. The alteration between positive and negative charges allows electrons to flow from one atom to the next, and that flow causes a negative charge, which creates what we call electricity.

Our bodies are made up of large numbers of atoms; therefore, we have the potential to generate huge amounts of electricity that can be measured. A few good examples: an electrocardiogram (EKG) measures the electrical activity of our heart, and an electroencephalogram (EEG) measures the electrical activity of our brain.

We are electrical beings, and this electricity is crucial for controlling many functions in our bodies, such as heart rate and neurotransmitter production. Negative ions can also alter our moods. Just walking in the forest or on the beach, where the level of negative ions in the air is high, helps to create a sense of renewed vigor and well-being in people.[1]

The earth is electrically charged, with a net negative charge. There is ongoing research on how direct contact with the earth through grounding and exposure to high levels of negative ions are important to our health. For example, high exposure to negative ions is important for proper cortisol secretion, maintaining a strong immune system, reducing inflammation, boosting moods, achieving restful sleep, balancing neurotransmitters and hormones, reducing cardiovascular disease and improving concentration.[2]

The good news is that you can increase your exposure to negative ions without having to buy special machines. Below are a few ideas and resources for learning more about improving your health by charging your body.

How to Charge Your Body with Negative Ions

Earthing (aka Grounding)

Go barefoot outside, optimally 40 minutes daily, in the dirt, grass or sand. If you cannot go outside, a concrete basement floor will also work. Wood and vinyl are not conductive and will not connect you to the earth.

There are also earthing products available; see https://www.earthing.com.

Diet

- Stay properly hydrated.
- Drink spring water.
- Juice vegetables.
- Eat a diet rich in antioxidants; these help our bodies to maintain a negative charge.
- Eat high-quality pure salt (for example, Redmond's Real Salt and Premier Research Lab's Pink Salt)
- Go out in the sunshine.
- Expose yourself to infrared light. (You can do this by sitting in an infrared sauna or lying on a Biomat.)
- Place salt lamps around your home.
- Use a negative ionizer in your home, car and office.

Chapter 11
Herbal and Supplemental Treatments

In this chapter, we outline some preferred supplements and herbs for women with endometriosis and explain how they support detoxification and provide help for inflammation, stress, pain and much more. The dosages suggested are based on general guidelines. Please discuss taking any of these herbs and supplements with a qualified practitioner before using.

Detoxification Support
Milk Thistle

> **Protecting the liver and optimizing liver function is important with endometriosis, as impaired liver function will decrease estrogen detoxification.**

Milk thistle has been used for some 2,000 years as an herbal remedy for several health problems, including poor detoxification and liver inflammation. The flavonoid silymarin in milk thistle protects the liver from toxins that can lead to liver damage and inflammation. Protecting the liver and optimizing liver function are important with endometriosis, as impaired liver function will decrease estrogen detoxification. There have been no studies conducted on the use of milk thistle for management or treatment of endometriosis. However, research does show you can improve liver health and reduce inflammation with dosages of milk thistle ranging from 70 to 420 mg daily.[1]

N-acetyl Cysteine (NAC)

NAC is an anti-inflammatory that supports phase II detoxification in the liver. Clinical studies on humans have not been done to determine dosages for endometriosis relief. However, studies have been done using endometriotic cells from women who have endometriosis. In these studies, NAC appears to aid in reduction of free radicals, decrease inflammation and slow the progression of the disease.[2] In addition, research shows it improves insulin sensitivity for women with polycystic ovary syndrome (a hormonal condition involving insulin resistance).[3] NAC is accepted as an effective detoxification nutrient through its ability to increase glutathione (a strong antioxidant and an important molecule in estrogen and general detoxification in the liver). Glutathione may be helpful in controlling endometriosis symptoms and progression. In several human studies, doses of 1,200 to 1,800 mg have been used for treatment.

Methylation Support

Methylation is an important biochemical process. It turns genes on and off, repairs DNA, strengthens the immune system, modulates inflammation and much more (see page 93). Healthy methylation supports detoxification. In order to optimize methylation, you may benefit from the following supplements. However, methylation supplementation is best if individualized. No studies have yet been done on endometriosis and methylation support. Recommended dosages are based on clinical practice and industry-recommended doses.

Magnesium

Magnesium is involved in several detoxification processes. It is necessary for neutralizing toxins, maintaining acid/base balance in the body and protecting the body from heavy metals. Magnesium is required for the synthesis of glutathione, a potent antioxidant and detoxifier. Research suggests that magnesium competes with heavy metals for entry into the brain and small intestine. In addition, magnesium supports important enzymes such as catechol-O-methyltransferase (COMT), which metabolizes estrogen for elimination.

We often measure magnesium levels in addition to performing a physical assessment and detailed medical history for signs of magnesium deficiency. We frequently start with 400 mg of magnesium glycinate and increase as needed. If someone has severe constipation, we may suggest magnesium citrate, starting with 400 mg and increasing by 100 to 200 mg every night until a soft, formed bowel movement is achieved the following morning. If someone has poor absorption, we may suggest the use of a magnesium cream on the feet or Epsom salt baths.

B Vitamins

Folate (5-formyltetrahydrofolate)

Folate is central to the methylation cycle. Up to 50% of the population has a defect in the enzyme involved in the conversion of inactive to active folate. We recommend a dose of 200 mcg to 1 mg daily. Some people do not tolerate folate right away and may need to address other issues such as gut dysbiosis, infections and liver function before working on methylation. Supplementing with other B vitamins before folate may improve tolerance. We do not recommend folic acid, which is a synthetic vitamin that is difficult for many people's bodies to utilize.

Did You Know?

B Complex Supplementation

B vitamins work in synergy, and in general we recommend supplementing with a B complex or a multivitamin with a wide range of activated B vitamins. Especially important B vitamins for methylation are folate, B_{12}, B_6 and riboflavin.

✍ *Vitamin B₆ (Pyridoxal-5-phosphate)*

Vitamin B_6 is involved in the methylation cycle and is critical to the formation of glutathione. We recommend a dose of 2 to 5 mg a day, although some people require higher doses. In general, we do not recommend doses higher than 100 mg per day, as high doses can cause irreversible nerve damage.

Vitamin B₁₂ (Methylcobalamin)

As we age we naturally absorb less B_{12} from our diet. In addition, low stomach acid drastically decreases B_{12} absorption. B_{12} is intimately involved with folate in the methylation cycle. If you have low stomach acid or poor nutrient absorption, you may require injections of B_{12}. We typically recommend doses of 500 to 2,000 mcg of B_{12} daily. In general, we recommend supplementing with either methylcobalamin or hydroxocobalamin, depending on genetics and tolerance.

Betaine

The main physiologic role of betaine is as an osmolyte and a methyl donor. As an osmolyte, betaine works to protect cells, proteins and enzymes from environmental stress. As a methyl donor, betaine assists in converting homocysteine (elevated levels of it damage the inner arterial lining and contribute to the development of many chronic diseases) into methionine, which helps with cystitis and urinary tract infections. It also lowers depression, removes heavy metals and detoxifies.

Phosphatidylserine

As with betaine, phosphatidylserine (PS) aids in the conversion of homocysteine to methionine. It can also be helpful with high cortisol levels resulting from chronic infection, chronic stress and inflammation. We generally recommend 100 mg twice daily.

● Zinc

A zinc deficiency can decrease the body's ability to use methyl groups from methyl donors such as SAMe (S-adenosylmethionine). Overall, this results in under-methylation of DNA, which can negatively alter gene expression. We typically recommend 30 mg of zinc picolinate. A dose of more than 30 mg daily can create a copper deficiency. We prefer measuring red blood cell zinc and copper levels before supplementing with either zinc or copper.

Antioxidants: More Support for Methylation

We generally recommend getting antioxidants from foods. However, when supplementing is needed, we recommend a group of antioxidants versus only one, as they act together.

Antioxidants, including vitamins C and E, selenium and beta-carotene (vitamin A), are important for protecting cells from free radical damage. As well, they act as important cofactors for liver enzymes involved in detoxification. Selenium is particularly important, as it recycles and helps to increase production of glutathione and also inhibits a methylating enzyme called DNA methyltransferase, which is located in cancer genes. Methylation of this enzyme turns the gene off, which decreases cancer growth. In addition, selenoproteins protect DNA and aid in proper metabolism of methionine. Here are some other key antioxidants.

- **Melatonin.** Most people think of a sleep aid when they hear the word *melatonin*. However, melatonin is also a powerful antioxidant. Research on women with endo who use 10 mg of melatonin at 8 p.m. each night demonstrated a reduction in pain and the regression and atrophy of endometriotic lesions.[4] We recommend between 0.5 and 10 mg taken at 8 p.m. each night, as higher doses can cause fatigue the following day.

- **Alpha-lipoic acid.** Alpha-lipoic acid is a powerful antioxidant. It regenerates other antioxidants (vitamin C and E, CoQ10 and glutathione) and has heavy metal chelating activity. It is both fat and water soluble, and therefore is highly absorbable from the gut and can easily cross the blood-brain membrane barrier. Small amounts of lipoic acid can be found in food sources such as dark leafy greens, beef and organ meats. No specific studies on endometriosis have been done to date; however, its use as an antioxidant is well known. The most potent form of lipoic acid is R-dihydro-lipoic acid.[5] Because of the potential for redistribution of heavy metals, it is best used in moderation. We recommend starting with 300 to 800 mg daily in divided doses.

- **Resveratrol.** Resveratrol is a potent antioxidant and aromatase inhibitor. It has been studied for use with endometriosis and appears to reduce pain significantly and suppress the development of new microvessel growth in endo lesions.[6] The dosage used in research was 30 mg daily.

- **Pycnogenol.** Pycnogenol is a powerful antioxidant that has been studied for its pain-reducing effect in women with endo and dysmenorrhea.[7] The dosage used in research was 60 mg daily (30 mg taken twice daily).

Inflammation Support
Turmeric/Curcumin

Eaten as an herb or taken as a supplement, curcumin, the most potent part of turmeric, is a natural COX-2 inhibitor (meaning it's anti-inflammatory). It's an antioxidant and it improves liver detoxification. It has also been shown to reduce estradiol production and may slow the progression of endometriosis.[8] No human studies have been done specifically to test curcumin's effect on endometriosis; however, studies on humans for its use for inflammation have used doses of 500 to 1,000 mg or more daily.[9] Absorption is improved if ingredients such as black pepper extract are present.

Boswellia serrata

Boswellia is a natural inhibitor of 5-LOX, a potent enzyme involved in the induction of the inflammatory process. Boswellia works as a strong anti-inflammatory. More potent forms of boswellia have become available, containing at least 30% of an acid known as AKBA.[10] AKBA binds directly to the 5-LOX enzyme and inhibits its activity. Products such as 5-Loxin, Aflapin and AprèsFLEX are all high in AKBA. No specific studies have been done on boswellia and its use for endometriosis. Other studies done to observe pain reduction used dosages ranging from 600 to 6,000 mg of boswellia serrata resin with meals or 100 to 250 mg of 5-Loxin/AprèsFLEX taken before the first meal of the day.[11]

Blood Sugar Support
Berberine

Berberine improves the metabolism of glucose (which will in turn lower inflammation).[14] In addition, it may help to prevent post-surgery intestinal adhesions and inflammation.[15] No human studies have been done using berberine to treat endometriosis. We recommend 500 mg one to three times daily, as this is supported by the literature using berberine to improve glycemic control.

Immune Support

Astragalus

Astragalus stimulates the body's production of macrophages (for more on macrophages, see page 42) and regulates the production of T cells.[16] A study on rats showed that oral administration of astragalus decreased uterine endo implants and lowered estradiol and inflammation.[17] No human studies have been done using astragalus for endometriosis care. However, studies conducted on humans to increase macrophage production have used doses of 250 to 500 mg of a standardized extract (standardized to 0.4% 4-hydroxy-3-methoxy isoflavone 7-sug) taken three to four times daily.[18]

Cat's Claw (*Uncaria tomentosa*)

Cat's claw activates macrophages.[19] A study done on rats demonstrated a reduction in endo lesion growth after 14 days.[20] There are reports of several Indigenous tribes using cat's claw as a contraceptive, but no human studies have been done to confirm this, and the dosage for this usage was much higher than most recommended doses. The antiproliferative effects and induction of apoptosis appear to be related to its contraceptive effects.[21] We recommend doses of 250 to 350 mg daily for immune support in products that contain only *Uncaria tomentosa* and are free of tetracyclic oxindole alkaloid (TOA).[22]

Reishi Mushrooms (*Ganoderma lucidum*)

Reishi mushrooms have a long history of enhancing immune function. They are considered adaptogens and not only strengthen the immune system but also balance it. The polysaccharide beta (1,3)-D glucan in reishi helps to boost the immune system by increasing the amount of macrophages and T cells, and enhancing their activity.[23] Reishi helps to boost levels of supoeroxide dismutase (SOD), a powerful antioxidant,[24] and increase beneficial gut bacteria, which is critical for a strong immune system, since 80% of the immune system resides in the gut.[25] In addition, reishi helps to support and heal the liver and repair the gastrointestinal lining.[26] As a bonus, reishi is anti-inflammatory!

There are different types of reishi. However, most herbalists consider red reishi to have the highest potency. The best time to take reishi is in the morning on an empty stomach with lots of water and a source of vitamin C. One study observing the effect of reishi mushroom supplementation on dysmenorrhea

> **Reishi mushrooms have a long history of enhancing immune function. They are considered adaptogens and not only strengthen the immune system but also balance it.**

demonstrated a reduction or elimination of symptoms after 2 to 3 cycles using 1,500 mg of *Ganoderma lucidum* extract taken three times daily.[27] The most common dosage for the basic extract of reishi is 1,800 mg taken three times daily (total daily dosage: 5.2 g).[28]

Probiotics

The beneficial bacteria in your gut are responsible for approximately 80% of your immune function. We have dedicated an entire section of this book to gut health (see page 44). We recommend getting probiotics from your diet by consuming fermented foods, but we also often recommend specific strains or combinations of probiotic supplements depending on an individual's needs. For example, *Bifidobacterium infantis* has prokinetic effects, which may help with SIBO — or small intestinal bacterial overgrowth, a syndrome resulting from an elevated number and/or abnormal type of bacteria that have overgrown in the small intestine (see pages 45–47 for more) — and constipation, as it helps with motility. [29]

Intestinal Support

Betaine HCl

Betaine HCl is often used to increase stomach acid. Low stomach acid is a common cause of indigestion, constipation, bacterial and yeast overgrowth, and intestinal infections.[30] Betaine HCl is usually taken at the start of a meal containing protein. We recommend starting with a single 750 to 1,000 mg capsule with each meal and adjusting until you feel discomfort (burning, heartburn, warmth in your stomach or burping), then reducing the dosage back to the maximum amount taken before discomfort. If you experience discomfort, have 1 teaspoon (5 mL) of baking soda in 1 cup (250 mL) of water to neutralize the acid.

Digestive Bitters

Bitters have been used since ancient times to aid in digestion. They stimulate the body's natural digestive response, triggering the production and release of digestive enzymes, bile and hydrochloric acid (HCl). In addition, bitters can aid in healing the gut. Examples include dandelion root and leaf, burdock root, yellow dock root, salad greens and green tea. You can purchase digestive bitters, make your own, or include bitter foods in your meals. Iberogast is a bitters product that also works as a fantastic prokinetic (helps with intestinal motility).[31] Take this at the end of meals. In addition, if you have SIBO, we recommend 20 drops before bed.

Digestive Enzymes

Digestive enzymes are necessary to break down food into absorbable nutrients. Protein is broken down into amino acids, carbohydrates are broken down into simple sugars (glucose, fructose and galactose) and fats are broken down into fatty acids. Most of our digestive enzymes are produced in the pancreas and small intestine, with a small amount also made in the mouth and stomach. When we are chronically ill, chronically stressed or have intestinal damage, our bodies are sometimes unable to produce adequate digestive enzymes to properly digest the food we eat. This can result in digestive symptoms such as constipation, heartburn, bloating, intestinal inflammation, food sensitivities and malabsorption. We recommend supplementation with digestive enzymes until the underlying issues are corrected, and you once again produce adequate digestive enzymes on your own.[32] When purchasing a digestive enzyme product, look for a multi-enzyme that includes proteases, lipases and amylase. As with bitters, we recommend taking digestive enzymes at the end of a meal.

When we are chronically ill, chronically stressed or have intestinal damage, our bodies are sometimes unable to produce adequate digestive enzymes to properly digest the food we eat.

DGL, Slippery Elm, Marshmallow Root, Aloe Vera

These all help to soothe the intestinal lining, enhance mucus production and form a protective barrier. This can expedite natural body repair. The dosage varies depending on the product and the needs of the individual. You can also make teas with slippery elm and marshmallow root, and drink aloe vera gel mixed with water.

Zinc Carnosine

Zinc carnosine is a micronutrient mineral that aids in protecting the cells from free radical damage. In addition, it has anti-inflammatory effects and helps stabilize mast cells, kills *H. pylori* and enhances cellular repair in the intestines.[33] Based on research using zinc carnosine for intestinal repair, we recommend 30 to 50 mg be taken two to three times daily for a month.

Butyrate

Butyrate is a short-chain fatty acid produced by bacteria when they digest fiber in the large intestine. It is critical for a healthy gut, especially the health of the intestinal lining. It balances the growth and death of cells that line the gut, provides fuel for the cells lining the gut and acts to decrease inflammation in the gut.[34] Not having enough of this beneficial bacteria in the gut can lead to inflammation. In addition, butyrate plays a large role in the immune system by regulating the production and development of T cells in the colon (remember, T cells act as your body's "dimmer" to regulate the immune response).[35] Luckily, butyrate can be obtained in foods and by supplementation; it's found in large amounts in butter and ghee. This is one reason we recommend 1 to 2 tablespoons (15 to 30 mL) of ghee during phase 1 of the Endometriosis Diet Plan. Occasionally, we recommend supplementing with butyrate and/or doing butyrate enemas.

L-Glutamine

L-glutamine is an amino acid used in huge amounts by the body. In fact, the cells in the intestines use this amino acid as their primary fuel. If there is intestinal lining damage, taking L-glutamine can expedite the healing process.[36] Glutamine dosages vary depending on therapeutic needs. Based on research and clinical use we recommend taking 5 g of L-glutamine with food twice daily for 1 to 2 months.[37]

Probiotics

Probiotics help to increase beneficial bacteria and encourage a healthy microbial balance. A robust amount of beneficial bacteria helps maintain healthy gastrointestinal function. In general, we recommend getting probiotics from fermented foods. However, during phase 1 of the Endometriosis Diet Plan, you may not tolerate fermented foods well. In the beginning, our favorite supplement to try is MegaSporeBiotic. Start with one daily with a meal and see how you feel. If it worsens your symptoms, stop and try it again in phase 2 of the diet. In addition, specific strains of probiotics may be helpful. For example, *Bifidobacterium infantis* has prokinetic effects, which may help with SIBO and constipation (as it helps with motility).[38]

Herbal SIBO Treatment

There are several practitioners using herbal treatments with great success. We recommend trying dietary changes, stress reduction, digestive aids and 450 mg of garlic taken three times daily as a first line defense. If this doesn't work, you may want to try an herbal protocol. We prefer a month-long protocol with neem, allicin, berberine and oregano oil. In addition, there is a new supplement called Atrantil (https://atrantil.com), which is designed specifically for the management of SIBO.

Did You Know?

Restore

Restore is a carbon-rich, alkaline-liquid product with specific amino acids. It is not a probiotic or a prebiotic. It has been shown to clinically repair the intestinal lining, support the immune system and support beneficial bacteria. For more information, visit http://restore4life.com.

Mitochondrial Support

CoQ10

The process of converting carbohydrates, protein and fats into adenosine triphosphate (or ATP, the body's energy currency) requires electrons to move back and forth across the mitochondrial cell membrane. This can cause considerable free radical production, which, as we have learned, causes cell and DNA damage. The result is mitochondrial death, a decrease in ATP production, accelerated aging, inflammation and, ultimately, disease.

CoQ10 is an important antioxidant and also a critical player in ATP production in the mitochondria. It is found in large amounts in the inner membrane of the mitochondria where the final phase of ATP production takes place. Low levels of CoQ10 are strongly correlated with fatigue.[39] CoQ10 is naturally produced in our bodies, but if you have a deficient quantity of mitochondria or damaged mitochondria, you may benefit from supplementation.

There have not been any specific studies conducted on CoQ10 and its use for endometriosis; however, research in similar low-mitochondrial conditions have used a range of 100 to 300 mg.[40] CoQ10 is poorly absorbed, but increased when consumed with a high-fat meal. The form of CoQ10 called ubiquinol appears to have superior absorption.

Magnesium

Magnesium is required for more than 300 different enzymes in the body. The mitochondria are intracellular magnesium storage areas. This makes sense, because magnesium is a critical cofactor in the pathway to generate ATP in the mitochondria. Without it, ATP cannot be made and your mitochondria cannot function properly. It is also an important cofactor in glutathione production. Magnesium tends to be lacking in our diet and it's estimated that 80% of Americans are magnesium deficient. The most common symptom of magnesium deficiency is muscle cramping (for example, "Charley horses" and eye twitching).

There are plenty of good food sources of magnesium (see sidebar), but some people require magnesium supplementation. Doses vary based on the condition and on needs. It is difficult to overdose on oral magnesium; if you take too much, you will develop loose stools. We recommend starting with 200 mg of magnesium glycinate daily and increasing every few days until your stools become soft, but well formed; then stay with that dosage. If you suffer from constipation, you may benefit from magnesium citrate, which has laxative properties.[41]

> ### Did You Know?
>
> **Foods with Magnesium**
> - dried seaweed
> - herbs such as basil, coriander, parsley and fennel
> - nuts such as cashews and almonds
> - seeds such as flax, sesame and pumpkin
> - whey protein
> - squash
> - berries
> - leafy greens

R-alpha-lipoic acid (ALA)

Alpha-lipoic acid is a potent antioxidant. It appears to protect mitochondria from oxidation, assist in repairing mitochondria from oxidative damage, decrease the amount of free radicals produced by the mitochondria during ATP production, and increase mitochondrial biogenesis (increasing the number of mitochondria).[42] The most potent form of ALA appears to be R-alpha-lipoic acid, which is the biologically active form.[43] No specific studies have been done using ALA for endometriosis; however, human studies using ALA have demonstrated a reduction in inflammation and free radicals with a dosage of 600 mg of R-ALA taken daily on an empty stomach.[44]

Resveratrol

Resveratrol appears to activate AMP-activated protein kinase (AMPK), thereby increasing the number of mitochondria in cells.[45] In addition to AMPK induction, resveratrol increases other pathways important for mitochondrial production, such as peroxisome proliferator-activator gamma coactivator 1-alpha (PGC-1 alpha) — which is considered the master regulator of mitochondrial biogenesis. In addition to resveratrol's powerful impact on the mitochondria, it has also been studied as a therapy for endometriosis.[46] The dosage used in endo studies was 30 mg daily.[47]

Hormone Balancing
Chasteberry Fruit Extract (Vitex)

Chasteberry works by reducing the amount of prolactin, lowering estrogen and increasing progesterone. There are a handful of studies on chasteberry supporting its use for PMS, menstrual irregularities, dysmenorrhea, infertility and cyclical breast discomfort.[48] In a small study, chasteberry was shown to be as effective as the birth control pill in reducing dysmenorrhea.[49] It is generally recommended to try chasteberry for 6 to 12 months to see its effect. Research doses vary, but a typical dosage is 40 mg of vitex fruit extract daily.

•Diindolylmethane (DIM)

DIM is a phytonutrient found in cruciferous vegetables such as broccoli. It assists with healthy estrogen metabolism in the liver.[50] No human trials on the use of DIM for endometriosis have yet been done to determine appropriate doses. However, studies on other estrogen-related health conditions using human subjects have demonstrated improved estrogen metabolism with the use of DIM supplementation.[51] Dosages used in research range from 100 to 300 mg daily.

Probiotics

Probiotics help to increase beneficial bacteria and encourage a healthy microbial balance. A robust amount of beneficial bacteria helps to inhibit the activity of beta-glucuronidase, thereby reducing the amount of estrogen reabsorbed from the intestines. In general, we recommend getting probiotics from fermented foods; however, during phase 1 of the Endometriosis Diet Plan, you may not tolerate fermented foods well. In the beginning, our favorite supplement to try is MegaSporeBiotic. Start with one daily with a meal and see how you feel. If it worsens your symptoms, stop, and try it again in phase 2 of the diet. In addition, specific strains of probiotics may be helpful. For example, *Bifidobacterium infantis* has prokinetic effects, which may help with SIBO and constipation (as it helps with motility).[52]

Resveratrol

Resveratrol is a potent antioxidant and aromatase inhibitor. It has been studied for use with endometriosis and appears to significantly reduce pain and suppress the development of new microvessel growth in endo lesions.[53] The dosage used during research was 30 mg daily.

Pycnogenol

Pycnogenol is a powerful antioxidant that has been studied for its pain-reducing effect on women with endo and dysmenorrhea.[54] The dosage used during research was 60 mg daily (30 mg taken twice daily).

Calcium D-Glucarate

Calcium D-glucarate inhibits beta-glucuronidase in the gut from reassembling estrogen for reabsorption. In addition, it increases glucuronidation (metabolism of estrogen) in the liver.[55] No human studies for endometriosis have been done. In animal studies, it has been shown to reduce estrogen by 23%; however, large doses were used. The human equivalent to the amount used in animal studies is a minimum of 100 mg/kg with maximum effects at 200 mg/kg.[56] (For example, if you weighed 50 kg you would need 5,000 mg of calcium D-glucarate daily. The usual dosage per pill is 500 mg.)

Stress Support

B Vitamins

B vitamins can become depleted during episodes of chronic stress. They also become depleted with use of oral contraceptives, which many women with pelvic pain and endometriosis are prescribed. Supplementation with B vitamins has been shown to support individuals under chronic stress.[57] Pantothenic acid (vitamin B₅) may be especially helpful. Animal and human studies have provided evidence that pantothenic acid supports the adrenal response in stressful situations, and supplementation may improve the stress response. We typically recommend a daily multivitamin or B-complex with activated B vitamins. We may recommend additional pantothenic acid at a dose of 500 mg taken twice daily to help with stress.

Vitamin C

A study on rats found that supplementation with vitamin C reduced the levels of stress hormones in the blood.

Vitamin C is another nutrient that can become depleted under chronic stress. In addition, stress also suppresses the immune system. Researchers placed rats under stress and fed them 200 mg of vitamin C daily (the equivalent to several grams daily for humans) and found that supplementation with vitamin C reduced the levels of stress hormones in the blood.[58] They also found that other common indicators of stress such as loss in body weight, enlargement of the adrenal glands and a reduction in the size of the thymus gland and spleen were reduced with vitamin C supplementation.

These results were demonstrated in humans, too. Vitamin C at a dosage of 500 mg and 1,500 mg daily was given to marathon runners 7 days before their marathon, on the day of the race, and 2 days after the race.[59] Researchers observed significantly lower post-race cortisol levels after both the 500 and 1,500 mg dosage. Another study observing cortisol levels brought about by psychological stress showed that supplementation of 3,000 mg of vitamin C lowered cortisol.[60] Based on these studies, we typically recommend between 500 and 3,000 mg of vitamin C daily from dietary sources or supplementation. Higher amounts may be required for those experiencing greater amounts of stress.

Magnesium

Magnesium is involved in more than 300 biochemical reactions in the body, including protein synthesis, muscle and nerve function, blood-glucose control, blood pressure regulation, energy production, detoxification and synthesis of DNA and RNA, yet many Americans are deficient in magnesium.[61] Magnesium is a natural muscle relaxant. Many women with endometriosis and pelvic pain have spasms in their pelvic muscles, which can result in pain and discomfort.

Magnesium is also useful for calming the nervous system. In fact, a deficiency in magnesium has been shown to cause dysfunction in the hypothalamus-pituitary-adrenal system, resulting in anxiety.[62] Based on research, we recommend doses of magnesium ranging from 400 to 1,200 mg daily, depending on individual needs. We base specific recommendations on symptoms as well as blood nutrient analysis using red blood cell stores.

Omega-3 Fatty Acids

Omega-3 fatty acids, including eicosapentaenoic acid (EPA) and docosahexaenoic acid (DHA), may help modulate the effects of stress on the body. Psychological stress has repeatedly been demonstrated to increase the production of cytokines (leading to inflammation) in the blood,[63] and omega-3 fatty acids have been shown to reduce levels of inflammatory cytokines in the blood. This may help with pain reduction in women with pelvic pain and endometriosis. In addition, supplementation with omega-3 fatty acids may lower cortisol levels by inhibiting the adrenal activation elicited by stress.[64] Based on available research, we generally recommend between 500 and 4,000 mg of omega-3 fatty acids daily.

Phosphatidylserine (PS)

PS is a glycerophospholipid in the cell membrane. It functions as a signaling lipid, playing an important role in neuronal cell structure and functioning, and it may enhance memory, learning, mood and a person's ability to handle stress.[65] PS has been shown to decrease the adrenocorticotropic hormone (ACTH) and cortisol release from the adrenals, thus blunting the stress response. A daily dose of 400 mg of PS has been shown to reduce cortisol levels effectively in subjects under chronic and acute stress.

L-theanine

A derivative of green tea, L-theanine calms the nervous system, promoting relaxation, boosting cognitive function and supporting brain health.[66] L-theanine works by decreasing excitatory neurotransmitters and increasing the release of inhibitory neurotransmitters such as serotonin.[67] L-theanine has been tested against popular prescribed anti-anxiety medications, such as alprazolam (Xanax), and has been shown to demonstrate superior relaxing effects at a dosage of 200 mg daily.[68]

L-theanine has been tested against popular prescribed anti-anxiety medications, such as alprazolam (Xanax), and has been shown to demonstrate superior relaxing effects.

Lemon Balm (Melissa)

Lemon balm was used in ancient Greece for relief from anxiety and insomnia. Several animal and human studies have demonstrated this natural botanical's impressive results for stress reduction. A dose of both 300 and 600 mg were shown to promote calmness and alertness in subjects exposed to laboratory-induced stress.[69] In addition, use of lemon balm for treatment of premenstrual syndrome symptoms in high-school girls was found to be effective in reducing the severity of symptoms. Based on research, we recommend a dosage of 300 mg taken once to twice daily to address daytime anxiety and promote relaxation and sleep.

Ashwagandha

> ## Caution
>
> If you are sensitive to nightshades, as some women with pelvic pain are, avoid ashwagandha, as it is in the nightshade family.

Ashwagandha is known as an adaptogen, which is an agent used to increase a person's resistance to biological, chemical and physical stressors. Ashwagandha has powerful effects on the nervous system, aiding in the management of stress-related anxiety and depression. Its results for relieving anxiety and depression are similar to those of the drugs lorazepam (Ativan) and imipramine (Tofranil).[70] In addition, ashwagandha protects the brain from negative side effects of stress.[71] Taking doses of 300 mg of ashwagandha root twice daily successfully reduces cortisol levels and anxiety in chronically stressed individuals.[72] Based on research, we recommend dosages of 300 to 1,000 mg daily.

Rhodiola rosea

Like ashwagandha, rhodiola is considered an adaptogen. It was used in traditional folk medicine to fight fatigue and depression, increase physical endurance, enhance work productivity, treat impotence and assist in the prevention of altitude sickness.[73] Rhodiola has been shown in several studies to reduce anxiety, depression and fatigue resulting from stress.[74] In one study, physicians working the night shift were given 170 mg of rhodiola daily, and a statistically significant improvement in mental acuity was observed.[75] Even a single dose of rhodiola has demonstrated a reduction in fatigue.[76] Rhodiola can be either calming or stimulating, depending on the dosage used. Based on research, recommended doses are between 100 to 400 mg daily, taken no later than lunchtime.

Sleep Support

Magnesium Glycinate

Magnesium is involved with over 300 biochemical reactions in the body, including protein synthesis, muscle and nerve function, blood glucose control, blood pressure regulation, energy production, detoxification and synthesis of DNA and RNA.[77] Magnesium is a natural muscle relaxant that many Americans are deficient in; women with endometriosis and pelvic pain often have pelvic muscle spasms, which can result in pain and discomfort. In addition, magnesium is useful for calming the nervous system. In fact, a deficiency in magnesium has been shown to cause dysfunction in the hypothalamus-pituitary-adrenal system, resulting in anxiety.[78]

Based on research, we recommend doses of magnesium ranging from 400 to 1,200 mg daily depending on individual needs. We base specific recommendations on symptoms as well as on blood nutrient analysis using red blood cell stores.

Melatonin

Melatonin is a hormone that naturally increases in your body at night to help you fall asleep. It is also a powerful antioxidant, and there are some studies to support the pain-lowering effects for endo.[79] Based on studies, we recommend starting with a dose of 0.5 to 2 mg at 8 p.m. each night. You can increase slowly, but we do not recommend taking more than 10 mg daily. Taking an extended-release form can help with sleeping through the night. Quick-release forms in small doses (0.5 to 1 mg) can be taken during the night to help you fall back to sleep after waking. Take melatonin in a dark room or while wearing amber/yellow glasses 1 hour before bed (preferably at the same time each night).

L-theanine

L-theanine is an amino acid derived from green tea. It can be helpful for anxiety and sleep, especially if your sleeping problems are due to an overactive, stressed mind. Based on research we recommend taking 50 to 200 mg at bedtime with a maximum dosage of 1,200 mg daily.[80] You can also take L-theanine during the night if you wake up feeling anxious.

> ### Caution
> Before taking any supplements, talk to your doctor or pharmacist about potential contra-indications.

Hops

Hops, commonly known as an ingredient in beer, have been traditionally used as a mild sedative for anxiety and insomnia. Based on research, we recommend taking 300 to 400 mg 30 minutes before bed.[81]

Aromatherapy

Lavender gently strengthens and calms the nervous system. We recommend diffusing it at night, putting a few drops on your pillow before bed or adding a few drops to your evening bath water. Other calming essential oils include ylang ylang, bergamot and chamomile.

Valerian (*Valeriana officinalis*)

Valerian works well when combined with California poppy, skullcap and passion flower.

Valerian is one of the most widely used and studied natural sleep remedies. It has also been used to help with dysmenorrhea.[82] Common in "sleep teas," it's known for its sedative action against insomnia, nervousness and restlessness, and may help to improve your ability to fall asleep quickly and to sleep more soundly. Valerian works well when combined with California poppy, skullcap and passion flower. Based on research, we recommend doses of 200 to 800 mg 30 to 60 minutes before bed.[83]

Lemon Balm (Melissa)

Lemon balm is known to reduce anxiety and promote sleep. Many studies have looked at the calming effects of this herb, but most have focused on lemon balm combined with other herbs. Lemon balm is also associated with calming digestive complaints related to emotional upset. Based on research, we recommend starting with doses of 300 to 900 mg at night.[84]

Pain Support
Valerian (*Valeriana officinalis*)

Valepotriates and valeric acid, compounds in valerian, bind to the same receptors in the brain as Valium does. This can reduce menstrual pain caused by muscle spasms. A 2011 study that used a dose of 225 mg of valerian three times a day starting on day 1 of the menstrual cycle and continuing for 2 more consecutive days demonstrated a significant reduction in menstrual cramp pain.[85]

Cramp Bark
(*Viburnum opulus*)

Cramp bark has been traditionally used as an antispasmodic and relaxant for uterine and ovarian spasms, which can result in painful cramping. No human studies have been done. However, animal studies have demonstrated a reduction in uterine spasms.[86] There is no scientifically tested dose at this time, but cramp bark appears to be a very safe herb. A safe daily amount appears to be 2 to 3 cups of tea (made with 1 gram of root steeped in 1 cup/250 mL of water) taken a few days before the menses and throughout the menstrual cycle.

Sample Endo Supplement Program

In general, we recommend starting with one supplement at a time and adding a new one every 5 to 7 days to test tolerance.

- **Pycnogenol:** 60 mg daily
- **NAC:** 1,200 mg daily
- **DIM:** 150 mg daily
- **Chasteberry/vitex:** 40 mg daily
- **Curcumin:** 500 mg with black pepper extract taken twice daily
- **Cramp bark and valerian root:** for pain as needed, see above and page 132 for dosing

Additional Supplements

- **Multivitamin and mineral supplement:** We often recommend the Metabolic Maintenance's The Big One with Vitamin D, once daily.
- **Magnesium glycinate:** The recommended starting dosage is 400 mg daily.
- **Milk thistle:** The recommended dosage is 300 mg daily.
- **Probiotic:** We recommend starting with MegaSporeBiotic. Recommended dosage is once daily with a meal.
- **High-quality omega-3:** We recommend Nordic Naturals ProOmega, in dosages of 2 to 8 capsules daily taken with meals. Store in the freezer and take frozen.
- **CoQ10:** We recommend 100 mg daily taken with a high-fat meal.

Part 3

Diet Plan for Endometriosis and Pelvic Pain

This part of the book focuses on food and its impact on endometriosis. Vital Health has developed the most up-to-date science-based diet — we call it the Endometriosis Diet Plan — targeted to specifically address several factors associated with the development of endo, and includes foods to decrease the severity of symptoms. The diet is designed to decrease inflammation, optimize gut health and function, balance and strengthen the immune system, stabilize blood sugar, improve energy, enhance the body's natural detoxification and optimize health.

The Endometriosis Diet Plan features three distinct phases. Phase 1, the Repair Phase, is a combination of low FODMAP (fermentable oligo-di-monosaccharides and polyols) foods, a modified elimination diet and a lower carbohydrate diet. We recommend following phase 1 for 1 to 2 months.

Phase 2, the Rebalance Phase, includes the slow addition of foods to increase beneficial bacteria in the gut and gastrointestinal function. In addition, foods that were eliminated in phase 1 are strategically reintroduced to test for tolerance. We recommend following phase 2 for 1 to 2 months. The 4-week menu plan includes instructions for when and how to reintroduce foods eliminated in phase 1.

Phase 3, the Rebuild Phase, builds on phase 2. Additional foods are included in the diet plan to further enhance gut health. In the beginning of this phase, there is a continued addition of previously eliminated foods. The goal of this phase is to liberalize your diet up to your tolerance, to allow more choices and freedom with eating. This is the maintenance phase of the diet — therefore, as you heal, you may continue to expand your dietary choices. Just as in phases 1 and 2, phase 3 includes foods to enhance the body's natural detoxification process, reduce inflammation and balance blood sugar.

For each phase of the diet, we have included a description of the phase, along with dietary recommendations, a list of allowable foods, a recipe list and a 2- or 4-week meal plan.

Chapter 12
Guidelines for the Endometriosis Diet Plan

Did You Know?

Supplements

In addition to making informed food choices, you may want to consider supplements to enhance and assist your body's natural function and expedite healing. See chapter 11 for more information.

Although there is no true "endo diet," there is some good literature to support various dietary strategies. The premise of our dietary recommendations is based on the available scientific evidence. We have described this information in detail in previous sections of the book. The dietary recommendations may not work for everyone; however, we have designed this diet to address most possible health conditions associated with endometriosis and pelvic pain.

The overall diet plan focuses on the pathophysiology and contributing factors of pelvic pain and endometriosis. The diet includes specific foods, spices, meal balancing and food preparation to reduce symptoms and encourage the body's own repair. Strategies to accomplish these goals include reducing environmental toxins, optimizing detoxification, reducing inflammation and oxidation, stabilizing blood sugar, regulating the immune system, rebalancing the gut microbiota, repairing the gut lining and function and balancing hormones.

The Endometriosis Diet Plan is split into three dietary phases. Each phase is followed for a loosely determined period of time. You may need more or less time in a particular phase depending on the severity of your symptoms and the reaction of your body to these dietary changes.

Phase 1: The Repair Phase

Phase 1 of the diet is the strictest, but don't worry, it only lasts for 1 to 2 months. The goal of this phase is to begin the process of rebalancing your gut microbiota, heal your gastrointestinal tract, lower inflammation, stabilize blood sugar, strengthen and rebalance your immune system, reduce toxins from your diet and encourage gentle detoxification.

Dietary Recommendations

Here are our dietary recommendations to help you achieve this phase's goals:

1. Start following a lower FODMAP (fermentable oligo-di-monosaccharides and polyols) menu to begin rebalancing your gut microbiota.

2. Stick to a lower-sugar and lower-carbohydrate diet to stabilize your blood sugar and reduce the overgrowth of yeast and non-beneficial bacteria in your gut.

3. Eliminate common food sensitivities — eggs, soy, dairy, gluten, nightshades (tomatoes, eggplant, peppers, potatoes), corn, peanuts, citrus and chocolate — for 4 weeks. (In phase 2, you will reintroduce these foods in a specific way to assess sensitivities, though you'll continue to avoid gluten).

4. Eliminate foods thought to worsen pelvic pain and endometriosis symptoms.

5. Prepare meals designed to balance blood sugar and reduce inflammation.

6. Eat foods that encourage the body's natural detoxification processes.

7. Consume foods and spices that are rich in antioxidants.

8. Enjoy foods and spices known to reduce inflammation.

9. Eat mostly cooked foods, for easy digestion.

10. Purchase non-GM, organic foods.

> **Did You Know?**
>
> **Food Sensitivities and Inflammation**
>
> Eating foods you are sensitive to can increase inflammation in your body and worsen your endo symptoms. Eating these foods triggers the release of pro-inflammatory mediators, such as cytokines, leukotrienes and prostaglandins, and your body reacts with increased pain.

Phase 1 Allowable Foods

Avoid legumes, grains and dairy (except for ghee) in this phase, and limit fruit to 1 to 2 servings per day. Where amounts are given for the foods listed below, limit your serving size to that amount per meal.

Category	Phase 1 Foods
Vegetables (raw)	• cucumber (peeled and seeded) • radish
Vegetables (cooked, juiced or strained from broth)	• acorn squash ($\frac{1}{4}$ cup/60 mL chopped) • arugula • bamboo shoots • beets (2 tbsp/30 mL chopped) • bok choy (1 cup/250 mL chopped) • broccoli ($\frac{1}{2}$ cup/125 mL chopped) • butternut squash ($\frac{1}{4}$ cup/60 mL chopped) • cabbage ($\frac{1}{2}$ cup/125 mL shredded) • carrots • celery (juiced or strained only) • celery root ($\frac{1}{4}$ cup/60 mL chopped) • chives • collard greens • endive • fennel bulb (juiced or strained only) • green onions (green part only) • kabocha squash ($\frac{1}{4}$ cup/60 mL chopped) • kale • radicchio (12 leaves) • rutabaga • spaghetti squash ($\frac{3}{4}$ cup/175 mL strands) • Swiss chard • yellow summer squash ($\frac{3}{4}$ cup/175 mL chopped) • zucchini ($\frac{3}{4}$ cup/175 mL chopped)
Fruits (fresh or frozen)	• banana ($\frac{1}{2}$ medium) • blueberries (1 cup/250 mL) • coconut butter (2 tbsp/30 mL) • lemon • lime • olives (in brine) • strawberries (1 cup/250 mL whole)
Meats	• beef • fish • game (buffalo, venison, quail, rabbit) • goat • lamb • organ meats • pork • poultry • seafood

Category	Phase 1 Foods
Fats	• coconut oil (okay for cooking) • duck fat (okay for cooking) • flaxseed oil (use cold only) • ghee (okay for cooking) • pure MCT oil (okay for cooking; see box, page xxx) • olive oil (use cold only)
Sweeteners	• stevia (liquid extract)
Herbs and spices	• all herbs (our favorites: rosemary, thyme, sage, oregano, basil) • all spices except onion powder and garlic powder
Flavorings	• apple cider vinegar
Fluids	• almond milk • broth (made with marrow bones only) • coconut milk (no thickeners added) • tea (herbal) • water (filtered flat)

Recipes for Phase 1

See the 4-week phase 1 meal plans in chapter 13 (pages 154–157) for help with combining these recipes into meals.

Breakfast Options

Coconut Milk (page 168)
Vanilla Almond Milk (page 169)
Power Smoothie 1 (page 170)
Turmeric Protein Tea (page 171)
Anti-Inflammatory Protein Bonbons (page 172)
Mouthwatering Sausage Patties (page 173)

Juices

Spicy Carrot and Ginger Juice (page 188)
Purple Haze Juice (page 188)
Refreshing Fennel, Cucumber and Ginger Juice (page 189)

Ghees

Basic Ghee (page 190)
Garlic-Infused Ghee (page 191)
Anti-Inflammatory Ghee (page 192)

Broths

Lunch and Dinner Options

Side Dish Options

Snacks, Dips, Sauces and Dressings

MCTs

Medium-chain triglycerides (MCTs) are a type of fat with a glycerol backbone and two or three fatty acid chains of medium length. Unlike other fatty acids with longer chain structures, which require a lengthy digestive process for absorption, MCTs pass easily through the intestines into circulation. This makes MCTs a fantastic fat for people with malnutrition and/or malabsorption. In addition, MCTs can withstand high cooking temperatures, so they are great for cooking. Coconut oil is high in MCTs, and pure MCT oil is also available.

Phase 2:
The Rebalance Phase

Phase 2 of the diet lasts 1 to 2 months. This phase is designed to strengthen your army of beneficial bacteria and slowly begin the reintroduction of foods to expand your dietary choices.

Dietary Recommendations

Here are our dietary recommendations to help you achieve this phase's goals:

1. Gradually begin adding probiotic and prebiotic foods into your daily diet, to encourage the proliferation of beneficial bacteria in your gut.

2. Strategically reintroduce commonly problematic foods to assess sensitivities (you'll continue to avoid gluten). Eat (challenge) one new food twice in the same day and then avoid that food again for 2 days. If you do not have any symptoms (see "Symptoms to Watch For," below), you can eat that food again. If you have any negative reactions to the challenged food, eliminate it from your diet for another 3 months, then try reintroducing it again in the same way.

3. Continue to prepare meals designed to balance blood sugar and reduce inflammation.

4. Continue to eat foods that encourage the body's natural detoxification processes, foods and spices that are rich in antioxidants, and foods and spices known to reduce inflammation.

5. Incorporate more raw foods into your diet as your digestion is strengthened.

6. Continue to purchase non-GM, organic foods.

Symptoms to Watch For

- gastrointestinal disturbances or changes in bowel habits
- skin changes
- rashes
- headaches
- tingling on tongue or lips
- congestion
- changes in sleep or anxiety
- worsening joint or muscle pain

Phase 2 Allowable Foods

Reintroduce the foods listed in bold below. Continue to limit fruit to 1 to 2 servings per day. Where amounts are given for the foods listed below, limit your serving size to that amount per meal.

Category	Phase 2 Foods
Vegetables (raw or cooked)	<ul><li>acorn squash (¼ cup/60 mL chopped)</li><li>arugula</li><li>asparagus (2 spears)</li><li>bamboo shoots</li><li>beets (¼ cup/60 mL)</li><li>bok choy (1 cup/250 mL chopped)</li><li>broccoli (½ cup/125 mL chopped)</li><li>Brussels sprouts (3 medium)</li><li>butternut squash (¼ cup/60 mL chopped)</li><li>cabbage (½ cup/125 mL shredded)</li><li>carrots</li><li>cauliflower (½ cup/125 mL chopped)</li><li>celery (juiced or strained from broth only)</li><li>celery root (¼ cup/60 mL chopped)</li><li>chives</li><li>collard greens</li><li>cucumber (peeled)</li><li>**eggplant**</li><li>endive</li><li>fennel bulb (juiced or strained only)</li><li>garlic (1 clove)</li><li>green onions (green part only)</li><li>kabocha squash (¼ cup/60 mL chopped)</li><li>kale</li><li>onions (1 tbsp/15 mL minced)</li><li>parsnips</li><li>**peppers (bell, chile)**</li><li>pumpkin (2½ cups/625 mL chopped)</li><li>radicchio (12 leaves)</li><li>radishes</li><li>rutabaga</li><li>spaghetti squash (¾ cup/175 mL strands)</li><li>spinach</li><li>Swiss chard</li><li>**tomatoes**</li><li>watercress</li><li>yellow summer squash (¾ cup/175 mL chopped)</li><li>zucchini (¾ cup/175 mL chopped)</li></ul>

Category	Phase 2 Foods
Fruits (fresh or frozen)	• banana (½ medium) • blueberries (1 cup/250 mL) • cantaloupe (½ cup/125 mL chopped) • coconut • coconut butter (2 tbsp/30 mL) • grapes (10) • guava (½ cup/125 mL chopped) • honeydew melon (½ cup/125 mL chopped) • kiwifruit (1 medium) • lemon • lime • olives (in brine) • **other citrus fruits (½ medium)** • papaya (½ cup/125 mL) • pineapple (½ cup/125 mL) • pomegranate (½ medium) • prickly pear (1 medium) • raspberries (15) • rhubarb (1 cup/250 mL chopped) • strawberries (1 cup/250 mL whole)
Legumes	• lentils (½ cup/125 mL cooked; soak dried lentils for 8 hours, rinse and cook, or cook sprouted lentils)
Grains	• gluten-free grains (amaranth, buckwheat, millet, quinoa, rice, teff), soaked 8 hours, rinsed and cooked • sprouted gluten-free grains
Nuts and seeds	• almond flour (2 tbsp/30 mL) • almonds (10) • cashews (5) • flax seeds, ground (2 tsp/10 mL) • hazelnuts (10) • **peanut butter (2 tbsp/30 mL)** • **peanuts (30)** • pecans (10) • pumpkin seeds (2 tbsp/30 mL) • sesame seeds (2 tbsp/30 mL) • walnuts (10)
Dairy	• **aged cheeses (made from goat's and cow's milk)** • **yogurt (homemade, fermented 24 hours)**

continued, next page...

Category	Phase 2 Foods
Meats	• beef • **eggs** • fish • game (buffalo, venison, quail, rabbit) • goat • lamb • organ meats • pork • poultry • seafood
Fats	• coconut oil (okay for cooking) • duck fat (okay for cooking) • flaxseed oil (use cold only) • ghee (okay for cooking) • pure MCT oil (okay for cooking; see box, page 140) • olive oil (use cold only)
Sweeteners	• honey (1 tbsp/15 mL) • molasses (1 tbsp/15 mL) • stevia (liquid extract)
Herbs and spices	• all herbs (our favorites: rosemary, thyme, sage, oregano, basil) • all spices
Flavorings	• apple cider vinegar • **chocolate and unsweetened cocoa powder** • hot pepper sauce • mustard • **tamari (or gluten-free soy sauce)** • wasabi • white vinegar • wine vinegar
Fluids	• almond milk • broth (made with marrow and/or cartilage bones) • coconut milk (no thickeners added) • tea (herbal) • water (filtered flat or carbonated)
Alcohol (in moderation)	• bourbon • gin • Scotch • vodka • whisky • wine (no sweet/dessert wines or sparkling wines)

Recipes for Phase 2

The 4-week phase 2 meal plans in chapter 13 (pages 158–161) will help guide you in properly reintroducing ingredients (such as dairy). In phase 2, you can include all phase 1 options plus:

Breakfast Options

Homemade Cow's Milk Yogurt (page 174)
Homemade Goat's Milk Yogurt (page 175)
Coconut Yogurt (page 176)
Power Smoothie 2 (page 177)
Grain-Free Granola (page 178)
Coconut Pancakes (page 179)
"The Bomb" Pancakes (page 180)

Lunch and Dinner Options

Mediterranean-Style Mahi-Mahi (page 209)
Grilled Salmon with Lemon and Oregano Pesto (page 210)
Pan-Roasted Trout with Fresh Tomato Basil Sauce (page 211)
Lemon Garlic Chicken (page 212)
Grilled Steak with Arugula and Parmesan (page 213)

Side Dish Options

Sautéed Bell Pepper and Eggplant (page 239)
Lemon Rosemary Glazed Parsnips (page 240)
Radish and Cucumber Salad (page 241)
Lentil-Stuffed Tomatoes (page 242)

Snacks, Dips, Sauces and Dressings

Salty Almonds with Thyme (page 259)
Anti-Inflammatory Cucumber Dip (page 260)
Goat's Milk Yogurt Dip (page 260)
Zucchini Garlic Hummus (page 261)
Lentil Tapenade (page 262)

Phase 3: The Rebuild Phase

Phase 3 of the diet is the maintenance phase. This phase is rich in prebiotic and probiotic foods to encourage growth of your beneficial bacteria. In addition, the dietary recommendations are designed to reduce your symptoms and help your body continue to heal.

Dietary Recommendations

Here are our dietary recommendations to help you achieve this phase's goals:

1. Continue adding probiotic and prebiotic foods into your daily diet, to increase and feed the beneficial bacteria in your gut.

2. Continue to reintroduce commonly problematic foods on a trial basis every 3 to 6 months to increase your dietary choices.

3. Continue to prepare meals designed to balance blood sugar and reduce inflammation.

4. Continue to eat foods that encourage the body's natural detoxification processes, foods and spices that are rich in antioxidants, and foods and spices known to reduce inflammation.

5. Continue to purchase non-GM, organic foods.

Phase 3 Allowable Foods

Reintroduce the foods listed in bold below. Continue to limit fruit to 1 to 2 servings per day. Where amounts are given for the foods listed below, limit your serving size to that amount per meal.

Category	Phase 3 Foods	
Vegetables (raw or cooked)	• acorn squash • artichoke • arugula • asparagus • avocado • bamboo shoots • beets • bok choy • broccoli • Brussels sprouts • butternut squash	• cabbage • carrots • cauliflower • celery • celery root • chives • collard greens • cucumber • endive • fennel bulb • garlic

Category	Phase 3 Foods	
Vegetables (raw or cooked, continued)	• green onions • jicama • kale • kabocha squash • mushrooms • okra • onions • parsnips • peas • potato • peppers (bell, chile) • radicchio • radishes • rutabaga • seaweeds	• spaghetti squash • spinach • Swiss chard • sugar snap peas • sweet potato • taro • tomatoes • turnip • water chestnuts • watercress • yam • yellow summer squash • yucca • zucchini
Fruits (fresh or frozen)	• apple (1 small) • apricots (2) • banana ($\frac{1}{2}$ medium) • blackberries ($\frac{1}{2}$ cup/125 mL) • blueberries (1 cup/250 mL) • cantaloupe ($\frac{1}{2}$ cup/125 mL chopped) • cherries (6 each) • coconut • coconut butter ($\frac{1}{4}$ cup/60 mL) • cranberries (2 tbsp/30 mL) • grapes (10) • guava ($\frac{1}{2}$ cup/125 mL chopped) • honeydew melon ($\frac{1}{2}$ cup/125 mL chopped) • kiwifruit (1 medium) • lemon • lime • olives (in brine)	• other citrus fruits ($\frac{1}{2}$ medium) • papaya ($\frac{1}{2}$ cup/125 mL chopped) • peach (1 medium) • pear (1 medium) • persimmon (1 medium) • pineapple ($\frac{1}{2}$ cup/125 mL chopped) • plantain ($\frac{1}{2}$ medium) • plum (1 medium) • pomegranate ($\frac{1}{2}$ medium) • prickly pear (1 medium) • pumpkin • raspberries (1 cup/250 mL) • rhubarb (1 cup/250 mL chopped) • strawberries (1 cup/250 mL whole) • watermelon ($\frac{1}{2}$ cup/125 mL chopped)

continued, next page...

Category	Phase 3 Foods
Legumes	• black beans (½ cup/125 mL cooked) • butter beans (½ cup/125 mL cooked) • cannellini (white kidney) beans (½ cup/125 mL cooked) • chickpeas (½ cup/125 mL cooked) • **edamame (½ cup/125 mL cooked)** • fava beans (½ cup/125 mL cooked) • lentils (½ cup/125 mL cooked) • lima beans (½ cup/125 mL cooked) • navy beans (½ cup/125 mL cooked) • pinto beans (½ cup/125 mL cooked) • red beans (½ cup/125 mL cooked) • split peas (½ cup/125 mL cooked) • tofu (4 oz/125 g)
Grains and starches	• arrowroot starch • **corn** • cornstarch • potato starch • rice flour • tapioca starch • gluten-free grains (amaranth, buckwheat, millet, quinoa, rice, teff), soaked 8 hours, rinsed and cooked • sprouted gluten-free grains
Nuts and seeds	• almond butter (2 tbsp/30 mL) • almond flour (¼ cup/60 mL) • almonds (¼ cup/60 mL) • cashews (5) • chia seeds (2 tbsp/30 mL) • flax seeds, ground (3 tbsp/45 mL) • hazelnuts (10) • peanut butter (2 tbsp/30 mL) • peanuts (20) • pecans (10) • pine nuts (1 tbsp/15 mL) • pistachios (10) • pumpkin seeds (2 tbsp/30 mL) • sesame seeds (2 tbsp/30 mL) • sunflower seeds (2 tbsp/30 mL) • walnuts (10)
Dairy	• aged cheeses (all) • kefir • milk (cow's and goat's) • sour cream • yogurt (homemade, fermented 24 hours)

Category	Phase 3 Foods	
Meats	• beef • eggs • fish • game (buffalo, venison, quail, rabbit) • goat	• lamb • organ meats • pork • poultry • seafood
Fats	• coconut oil (okay for cooking) • duck fat (okay for cooking) • flaxseed oil (use cold only) • ghee (okay for cooking) • pure MCT oil (okay for cooking; see box, page xxx) • olive oil (use cold only)	
Sweeteners	• coconut sugar (1 tbsp/15 mL) • honey (1 tbsp/15 mL) • maple syrup (1 tbsp/15 mL) • molasses (1 tbsp/15 mL) • stevia (liquid extract) • xylitol (1 tbsp/15 mL)	
Herbs and spices	• all herbs (our favorites: rosemary, thyme, sage, oregano, basil) • all spices	
Flavorings	• apple cider vinegar • asafoetida powder • balsamic vinegar • chocolate/cocoa (unsweetened) • gums/thickeners • hot pepper sauce	• mustard • tamari (or gluten-free soy sauce) • wasabi • white vinegar • wine vinegar
Fluids	• almond milk • broth • coconut milk (thickener okay) • coffee • hemp milk • tea (herbal and caffeinated) • water (filtered flat or carbonated)	
Alcohol (in moderation)	• beer (gluten-free) • bourbon • brandy • cider • gin • rum	• Scotch • sherry • tequila • vodka (potato) • whisky • wine

Recipes for Phase 3

The 2-week phase 3 meal plans in chapter 13 (pages 162–163) will help guide you in properly reintroducing ingredients such as edamame and corn. In phase 3, you can include all phase 1 and 2 options plus:

Breakfast Options

Goat's Milk Kefir (page 181)
Power Smoothie 3 (page 182)
Mixed Fruit, Chia and Flaxseed Porridge (page 183)
Skillet-Roasted Cauliflower Omelet (page 184)
Garlicky Kale Frittata (page 185)
Red Lentil Frittata (page 186)

Lunch and Dinner Options

Green Thai Curry with Spinach and Sweet Potatoes (page 214)
Coconut Squash Pizza (page 215)
Stuffed Portobellos (page 216)
Black Bean Coconut Burgers (page 217)
Black Cod with Fresh Herb Sauce (page 218)
White Fish with Mediterranean Flavors (page 219)
Grilled Salmon with Mustard Maple Vinaigrette (page 220)
Swedish Salmon, Asparagus and Potato Omelet (page 221)
Mediterranean Quinoa-Stuffed Chicken Breasts (page 222)
Herbed Chicken and Pomegranate Salad (page 223)
Japanese Sesame Chicken Skewers (page 224)
Roasted Pork Tenderloin with Pear Slaw (page 225)
Beef and Quinoa Soup (page 226)
Persian Ground Beef Kebabs (page 227)
Bison Stew with Kumquats (page 228)

Side Dish Options

Beet Soup with Lemongrass and Lime (page 243)
Thai-Style Pumpkin Soup (page 244)
Garlic Soup (page 245)
Gingered Carrot and Coconut Soup (page 246)
Gut-Building Blended Vegetable Soup (page 247)
Mexican Jicama Slaw (page 248)
Crunchy, Colorful Thai Cabbage Slaw (page 249)
Fast and Easy Greek Salad (page 250)
Pan-Braised Brussels Sprouts (page 251)
Sugar Snap Peas in Ginger Butter (page 252)
Roasted Butternut Squash with Onion and Sage (page 253)
Baked Sweet Potato Fries (page 254)
Veggie Kabobs (page 255)
Coconut Flax Tortillas (page 256)

Snacks, Dips, Sauces and Dressings

Spicy Tamari Almonds (page 263)
Spicy Cashews (page 264)
Artichoke and White Bean Spread (page 265)
Basic Pesto (page 266)
Parsley Pesto Sauce (page 267)
Artichoke Salsa (page 267)
Green Goddess Salad Dressing (page 268)

Making Lifestyle Changes

Each phase of the diet includes a meal plan and recipes that comply with all dietary guidelines for that phase. The goal is to make this transition into optimizing your health as simple as possible. We know how hard lifestyle changes are, and we want to support you as best we can in this transition. Here are some techniques that our clients have found helpful:

- Find a motivated buddy or family member to join you on this journey.

- Explain to your family and friends that you are making some major lifestyle changes to optimize your health and happiness and that you would love their support.

- Write down some goals. We typically recommend one weekly goal and one monthly goal. Make sure your goals are easy to measure and specific. We also encourage having a set reward for each weekly and monthly goal. Make sure to give yourself this reward!

Weekly and Monthly Goals

Some examples of these goals include:

Weekly

- "I will prepare for my weekly meals every Sunday by shopping for everything needed on my menu and prepping as much of my meals as possible."

- "I will try two new foods this week."

- "I will add one new detox food and one new anti-inflammatory food each week."

Planning Ahead

Journal about potential challenges you may encounter on your new lifestyle journey. Brainstorm ways you could overcome these hurdles. Be realistic and honest. We all have perceived and real barriers that can sometimes make it difficult to put our own health first or make healthy changes. Planning ahead for how to stay on course with your health goals can often keep you on track.

Monthly

- "By making these lifestyle changes, I will decrease my pain medications by one a day by the end of the month."
- "By making these lifestyle changes, I will reduce my weight by 5 pounds by the end of the month."
- "By making these lifestyle changes, I will decrease my pain levels from a 10 to a 5."

Rewards

Some examples of a reward for achieving your goals include:

- Put $2 to $5 in a jar every day you follow your menu plan. At the end of the week, use that money to do something special (and non-food-related) for yourself, or save the money until the end of the month and take yourself shopping or get a massage.
- At the end of the week, reward yourself by enjoying some relaxing time. Examples of activities include taking a bath with candles and music, having a 15-minute foot rub, taking a walk on the beach, or doing something you enjoy but seldom take the time to do.

Chapter 13
Meal Plans for the Endometriosis Diet Plan

Use these meal plans as a guide to a balanced diet. We have included a 4-week meal plan for phases 1 and 2 and a 2-week meal plan for phase 3. All phases are carbohydrate-controlled (20 grams or less per meal) and moderate in protein and healthy fats.

The goal is to eat every 3 to 5 hours and minimize snacking between meals. This may equate to 2 to 4 meals a day, depending on your schedule and hunger. Eat only when you are hungry, and eat until you are satisfied but not full. You should take at least 20 minutes to eat a meal. Set a timer if needed to avoid eating too quickly. Chew, chew and chew some more.

You may want to try eating foods that are typically eaten at lunch and dinner for breakfast, especially in phase 1, for more options and variety for your first meal of the day.

The portions indicated in the meal plans are only general recommendations. Eat as much or as little as you need to feel strong and achieve a healthy weight. If you are hungry or losing weight rapidly (more than 1 to 2 pounds/0.5 to 1 kg per week), or you do not need to lose weight), eat larger servings or add a meal.

All of the recipes mentioned in the meal plans are included in Part 4. Flipping through Part 4, you will see that each recipe is labeled "Phase 1," "Phase 2" or "Phase 3" to assist you in meal planning. If you dislike a recipe in the meal plan, simply replace it with another recipe that is allowed in that phase of the diet.

> ### Did You Know?
> **Using Time Wisely**
> If you have limited time, cook enough the night before for leftovers the following day (for example, eat leftovers from Monday's dinner for lunch on Tuesday), subbing the leftovers in for the meal specified in the menu for that day. Alternatively, when you have time on your hands, make big batches of recipes that will freeze well (such as soups and broths), so that you always have options ready to take with you to work or heat up for an easy dinner when you're too exhausted to cook.

Meal	Breakfast	Lunch	Snack	Dinner
SUNDAY	Turmeric Protein Tea 1 serving allowed fruit	Easy Herbed Shrimp Sautéed Kale Baked Acorn Squash	Bone Marrow Broth	Homemade Chicken Soup Roasted Vegetables
MONDAY	Spicy Carrot and Ginger Juice 2 or 3 Anti-Inflammatory Protein Bonbons	Homemade Chicken Soup Roasted Vegetables	Bone Marrow Broth	Anti-Inflammatory Baked Cod Cinnamon-Roasted Kabocha Squash and Carrots
TUESDAY	Refreshing Fennel, Cucumber and Ginger Juice 2 or 3 Anti-Inflammatory Protein Bonbons 1 serving allowed fruit	Turkey Wraps Cinnamon-Roasted Kabocha Squash and Carrots	Bone Marrow Broth	Slow Cooker Chicken Wraps Blended Vegetable Soup 1 serving allowed fruit
WEDNESDAY	Power Smoothie 1	Slow Cooker Chicken Wraps Roasted Vegetables	Bone Marrow Broth	Bone Marrow Soup Rutabaga Mash
THURSDAY	Mouthwatering Sausage Patties Roasted Vegetables	Bone Marrow Soup Rutabaga Mash	Bone Marrow Broth	Chinese Chicken and Greens Roasted Vegetables
FRIDAY	Purple Haze Juice 2 or 3 Anti-Inflammatory Protein Bonbons 1 serving allowed fruit	Chinese Chicken and Greens Roasted Vegetables	Bone Marrow Broth	Baked Salmon Sautéed Kale Rutabaga Mash
SATURDAY	Refreshing Fennel, Cucumber and Ginger Juice 2 or 3 Anti-Inflammatory Protein Bonbons 1 serving allowed fruit	Anti-Inflammatory Meatballs Spaghetti Squash Noodles	Bone Marrow Broth	Easy Baked Chicken Breasts over Arugula Cinnamon-Roasted Kabocha Squash and Carrots

Meal	Breakfast	Lunch	Snack	Dinner
SUNDAY	Turmeric Protein Tea 1 serving allowed fruit	Carrot Bone Broth Soup Roasted Vegetables	Bone Marrow Broth	Homemade Chicken Soup Roasted Vegetables
MONDAY	Spicy Carrot and Ginger Juice 2 Anti-Inflammatory Protein Bonbons	Homemade Chicken Soup Roasted Vegetables	Bone Marrow Broth	Turmeric Ginger Chicken Skewers Cinnamon-Roasted Kabocha Squash and Carrots
TUESDAY	Refreshing Fennel, Cucumber and Ginger Juice 2 or 3 Anti-Inflammatory Protein Bonbons 1 serving allowed fruit	Anti-Inflammatory Meatballs Spaghetti Squash Noodles 1 serving allowed fruit	Bone Marrow Broth	Slow Cooker Chicken Wraps Blended Vegetable Soup 1 serving allowed fruit
WEDNESDAY	Power Smoothie 1	Slow Cooker Chicken Wraps Roasted Vegetables	Bone Marrow Broth	Bone Marrow Soup Rutabaga Mash
THURSDAY	Mouthwatering Sausage Patties Roasted Vegetables	Bone Marrow Soup Rutabaga Mash	Bone Marrow Broth	Chinese Chicken and Greens Roasted Vegetables
FRIDAY	Power Smoothie 1	Turkey Wraps Carrot Chips 1 serving allowed fruit	Bone Marrow Broth	Anti-Inflammatory Baked Cod Rutabaga Mash
SATURDAY	Refreshing Fennel, Cucumber and Ginger Juice 2 or 3 Anti-Inflammatory Protein Bonbons 1 serving allowed fruit	Baked Salmon Sautéed Kale Rutabaga Mash	Bone Marrow Broth	Easy Baked Chicken Breasts over Arugula Cinnamon-Roasted Kabocha Squash and Carrots

Meal	Breakfast	Lunch	Snack	Dinner
SUNDAY	Turmeric Protein Tea 1 serving allowed fruit	Easy Herbed Shrimp Sautéed Kale Baked Acorn Squash	Bone Marrow Broth	Homemade Chicken Soup Roasted Vegetables
MONDAY	Spicy Carrot and Ginger Juice 2 or 3 Anti-Inflammatory Protein Bonbons	Homemade Chicken Soup Roasted Vegetables	Bone Marrow Broth	Turmeric Ginger Chicken Skewers Cinnamon-Roasted Kabocha Squash and Carrots
TUESDAY	Refreshing Fennel, Cucumber and Ginger Juice 2 or 3 Anti-Inflammatory Protein Bonbons 1 serving allowed fruit	Turmeric Ginger Chicken Skewers Cinnamon-Roasted Kabocha Squash and Carrots	Bone Marrow Broth	Slow Cooker Chicken Wraps Blended Vegetable Soup 1 serving allowed fruit
WEDNESDAY	Mouthwatering Sausage Patties Roasted Vegetables	Slow Cooker Chicken Wraps Roasted Vegetables	Bone Marrow Broth	Bone Marrow Soup Rutabaga Mash
THURSDAY	Purple Haze Juice 2 or 3 Anti-Inflammatory Protein Bonbons 1 serving allowed fruit	Bone Marrow Soup Rutabaga Mash	Bone Marrow Broth	Chinese Chicken and Greens Roasted Vegetables
FRIDAY	Power Smoothie 1	Chinese Chicken and Greens Roasted Vegetables	Bone Marrow Broth	Baked Salmon Sautéed Kale Rutabaga Mash
SATURDAY	Refreshing Fennel, Cucumber and Ginger Juice 2 or 3 Anti-Inflammatory Protein Bonbons 1 serving allowed fruit	Anti-Inflammatory Meatballs Spaghetti Squash Noodles	Bone Marrow Broth	Easy Baked Chicken Breasts over Arugula Cinnamon-Roasted Kabocha Squash and Carrots

Meal	Breakfast	Lunch	Snack	Dinner
SUNDAY	Turmeric Protein Tea 1 serving allowed fruit	Baked Salmon Baked Acorn Squash	Bone Marrow Broth	Homemade Chicken Soup Roasted Vegetables
MONDAY	Spicy Carrot and Ginger Juice 2 or 3 Anti-Inflammatory Protein Bonbons 1 serving allowed fruit	Homemade Chicken Soup Roasted Vegetables	Bone Marrow Broth	Turmeric Ginger Chicken Skewers Cinnamon-Roasted Kabocha Squash and Carrots
TUESDAY	Refreshing Fennel, Cucumber and Ginger Juice 2 or 3 Anti-Inflammatory Protein Bonbons	Anti-Inflammatory Meatballs Spaghetti Squash Noodles	Bone Marrow Broth	Slow Cooker Chicken Wraps Blended Vegetable Soup 1 serving allowed fruit
WEDNESDAY	Mouthwatering Sausage Patties Roasted Vegetables	Slow Cooker Chicken Wraps Roasted Vegetables	Bone Marrow Broth	Easy Herb Shrimp Sautéed Kale Roasted Vegetables
THURSDAY	Purple Haze Juice 2 or 3 Anti-Inflammatory Protein Bonbons 1 serving allowed fruit	Bone Marrow Soup Rutabaga Mash	Bone Marrow Broth	Bone Marrow Soup Rutabaga Mash
FRIDAY	Power Smoothie 1	Turkey Wraps Carrot Chips 1 serving allowed fruit	Bone Marrow Broth	Anti-Inflammatory Baked Cod Rutabaga Mash Sautéed Kale
SATURDAY	Refreshing Fennel, Cucumber and Ginger Juice 2 or 3 Anti-Inflammatory Protein Bonbons 1 serving allowed fruit	Chinese Chicken and Greens Roasted Vegetables	Bone Marrow Broth	Easy Baked Chicken Breasts over Arugula Cinnamon-Roasted Kabocha Squash and Carrots

Introduce bold foods to check for sensitivities. It is important to follow the food introductions as specified.

Meal	Breakfast	Lunch	Snack	Dinner
SUNDAY	Coconut Pancakes **1 soft-cooked egg** with 1 tsp (5 mL) ghee, fine sea salt and pepper 1 serving allowed fruit	Easy Herbed Shrimp Sautéed Kale topped with 1 chopped **hard-cooked egg** Carrot Chips	Bone Marrow Broth	Homemade Chicken Soup Radish and Cucumber Salad Lemon Rosemary Glazed Parsnips
MONDAY	Power Smoothie 2	Homemade Chicken Soup Radish and Cucumber Salad Lemon Rosemary Glazed Parsnips	Bone Marrow Broth	Grilled Salmon with Lemon and Oregano Pesto Blended Vegetable Soup
TUESDAY	Turmeric Protein Tea A handful of Salty Almonds with Thyme 1 serving allowed fruit	Turkey Wraps Cinnamon-Roasted Kabocha Squash and Carrots	Bone Marrow Broth	Slow Cooker Chicken Wraps Cinnamon-Roasted Kabocha Squash and Carrots
WEDNESDAY	Mouthwatering Sausage Patties Roasted Vegetables	Slow Cooker Chicken Wraps Roasted Vegetables ½ tomato, sliced Anti-Inflammatory Cucumber Dip	Bone Marrow Broth	Bone Marrow Soup Rutabaga Mash **½ tomato, sliced**
THURSDAY	Spicy Carrot and Ginger Juice 2 or 3 Anti-Inflammatory Protein Bonbons 1 serving allowed fruit	Bone Marrow Soup Rutabaga Mash	Bone Marrow Broth	Easy Herbed Shrimp Sautéed Kale Carrot Chips
FRIDAY	Purple Haze Juice "The Bomb" Pancakes	Turkey Wraps spread with Zucchini Garlic Hummus Carrot Chips	Bone Marrow Broth	Grilled Salmon with Lemon and Oregano Pesto Rutabaga Mash
SATURDAY	Power Smoothie 1	Lemon Garlic Chicken **Sautéed Bell Pepper and Eggplant** Baked Acorn Squash	Bone Marrow Broth	Mediterranean-Style Mahi-Mahi Roasted Vegetables **Sautéed Bell Pepper and Eggplant**

Introduce bold foods to check for sensitivities. It is important to follow the food introductions as specified.

Meal	Breakfast	Lunch	Snack	Dinner
SUNDAY	½ cup (125 mL) Coconut Yogurt ¼ cup (60 mL) Grain-Free Granola 1 Anti-Inflammatory Protein Bonbon	Brined and Tender Lemon Roast Chicken Carrot Chips Radish and Cucumber Salad 1 tsp (5 mL) raw sauerkraut juice	Bone Marrow Broth	Pan-Roasted Trout with Fresh Tomato Basil Sauce Lemon Rosemary Glazed Parsnips
MONDAY	Spicy Carrot and Ginger Juice 2 hard-cooked eggs ½ cup (125 mL) blueberries	Bone Marrow Soup Lemon Rosemary Glazed Parsnips 1 tsp (5 mL) raw sauerkraut juice	Bone Marrow Broth	Easy Baked Chicken Breasts over Arugula Cinnamon-Roasted Kabocha Squash and Carrots
TUESDAY	½ cup (125 mL) **Homemade Goat's Milk Yogurt** ¼ cup (60 mL) Grain-Free Granola ½ cup (125 mL) blueberries	Turkey Wraps Cinnamon-Roasted Kabocha Squash and Carrots 1 tsp (5 mL) raw sauerkraut juice	Bone Marrow Broth	Baked Salmon Lentil-Stuffed Tomatoes ¼ cup (60 mL) **Goat's Milk Yogurt Dip** (dip salmon or add on top after cooking)
WEDNESDAY	Turmeric Protein Tea ¼ cup (60 mL) Grain-Free Granola	Turmeric Ginger Chicken Skewers Lentil-Stuffed Tomatoes 1 tsp (5 mL) raw sauerkraut juice	Bone Marrow Broth	Anti-Inflammatory Meatballs Spaghetti Squash Noodles 1 serving allowed fruit
THURSDAY	Power Smoothie 2 ¼ cup (60 mL) Grain-Free Granola	Anti-Inflammatory Meatballs Spaghetti Squash Noodles 1 tsp (5 mL) raw sauerkraut juice	Bone Marrow Broth	Mediterranean-Style Mahi-Mahi Sautéed Kale Roasted Vegetables
FRIDAY	Coconut Pancakes 1 or 2 poached eggs with 1 tsp (5 mL) ghee, fine sea salt and pepper 1 serving allowed fruit	Slow Cooker Chicken Wraps spread with **1 tsp (5 mL) tamari** Carrot Chips 1 tsp (5 mL) raw sauerkraut juice	Bone Marrow Broth	Slow Cooker Chicken Wraps spread with **1 tsp (5 mL) tamari** Carrot Chips
SATURDAY	"The Bomb" Pancakes Refreshing Fennel, Cucumber and Ginger Juice	Turkey Wraps spread with Zucchini Garlic Hummus Carrot Chips 1 tsp (5 mL) raw sauerkraut juice	Bone Marrow Broth	Grilled Steak with Arugula and Parmesan (but omit the Parmesan) Rutabaga Mash Blended Vegetable Soup

Introduce bold foods to check for sensitivities. It is important to follow the food introductions as specified.

Meal	Breakfast	Lunch	Snack	Dinner
SUNDAY	Coconut Pancakes 1 or 2 poached eggs with 1 tsp (5 mL) ghee, fine sea salt and pepper	Chinese Chicken and Greens Carrot Chips 1 serving allowed fruit 1 tbsp (15 mL) raw sauerkraut	Bone Marrow Broth	Anti-Inflammatory Meatballs Spaghetti Squash Noodles 1 serving allowed fruit
MONDAY	Power Smoothie 2	Anti-Inflammatory Meatballs Spaghetti Squash Noodles 1 tbsp (15 mL) raw sauerkraut **1 oz (30 g) dark chocolate**	Bone Marrow Broth	Mediterranean-Style Mahi-Mahi Blended Vegetable Soup **1 oz (30 g) dark chocolate**
TUESDAY	½ cup (125 mL) Homemade Goat's Milk Yogurt ¼ cup (60 mL) Grain-Free Granola ½ cup (125 mL) blueberries	Turkey Wraps ¼ cup (60 mL) Goat's Milk Yogurt Dip Roasted Vegetables 1 tbsp (15 mL) raw sauerkraut	Bone Marrow Broth	Slow Cooker Chicken Wraps Roasted Vegetables
WEDNESDAY	Mouthwatering Sausage Patties Roasted Vegetables	Slow Cooker Chicken Wraps Roasted Vegetables 1 tbsp (15 mL) raw sauerkraut	Bone Marrow Broth	Anti-Inflammatory Baked Cod Carrot Chips 1 serving allowed fruit
THURSDAY	"The Bomb" Pancakes spread with **1 tbsp (15 mL) peanut butter** Refreshing Fennel, Cucumber and Ginger Juice	Turkey Wraps Carrot Chips 1 oz (30 g) dark chocolate **1 tbsp (15 mL) peanut butter** 1 tbsp (15 mL) raw sauerkraut	Bone Marrow Broth	Homemade Chicken Soup Baked Acorn Squash
FRIDAY	½ cup (125 mL) Homemade Goat's Milk Yogurt ¼ cup (60 mL) Grain-Free Granola ½ cup (125 mL) blueberries	Homemade Chicken Soup Baked Acorn Squash 1 tbsp (15 mL) raw sauerkraut	Bone Marrow Broth	Grilled Steak with Arugula and Parmesan (but omit the Parmesan) Roasted Vegetables
SATURDAY	Turmeric Protein Tea ¼ cup (60 mL) Grain-Free Granola	Leftover steak from Friday dinner Sautéed Kale Roasted Vegetables 1 tbsp (15 mL) raw sauerkraut	Bone Marrow Broth	Pan-Roasted Trout with Fresh Tomato Basil Sauce Carrot Chips Sautéed Kale

Introduce bold foods to check for sensitivities. It is important to follow the food introductions as specified.

Meal	Breakfast	Lunch	Snack	Dinner
SUNDAY	Refreshing Fennel, Cucumber and Ginger Juice "The Bomb" Pancakes spread with 1 tbsp (15 mL) peanut butter **½ pink grapefruit**	Turmeric Ginger Chicken Skewers Cinnamon-Roasted Kabocha Squash and Carrots **½ pink grapefruit** 2 tbsp (30 mL) raw sauerkraut	Bone Marrow Broth	Baked Salmon Sautéed Kale Rutabaga Mash
MONDAY	½ cup (125 mL) Homemade Goat's Milk Yogurt ¼ cup (60 mL) Grain-Free Granola ½ cup (125 mL) blueberries	Slow Cooker Chicken Wraps spread with 1 tsp (5 mL) tamari Carrot Chips 1 oz (30 g) dark chocolate 2 tbsp (30 mL) raw sauerkraut	Bone Marrow Broth	Slow Cooker Chicken Wraps spread with 1 tsp (5 mL) tamari Carrot Chips 1 serving allowed fruit
TUESDAY	Power Smoothie 2	Anti-Inflammatory Meatballs Spaghetti Squash Noodles tossed with Basic Pesto 1 serving allowed fruit 2 tbsp (30 mL) raw sauerkraut	Bone Marrow Broth	Carrot Bone Broth Soup Baked Acorn Squash
WEDNESDAY	**½ cup (125 mL) Homemade Cow's Milk Yogurt** ¼ cup (60 mL) Grain-Free Granola ½ cup (125 mL) blueberries	Turkey Wrap spread with Green Goddess Salad Dressing **½ cup (125 mL) Homemade Cow's Milk Yogurt** 1 serving allowed fruit 2 tbsp (30 mL) raw sauerkraut	Bone Marrow Broth	Homemade Chicken Soup Cinnamon-Roasted Kabocha Squash and Carrots
THURSDAY	Power Smoothie 2	Homemade Chicken Soup Cinnamon-Roasted Kabocha Squash and Carrots 2 tbsp (30 mL) raw sauerkraut	Bone Marrow Broth	Anti-Inflammatory Baked Cod Carrot Chips
FRIDAY	2 or 3 Anti-Inflammatory Protein Bonbons Spicy Carrot and Ginger Juice	Turkey Wrap spread with Green Goddess Salad Dressing Carrot Chips ½ cup (125 mL) blueberries 2 tbsp (30 mL) raw sauerkraut	Bone Marrow Broth	Chinese Chicken and Greens Baked Acorn Squash
SATURDAY	Coconut Pancakes 1 poached egg with 1 tsp (5 mL) ghee, fine sea salt and pepper 1 orange	Chinese Chicken and Greens Baked Acorn Squash 1 orange 2 tbsp (30 mL) raw sauerkraut	Bone Marrow Broth	Grilled Steak with Arugula and Parmesan Lentil-Stuffed Tomatoes

Introduce bold foods to check for sensitivities. It is important to follow the food introductions as specified.

Meal	Breakfast	Lunch	Snack	Dinner
SUNDAY	¼ cup (60 mL) Goat's Milk Kefir Skillet-Roasted Cauliflower Omelet 1 serving fruit	Anti-Inflammatory Meatballs Spaghetti Squash Noodles tossed with Basic Pesto 1 serving fruit 2 tbsp (30 mL) raw sauerkraut	Salty Almonds with Thyme	Persian Ground Beef Kebabs Gut-Building Blended Vegetable Soup Roasted Butternut Squash with Onion and Sage
MONDAY	¼ cup (60 mL) Goat's Milk Kefir Mouthwatering Sausage Patties Roasted Vegetables	Bone Marrow Soup topped with 2 tbsp (30 mL) raw sauerkraut Roasted Vegetables	Anti-Inflammatory Cucumber Dip with raw vegetables	Grilled Salmon with Mustard Maple Vinaigrette Sugar Snap Peas in Ginger Butter 1 serving fruit
TUESDAY	¼ cup (60 mL) Goat's Milk Kefir Mixed Fruit, Chia and Flaxseed Porridge	Easy Baked Chicken Breasts over Arugula 1 corn tortilla (made without hydrogenated oils, partially hydrogenated oils or shortening) 2 tbsp (30 mL) raw sauerkraut	Bone Marrow Broth	Bison Stew with Kumquats 1 ear corn on the cob or 1 corn tortilla
WEDNESDAY	Power Smoothie 3 made with ¼ cup (60 mL) Goat's Milk Kefir	Herbed Chicken and Pomegranate Salad Baked Sweet Potato Fries 2 tbsp (30 mL) raw sauerkraut	Lentil Tapenade with 5 gluten-free crackers	Thai-Style Pumpkin Soup Coconut Flax Tortillas
THURSDAY	¼ cup (60 mL) Goat's Milk Kefir ½ cup (125 mL) Homemade Cow's (or Goat's) Milk Yogurt ¼ cup (60 mL) Grain-Free Granola	Pork Tenderloin with Pear Slaw Sugar Snap Peas in Ginger Butter Sautéed Bell Pepper and Eggplant 2 tbsp (30 mL) raw sauerkraut	Salty Almonds with Thyme	Black Cod with Fresh Herb Sauce Garlic Soup 1 serving fruit
FRIDAY	Power Smoothie 2 made with ¼ cup (60 mL) Goat's Milk Kefir	Turkey Wraps ½ cup (125 mL) steamed edamame served with Green Goddess Salad Dressing Fast and Easy Greek Salad 2 tbsp (30 mL) raw sauerkraut	Bone Marrow Broth	Japanese Sesame Chicken Skewers Veggie Kabobs Fast and Easy Greek Salad ½ cup (125 mL) steamed edamame
SATURDAY	¼ cup (60 mL) Goat's Milk Kefir Red Lentil Frittata 1 serving fruit	Black Bean Coconut Burger Carrot Chips 2 tbsp (30 mL) raw sauerkraut	Zucchini Garlic Hummus with raw vegetables	Coconut Squash Pizza topped with cooked chicken or gluten-free chicken sausage Sautéed Kale

Introduce bold foods to check for sensitivities. It is important to follow the food introductions as specified.

Meal	Breakfast	Lunch	Snack	Dinner
SUNDAY	¼ cup (60 mL) Goat's Milk Kefir Garlicky Kale Frittata 1 serving fruit	Bison Stew with Kumquats Mexican Jicama Slaw 2 tbsp (30 mL) raw sauerkraut	Salty Almonds with Thyme	Grilled Salmon with Mustard Maple Vinaigrette Sautéed Kale
MONDAY	Power Smoothie 3 made with ¼ cup (60 mL) Goat's Milk Kefir	Stuffed Portobello Gut-Building Blended Vegetable Soup 2 tbsp (30 mL) raw sauerkraut	Anti-Inflammatory Cucumber Dip with raw vegetables	Japanese Sesame Chicken Skewers Pan-Braised Brussels Sprouts
TUESDAY	¼ cup (60 mL) Goat's Milk Kefir Coconut Pancakes 1 hard-cooked egg ½ to 1 serving fruit	Turkey Wraps made with Coconut Flax Tortillas or corn tortillas 2 tbsp (30 mL) raw sauerkraut	Bone Marrow Broth	Swedish Salmon, Asparagus and Potato Omelet Pan-Braised Brussels Sprouts
WEDNESDAY	¼ cup (60 mL) Goat's Milk Kefir Anti-Inflammatory Protein Bonbons 1 serving fruit	Lemon Garlic Chicken Carrot Fries 2 tbsp (30 mL) raw sauerkraut	Lentil Tapenade with 5 gluten-free crackers	Coconut Squash Pizza Fast and Easy Greek Salad (put half away without dressing and add dressing at lunch Thursday)
THURSDAY	¼ cup (60 mL) Goat's Milk Kefir ½ cup (125 mL) Homemade Goat's or Cow's Milk Yogurt ¼ cup (60 mL) Grain-Free Granola 1 serving fruit	Black Bean Coconut Burger Fast and Easy Greek Salad 2 tbsp (30 mL) raw sauerkraut	Salty Almonds with Thyme	Black Cod with Fresh Herb Sauce Sautéed Kale Baked Acorn Squash
FRIDAY	Power Smoothie 2 made with ¼ cup (60 mL) Goat's Milk Kefir	Easy Herbed Shrimp Baked Acorn Squash 2 tbsp (30 mL) raw sauerkraut	Bone Marrow Broth	Mediterranean Quinoa-Stuffed Chicken Breasts Sautéed Bell Pepper and Eggplant
SATURDAY	¼ cup (60 mL) Goat's Milk Kefir "The Bomb" Pancakes ½ to 1 serving fruit 1 soft-cooked egg with 1 tsp (5 mL) ghee, fine sea salt and pepper	Mediterranean Quinoa-Stuffed Chicken Breasts 2 tbsp (30 mL) raw sauerkraut	Zucchini Garlic Hummus with raw vegetables	Bison Stew with Kumquats Mexican Jicama Slaw

Part 4

Recipes for Endometriosis and Pelvic Pain

About the Nutrient Analyses

The nutrient analysis done on the recipes in this book was derived from the Food Processor SQL Nutrition Analysis Software, version 10.9, ESHA Research (2011). Where necessary, data was supplemented using the following references:

1. USDA National Nutrient Database for Standard Reference, Release #28 (2016). Retrieved November 2016 from the USDA Agricultural Research Service website: www.nal.usda.gov/fnic/foodcomp/search/.

2. Great Lakes Gelatin Company (2010). Collagen Hydrolysate Supplement. Retrieved November 2016 from www.greatlakesgelatin.com/consumer/supFacts.php.

3. Coconut Secret Coconut Aminos (2009). Coconut Secret, The Original Coconut Aminos, Soy-Free Seasoning Sauce. Retrieved November 2016 from www.coconutsecret.com/aminos2.html.

4. The Pure Wraps (2016). Pure Wraps, Paleo Coconut Wraps, Original Flavor. Retrieved November 2016 from www.thepurewraps.com/images/stories/nutrition-original-150507.jpg.

Recipes were evaluated as follows:

- The larger number of servings was used where there is a range.
- Where alternatives are given, the first ingredient and amount listed were used.
- The smaller quantity of an ingredient was used where a range is provided.
- Optional ingredients and ingredients that are not quantified were not included.
- Calculations were based on imperial measures and weights.
- The weight of an ingredient was used where a weight was provided.
- Homogenized milk was used where the ingredient is listed as cow's milk.
- Nutrient values were rounded to the nearest whole number for calories, fat, carbohydrate, fiber, sugar, protein, vitamin C, vitamin E, folate and magnesium.
- Nutrient values were rounded to one decimal point for vitamin B_6 and B_{12}.
- Recipes were analyzed prior to cooking.

It is important to note that the cooking method used to prepare the recipe may alter the nutrient content per serving, as may ingredient substitutions and differences among brand-name products.

Breakfasts

Coconut Milk

Not only is this coconut milk easy to make, but it is also delicious! It is important to avoid added thickeners in the first phase of the Endometriosis Diet Plan. Most store-bought coconut milks contain ingredients such as guar gum that may worsen your symptoms.

Tips

Use full-fat, not reduced-fat, coconut flakes.

It is best to use filtered water to avoid ingestion of chlorine and other contaminants. Chlorine can be irritating to your gut and add to your toxic load.

Makes about 4½ cups (1.125 L)

- Four 1-quart (1 L) mason jars
- Blender
- Nut bag or 2 to 3 layers of cheesecloth

1 cup	unsweetened coconut flakes (see tip)	250 mL
4 cups	boiling water	1 L
1 tsp	vanilla extract	5 mL

1. Divide coconut flakes between 2 jars and pour in boiling water. Let stand for at least 1 hour, until softened, or up to 4 hours.

2. Pour the contents of 1 jar into the blender and blend on high for 2 minutes. Strain through nut bag or cheesecloth into a clean jar. Repeat with the remaining jar.

3. Divide vanilla between jars, seal and shake to combine. Serve immediately or store in the refrigerator for up to 3 days.

Nutrients per ½ cup (125 mL)	
Calories	60
Fat	6 g
Carbohydrate	2 g
Fiber	2 g
Sugar	1 g
Protein	1 g
Vitamin C	0 mg
Vitamin E	0 IU
Folate	0 µg
Vitamin B$_6$	0.0 mg
Vitamin B$_{12}$	0.0 µg
Magnesium	9 mg

Vanilla Almond Milk

Almond milk is a delicious alternative to animal milks. Although store-bought almond milk is convenient, it is important to avoid added thickeners in the first phase of the Endometriosis Diet Plan. Most store-bought almond milks contain ingredients such as guar gum that may worsen your symptoms.

Tips

Save the almond meal that remains in the nut bag after step 2 to make "The Bomb" Pancakes (page 180). Store it in an airtight container for up to 3 days or dry it for longer storage. If you own a food dehydrator, simply spread the almond meal out on a tray and dehydrate until dried. To use your oven, line a baking sheet with parchment paper, spread the almond meal over the paper and bake at 200°F (100°C), stirring occasionally, for 2 to 3 hours or until dry and crumbly. Store dried meal in an airtight container at room temperature for up to 2 weeks or in the freezer for up to 3 months.

It is best to use filtered water to avoid ingestion of chlorine and other contaminants. Chlorine can be irritating to your gut and add to your toxic load.

Makes about 8½ cups (2.125 L)

- Four 1-quart (1 L) mason jars
- Blender
- Nut bag or 2 to 3 layers of cheesecloth

1 cup	raw almonds	250 mL
8 cups	water, divided	2 L
1 tsp	vanilla extract	5 mL
6	drops liquid stevia extract	6

1. Divide almonds between 2 jars. Add 2 cups (500 mL) water to each jar. Let stand for 8 to 12 hours. Pour out water and rinse almonds.

2. In blender, combine half the almonds and 2 cups (500 mL) water; blend on high for 2 minutes. Strain through nut bag or cheesecloth into a clean jar. Repeat with the remaining almonds and water.

3. Add ½ tsp (2 mL) vanilla extract and 3 drops of stevia to each jar; seal and shake to combine. Serve immediately or store in the refrigerator for up to 3 days.

Nutrients per ½ cup (125 mL)			
Calories	25	Vitamin C	0 mg
Fat	2 g	Vitamin E	2 IU
Carbohydrate	1 g	Folate	2 µg
Fiber	1 g	Vitamin B_6	0.0 mg
Sugar	0 g	Vitamin B_{12}	0.0 µg
Protein	1 g	Magnesium	12 mg

Power Smoothie 1

Power up your morning with an easy-to-digest anti-inflammatory smoothie. If you don't have time to cook in the morning, or don't have much of an appetite, this is the perfect breakfast for you.

Tips

We recommend using grass-fed hydrolyzed collagen powder or collagen peptides. A reputable brand that is easy to find is Great Lakes collagen hydrolysate. Use an amount that provides about 20 grams of protein (this may be more or less than 1/4 cup/60 mL, depending on the brand).

Use anywhere from 1 to 10 ice cubes, depending on how thick you want your smoothie to be.

If your smoothie is too thick, add water, a little bit at a time, until you achieve the desired consistency.

Makes 1 serving

- Blender

1 cup	Vanilla Almond Milk (page 169) or Coconut Milk (page 168)	250 mL
1 tbsp	coconut butter	15 mL
1	small (3- to 4-inch/7.5 to 10 cm) cucumber, peeled and seeded	1
1/2	banana	1/2
1/2 cup	fresh or frozen blueberries or strawberries	125 mL
1/4 cup	protein powder (see tip)	60 mL
1/2 tsp	ground cinnamon (see tip, page 172)	2 mL
	Ice cubes (see tip)	

1. In blender, combine almond milk, coconut butter, cucumber, banana, blueberries, protein powder, cinnamon, and ice cubes; blend until smooth.

Variation

You can add up to 1/2 cup (125 mL) cooked vegetables to increase alkalinity (see the Allowable Foods list for phase 1, page 138). Alternatively, you can use juiced vegetables in place of all or half of the almond milk.

Nutrients per serving

Calories	321	Vitamin C	17 mg
Fat	13 g	Vitamin E	4 IU
Carbohydrate	32 g	Folate	41 µg
Fiber	8 g	Vitamin B$_6$	0.0 mg
Sugar	17 g	Vitamin B$_{12}$	0.0 µg
Protein	22 g	Magnesium	63 mg

Turmeric Protein Tea

This tea is a quick, easy way to decrease inflammation. Satisfy your craving for a warm cup of tea in the morning or drink this as a snack. It is both filling and healing.

Tips

We recommend using grass-fed hydrolyzed collagen powder or collagen peptides. A reputable brand that is easy to find is Great Lakes collagen hydrolysate. Use an amount that provides about 20 grams of protein (this may be more or less than ¼ cup/60 mL, depending on the brand).

You can use 2 tsp (10 mL) grated turmeric root in place of the ground turmeric. Bring the tea mixture to a boil, then reduce heat to low and simmer for 5 minutes. Strain out the turmeric before pouring the tea.

Nutrients per serving	
Calories	315
Fat	23 g
Carbohydrate	12 g
Fiber	7 g
Sugar	3 g
Protein	20 g
Vitamin C	1 mg
Vitamin E	0 IU
Folate	4 µg
Vitamin B_6	0.0 mg
Vitamin B_{12}	0.0 µg
Magnesium	40 mg

Makes 1 serving

2 cups	Coconut Milk (page 168)	500 mL
¼ cup	protein powder (see tip)	60 mL
1 tsp	ground cinnamon (see tip, page 172)	5 mL
½ tsp	ground turmeric	2 mL
	Liquid stevia extract	

1. In a small saucepan, combine coconut milk, protein powder, cinnamon and turmeric. Heat over medium heat to the desired temperature.

2. Pour into a mug and stir in stevia to taste.

Anti-Inflammatory Protein Bonbons

These anti-inflammatory balls of goodness are filling and healing. They are great to have on hand for a quick breakfast, a snack or when you have a sugar craving. In later phases of the diet, you can experiment with adding other flavors, such as peppermint extract, unsweetened cocoa powder or orange extract.

Tips

For the protein powder, we recommend using grass-fed hydrolyzed collagen powder or collagen peptides. A reputable brand that is easy to find is Great Lakes collagen hydrolysate.

Choose Ceylon cinnamon (also called real cinnamon), not cassia cinnamon. Cassia contains much higher amounts of a compound called coumarin, which in higher doses can contribute to liver damage. Ceylon cinnamon contains only trace amounts of coumarin.

Makes about 20 bonbons

- 24-cup silicone mini muffin pan

1 cup	coconut butter	250 mL
2 tbsp	virgin coconut oil	30 mL
2/3 cup	protein powder (see tip)	150 mL
10 to 20	drops liquid stevia extract	10 to 20
2 tsp	ground cinnamon (see tip)	10 mL
Pinch	fine sea salt	Pinch
1 tsp	vanilla extract	5 mL

1. In a medium saucepan, heat coconut butter and coconut oil over low heat until softened. Whisk in protein powder and 10 drops stevia until blended. Whisk in cinnamon, salt and vanilla until blended. Taste and add more stevia as desired.

2. Pour into 20 muffin cups, dividing evenly and filling the cups about three-quarters full. Refrigerate for 30 minutes. Serve immediately or transfer bonbons to an airtight container and store in the refrigerator for up to 3 months.

Nutrients per bonbon			
Calories	92	Vitamin C	0 mg
Fat	8 g	Vitamin E	0 IU
Carbohydrate	3 g	Folate	0 µg
Fiber	2 g	Vitamin B$_6$	0.0 mg
Sugar	0 g	Vitamin B$_{12}$	0.0 µg
Protein	3 g	Magnesium	0 mg

Mouthwatering Sausage Patties

These easy, protein-packed sausages are delicious and will help decrease inflammation and fuel you for hours! They are great with Carrot Mash (page 234).

Tip

Natural salt contains over 50 minerals, which are all important for balancing blood pressure and other bodily functions. Table salt has been chemically stripped of all its natural minerals, except sodium and chloride, by the use of harsh chemicals. Table salt also contains additives that have been shown to be toxic to human health. We recommend using sea salt (look at the ingredients to ensure that the only ingredient is "sea salt").

Makes 4 patties

1 lb	ground turkey, beef, bison or other meat	500 g
1/2 tsp	fine sea salt	2 mL
1/2 tsp	ground fennel seeds	2 mL
1/2 tsp	chopped fresh thyme	2 mL
1/2 tsp	chopped fresh oregano	2 mL
1/2 tsp	chopped fresh basil	2 mL
1/4 tsp	ground turmeric	1 mL
1/2 tsp	Anti-Inflammatory Ghee (page 192)	2 mL

1. In a large bowl, combine turkey, salt, fennel, thyme, oregano, basil and turmeric until thoroughly mixed. Form into four 1/2-inch (1 cm) thick patties.

2. In a large skillet, melt ghee over medium heat. Add patties and cook, turning once, for 5 to 7 minutes per side or until well browned on both sides and no longer pink inside.

Nutrients per patty	
Calories	175
Fat	9 g
Carbohydrate	0 g
Fiber	0 g
Sugar	0 g
Protein	22 g
Vitamin C	0 mg
Vitamin E	0 IU
Folate	8 µg
Vitamin B$_6$	0.6 mg
Vitamin B$_{12}$	1.1 µg
Magnesium	28 mg

Homemade Cow's Milk Yogurt

Phase 2

Most store-bought yogurts are fermented for only 12 hours. By fermenting your homemade yogurt for 24 hours, you greatly increase the amount of beneficial bacteria. Enjoy it as a healing breakfast or as a snack.

Tip

If you don't have a yogurt maker, you can wrap the sealed jar in a towel and place it in a slow cooker on Low, then place another towel over the slow cooker.

Makes 4 servings

- Instant-read thermometer
- 1-quart (1 L) mason jar or jars to fit yogurt maker
- Yogurt maker (optional, see tip)

2 cups	cow's milk (preferably raw)	500 mL
2	broad spectrum probiotic capsules	2
1 to 2 tsp	liquid honey (optional)	5 to 10 mL
½ tsp	vanilla extract	2 mL

1. In a saucepan, bring milk to a boil over medium heat. Boil for 10 to 15 seconds. Remove from heat and let cool to 110°F (44°C).

2. Pour ½ cup (125 mL) cooled milk into a bowl. Empty probiotics from capsules into milk, discarding capsules, and whisk to combine. Add the remaining milk, then whisk in honey to taste (if using) and vanilla.

3. Pour into the jar(s), seal the lid(s) and incubate for 24 hours in the yogurt maker, following the manufacturer's instructions

4. Store, tightly sealed, in the refrigerator for up to 1 month.

Nutrients per serving	
Calories	76
Fat	4 g
Carbohydrate	6 g
Fiber	0 g
Sugar	6 g
Protein	4 g
Vitamin C	0 mg
Vitamin E	0 IU
Folate	6 µg
Vitamin B_6	0.0 mg
Vitamin B_{12}	1.0 µg
Magnesium	12 mg

Homemade Goat's Milk Yogurt

Goat's milk yogurt can be a great alternative to those sensitive to cow's milk.

Tip

If you don't have a yogurt maker, wrap the sealed jar in a towel and place it in a slow cooker on Low, then place another towel over the slow cooker.

- Instant-read thermometer
- 1-quart (1 L) mason jar or jars to fit yogurt maker
- Yogurt maker (optional, see tip)

2 cups	goat's milk (preferably raw)	500 mL
2	broad spectrum probiotic capsules	2
1 to 2 tsp	liquid honey (optional)	5 to 10 mL
1/2 tsp	vanilla extract	2 mL

1. In a saucepan, bring milk to a boil over medium heat. Boil for 10 to 15 seconds. Turn off heat and let cool to 110°F (44°C).

2. Pour 1/2 cup (125 mL) cooled milk into a bowl. Empty probiotics from capsules into milk, discarding capsules, and whisk to combine. Add the remaining milk, then whisk in honey to taste (if using) and vanilla.

3. Pour into the jar(s), seal the lid(s) and incubate for 24 hours in the yogurt maker, following the manufacturer's instructions

4. Store, tightly sealed, in the refrigerator for up to 1 month.

Nutrients per serving	
Calories	84
Fat	5 g
Carbohydrate	6 g
Fiber	0 g
Sugar	6 g
Protein	4 g
Vitamin C	2 mg
Vitamin E	0 IU
Folate	1 μg
Vitamin B_6	0.1 mg
Vitamin B_{12}	0.1 μg
Magnesium	17 mg

Coconut Yogurt

If you are dairy-sensitive, coconut yogurt is a great alternative way to get a tasty dose of probiotics!

Tips

If coconut cream is not available, you can make coconut cream from full-fat, high-quality coconut milk. Place the coconut milk in the refrigerator until cold. Avoid shaking when opening the can. Scoop out the solid coconut cream that settles on the top (reserve the remaining, thin coconut milk portion for smoothies or for any recipe calling for coconut water). You'll need about four 14-oz (398 mL) cans of coconut milk to get 2 cups (500 mL) of cream.

Probiotic capsules for yogurt-making are available at health and natural food stores, as well as in the health food sections of well-stocked supermarkets. We recommend ProbioMax DF or Ther-Biotic Complete probiotics.

You can use 2 tbsp (30 mL) of purchased probiotic coconut yogurt or kefir in place of the probiotic capsules. Once you have made a batch of coconut yogurt, you can use 2 tbsp (30 mL) of that in place of the probiotic capsules.

Makes 2 cups (500 mL)

- Electric yogurt maker

2 cups	coconut cream	500 mL
2	probiotic capsules	2

1. Place the coconut cream in a medium bowl. Empty the contents of the capsules over the cream, discarding the casings, then whisk until smooth.

2. Transfer coconut cream mixture into yogurt maker jars; place jars in yogurt maker. Follow the manufacturer's directions for processing the yogurt.

Variations

Coconut Yogurt Kefir: Use an equal amount of well-stirred coconut milk (full-fat) in place of the coconut cream. (Note that this is akin to dairy-style kefir; it is not like coconut kefir made from fermented coconut water).

Greek-Style Coconut Yogurt: After step 2, strain the yogurt through doubled layers of cheesecloth, or a coffee filter, overnight in the refrigerator. Reserve the drained liquid for use in smoothies or any recipe calling for coconut water.

Nutrients per ¼ cup (60 mL)

Calories	198	Vitamin C	2 mg
Fat	21 g	Vitamin E	0 IU
Carbohydrate	4 g	Folate	14 µg
Fiber	1 g	Vitamin B_6	0.0 mg
Sugar	0 g	Vitamin B_{12}	0.0 µg
Protein	2 g	Magnesium	17 mg

Power Smoothie 2

Power up your morning with this easy-to-make, healing smoothie. Ground flax seeds are added to help with healthy estrogen levels and add fiber and healthy fats.

Tips

For the protein powder, we recommend using grass-fed hydrolyzed collagen powder or collagen peptides. A reputable brand that is easy to find is Great Lakes collagen hydrolysate.

Use anywhere from 1 to 10 ice cubes, depending on how thick you want your smoothie to be.

If your smoothie is too thick, add water, a little bit at a time, until you achieve the desired consistency.

- Blender

1 cup	Coconut Milk (page 168)	250 mL
½	banana	½
½ cup	fresh or frozen blueberries	125 mL
2 tbsp	protein powder (see tip)	30 mL
2 tsp	ground flax seeds (flaxseed meal)	10 mL
1 to 2	kale leaves, stems removed	1 to 2
	Ice cubes (see tip)	

1. In blender, combine coconut milk, banana, blueberries, protein powder, flax seeds, kale and ice cubes; blend until smooth.

Variations

Replace the banana with 1 serving's worth of another fruit (see the Allowable Foods list for phase 2, page 142).

You can add more vegetables to further increase alkalinity.

Healing Help

For easier digestion, soak the flax seeds overnight in filtered water before adding them to the blender.

Nutrients per serving

Calories	241
Fat	14 g
Carbohydrate	19 g
Fiber	6 g
Sugar	8 g
Protein	14 g
Vitamin C	25 mg
Vitamin E	0 IU
Folate	21 µg
Vitamin B_6	0.3 mg
Vitamin B_{12}	0.0 µg
Magnesium	56 mg

Grain-Free Granola

Because this granola is grain-free, it is a great gluten-free alternative to store-bought granolas. It is also higher in protein and healthy fats. It's great with homemade Vanilla Almond Milk (page 169) or yogurt, or on its own as a crunchy snack!

Tip

For easier digestion, soak and dry the nuts and seeds before starting the recipe. Place the nuts and seeds in a pot and add enough purified drinking water to cover them by about 2 inches (5 cm). Cover the pot and let stand at room temperature for 12 to 24 hours. Drain and transfer nuts and seeds to a baking sheet, spreading them out in a single layer. Dry in a 150°F (70°C) oven for 12 to 24 hours. When nuts are dry, proceed with step 1.

Makes about 2½ cups (625 mL)

- Preheat oven to 300°F (150°C)
- Baking sheet, lightly greased

1 cup	raw almonds, finely chopped	250 mL
½ cup	raw cashews, finely chopped	125 mL
½ cup	raw green pumpkin seeds (pepitas)	125 mL
½ cup	unsweetened flaked coconut	125 mL
¼ cup	liquid honey	60 mL
¼ cup	virgin coconut oil	60 mL
2 tsp	ground cinnamon (see tip, page 172)	10 mL
½ tsp	fine sea salt	2 mL
½ tsp	gluten-free vanilla extract	2 mL

1. In a large bowl, combine almonds, cashews, pumpkin seeds and coconut.

2. In a small saucepan, melt honey and coconut oil over medium heat. Stir in cinnamon, salt and vanilla; bring to a boil.

3. Slowly pour honey mixture over nut mixture, stirring until well combined. Spread into a thin layer on prepared baking sheet.

4. Bake in preheated oven for 25 minutes, stirring every 5 to 10 minutes to keep mixture from burning, until golden brown. Let cool completely on a wire rack. As it cools, the mixture will harden. Once cool, break apart into smaller clusters. Store in an airtight container at room temperature for up to 2 weeks.

Nutrients per ¼ cup (60 mL)			
Calories	258	Vitamin C	0 mg
Fat	21 g	Vitamin E	6 IU
Carbohydrate	14 g	Folate	16 µg
Fiber	3 g	Vitamin B_6	0.1 mg
Sugar	8 g	Vitamin B_{12}	0.0 µg
Protein	6 g	Magnesium	98 mg

Coconut Pancakes

These delicious pancakes are packed full of anti-inflammatory, healing ingredients — and have no refined grains!

Tips

It is best to use filtered water to avoid ingestion of chlorine and other contaminants. Chlorine can be irritating to your gut and add to your toxic load.

Serve the pancakes brushed with Anti-Inflammatory Ghee, using 1 tsp (5 mL) ghee for every 2 pancakes.

You can make these in larger batches and freeze the cooled pancakes for up to 6 months. Just pop the frozen pancakes in the toaster to reheat.

Makes 12 small pancakes

4	large eggs	4
1¼ cups	water	300 mL
1 tbsp	dark (cooking) molasses	15 mL
1 tsp	vanilla extract	5 mL
½ cup	coconut flour	125 mL
1 tsp	baking soda	5 mL
1 tsp	ground cinnamon (see tip, page 172)	5 mL
1 tsp	Anti-Inflammatory Ghee (page 192) or virgin coconut oil (approx.)	5 mL

1. In a large bowl, whisk together eggs, water, molasses and vanilla. Stir in flour, baking soda and cinnamon until well combined.

2. Preheat a griddle or large skillet over medium heat and grease with a thin layer of ghee. Working in batches as necessary, drop batter by tablespoonfuls (15 mL) and cook until the edges look slightly dry. Turn the pancakes over and cook until the bottoms are golden brown. Regrease the griddle or skillet and adjust the heat between batches as necessary.

Nutrients per 2 pancakes

Calories	91
Fat	6 g
Carbohydrate	4 g
Fiber	1 g
Sugar	2 g
Protein	4 g
Vitamin C	0 mg
Vitamin E	1 IU
Folate	17 µg
Vitamin B$_6$	0.1 mg
Vitamin B$_{12}$	0.3 µg
Magnesium	15 mg

"The Bomb" Pancakes

	Makes 8 small pancakes	
4	large eggs	4
1/4 cup	Basic Ghee (page 190) or virgin coconut oil, melted	60 mL
1 tsp	vanilla extract	5 mL
10	drops liquid stevia extract	10
1/2 cup	almond flour (see tip)	125 mL
2 tbsp	protein powder (see tip)	30 mL
1 tsp	baking soda	5 mL
1 tsp	ground cinnamon (see tip, page 172)	5 mL
1/4 to 1/2 tsp	fine sea salt	1 to 2 mL
1 tsp	Basic Ghee (page 190) or virgin coconut oil (approx.)	5 mL

These pancakes really are "the bomb"! With each delicious bite, you can celebrate the gift you are giving your body with this healing breakfast. Serve with berries and ghee.

Tips

If you have leftover almond meal from making Vanilla Almond Milk (page 169), you can use it in place of the almond flour.

For the protein powder, we recommend using grass-fed hydrolyzed collagen powder or collagen peptides. A reputable brand that is easy to find is Great Lakes collagen hydrolysate.

You can make these in larger batches and freeze the cooled pancakes for up to 6 months. Just pop the frozen pancakes in the toaster to reheat.

1. In a large bowl, whisk together eggs, melted ghee, vanilla and stevia. Stir in flour, protein powder, baking soda, cinnamon and salt until well combined.

2. Preheat a griddle or large skillet over medium heat and grease with 1 tsp (5 mL) ghee. Working in batches as necessary, drop batter by tablespoonfuls (15 mL) and cook until the edges look slightly dry. Turn the pancakes over and cook until the bottoms are golden brown. Regrease the griddle or skillet and adjust the heat between batches as necessary.

Nutrients per 2 pancakes	
Calories	187
Fat	13 g
Carbohydrate	2 g
Fiber	1 g
Sugar	0 g
Protein	15 g
Vitamin C	0 mg
Vitamin E	3 IU
Folate	15 µg
Vitamin B$_6$	0.1 mg
Vitamin B$_{12}$	0.2 µg
Magnesium	19 mg

Goat's Milk Kefir

Unlike most probiotic supplements, which contain only a few different strains of beneficial bacteria, kefir is packed with over 50 different strains. Gut diversity (having several different strains of beneficial bacteria living in your gut) is strongly correlated to good health, so a little kefir a day may help keep the doctor away!

Tips

Either raw or pasteurized milk will work here, but avoid using ultra-pasteurized milk.

When you first start enjoying kefir, consume only a small amount each day. We recommend starting with 1 tbsp (15 mL) a day and working up to ½ cup (125 mL). This is strong stuff!

Makes 4 cups (1 L)

- Two 1-quart (1 L) mason jars

4 cups	goat's milk (see tip)	1 L
1 tbsp	milk kefir grains	15 mL

1. Combine milk and kefir grains in a jar, seal tightly and let stand in a dark place (such as in a cupboard) for 12 to 24 hours, opening the lid once or twice to release the gas then resealing, until the grains float to the top of the jar and the milk has a sour smell.

2. Strain the kefir through a colander into a clean jar, using a wooden spoon as needed to stir the grains and press out liquid. Serve immediately or store, tightly covered, in the refrigerator for up to 3 weeks.

Variation

Use cow's milk in place of the goat's milk.

Nutrients per 1 tbsp (15 mL)

Calories	10	Vitamin C	0 mg
Fat	1 g	Vitamin E	0 IU
Carbohydrate	1 g	Folate	0 µg
Fiber	0 g	Vitamin B_6	0.0 mg
Sugar	1 g	Vitamin B_{12}	0.0 µg
Protein	1 g	Magnesium	2 mg

Power Smoothie 3

Power up your morning with this healthy, filling smoothie! Chia seeds increase fiber, provide healthy fat and feed beneficial bacteria in your gut.

Tips

For the protein powder, try whey, grass-fed hydrolyzed collagen, pea or hemp. Use an amount that provides about 20 grams of protein (this may be more or less than 1/4 cup/60 mL, depending on the brand).

Use anywhere from 1 to 10 ice cubes, depending on how thick you want your smoothie to be.

If your smoothie is too thick, add water, a little bit at a time, until you achieve the desired consistency.

Nutrients per serving	
Calories	351
Fat	22 g
Carbohydrate	18 g
Fiber	9 g
Sugar	4 g
Protein	25 g
Vitamin C	62 mg
Vitamin E	9 IU
Folate	39 µg
Vitamin B$_6$	0.1 mg
Vitamin B$_{12}$	0.6 µg
Magnesium	95 mg

Makes 1 serving

1 cup	unsweetened hemp milk	250 mL
1 tbsp	natural almond butter	15 mL
1/2 cup	fresh or frozen strawberries	125 mL
1/4 cup	protein powder (see tip)	60 mL
1 1/2 tbsp	chia seeds	22 mL
1 to 2	kale leaves, stems removed	1 to 2
	Ice cubes (see tip)	

1. In blender, combine hemp milk, almond butter, strawberries, protein powder, chia seeds, kale and ice cubes; blend until smooth.

Variations

Use any other type of milk in place of the hemp milk.

Add 1 tbsp to 1/4 cup (15 to 60 mL) kefir.

Replace the almond butter with another natural nut butter or peanut butter.

Thank you for your order, Alexandra O'Connell!

Visit our stores to sell your books, music, movies games for cash.

SKU	ISBN/UPC	Title & Author/Artist	Shelf ID	Qty	OrderSKU
S327646213	9780778805625	The Endometriosis Health and Diet Program:.. Cook MS RD CDE, Danielle, Cook MD FACC	MED 1.5	1	

SHIPPED STANDARD TO:
Alexandra O'Connell
23121 CLARABELLE DR
CHARLOTTE NC 28273-4392
6t0h8xy82g9zq82@marketplace.amazon.com

ORDER# **113-7049593-4881862**
AmazonMarketplaceUS

Thank you

Mixed Fruit, Chia and Flaxseed Porridge

Phase 3

Makes 2 to 3 servings

This simple mixture is extremely nutritious. It is quick to prepare and will leave you feeling well satisfied throughout the morning. It is also full of healthy fiber to feed the beneficial bacteria in your gut.

3 tbsp	whole flax seeds, soaked (see tips)	45 mL
½ cup	Coconut Milk (page 168)	125 mL
¼ cup	chopped apple	60 mL
¼ cup	chopped banana	60 mL
¼ cup	chopped orange, skin and membrane removed (see tip)	60 mL
¼ cup	chopped hulled strawberries	60 mL
¼ cup	blueberries	60 mL
3 tbsp	chia seeds	45 mL
½ tsp	gluten-free vanilla extract	2 mL

1. In bowl, toss together coconut milk, apple, banana, orange, strawberries, blueberries, soaked flax seeds, chia seeds and vanilla. Set aside for 5 minutes so the chia seeds can swell and absorb some of the liquid.

Tips

To soak flax seeds, submerge them in double the amount of liquid. For this recipe, soak 3 tbsp (45 mL) flax seeds in 6 tbsp (90 mL) water. Set aside for 30 minutes. Drain and rinse under cold running water.

Flax seeds must be soaked or ground so your body can absorb the nutrients. In this recipe, soaked whole flax seeds add body to the porridge. Otherwise, it would be runny.

To remove the membrane from an orange, use a chef's knife to remove a bit of the skin from the top and the bottom. Using the tip of the knife, remove the skin and as much of the white pith as possible without losing flesh. Cut the orange in half and then cut into ½-inch (1 cm) cubes for this recipe.

Variations

For added protein, mix 1 scoop (or 15 to 20 grams of protein equivalent) of your preferred protein powder (whey, pea, hemp or beef collagen hydrolysate) into the porridge before serving.

Use ⅓ cup (75 mL) chia seeds and 1 tbsp (15 mL) flax seeds soaked in 2 tbsp (30 mL) water. The result will have a very similar texture and flavor but a higher content of omega-3 fatty acids, because the chia seeds contain more omega-3 fats than the flax seeds.

Nutrients per serving (1 of 3)

Calories	237	Vitamin C	20 mg
Fat	17 g	Vitamin E	0 IU
Carbohydrate	19 g	Folate	27 µg
Fiber	9 g	Vitamin B_6	0.1 mg
Sugar	8 g	Vitamin B_{12}	0.0 µg
Protein	5 g	Magnesium	64 mg

Skillet-Roasted Cauliflower Omelet

Phase 3		Makes 4 servings	

Turn your everyday omelet into a delicious, healing meal. Cauliflower and garlic not only taste great, but also help with detoxification, inflammation and feeding your healthy microbiome.

5	large eggs	5
1/4 tsp	fine sea salt	1 mL
1/4 tsp	freshly cracked black pepper	1 mL
2 tsp	extra virgin olive oil	10 mL
3 cups	coarsely chopped cauliflower florets	750 mL
2	cloves garlic, minced	2
1/2 cup	crumbled feta cheese	125 mL
1/4 cup	packed fresh flat-leaf (Italian) parsley leaves	60 mL

Tip

Natural salt contains over 50 minerals, which are all important for balancing blood pressure and other bodily functions. Table salt has been chemically stripped of all its natural minerals, except sodium and chloride, by the use of harsh chemicals. Table salt also contains additives that have been shown to be toxic to human health. We recommend using sea salt (look at the ingredients to ensure that the only ingredient is "sea salt").

1. In a large bowl, whisk together eggs, salt and pepper. Set aside.

2. In a large skillet, heat oil over medium-high heat. Add cauliflower and cook, stirring, for 7 to 10 minutes or until browned and tender. Reduce heat to medium, add garlic and cook, stirring, for 30 seconds.

3. Pour egg mixture over cauliflower. Cook, lifting edges to allow uncooked eggs to run underneath and shaking skillet occasionally to loosen omelet, for 4 to 5 minutes or until almost set. Slide out onto a large plate.

4. Invert skillet over omelet and, using pot holders, firmly hold plate and skillet together. Invert omelet back into skillet and cook for 1 to 2 minutes to set eggs. Slide out onto plate and sprinkle with cheese and parsley.

Nutrients per serving			
Calories	194	Vitamin C	44 mg
Fat	13 g	Vitamin E	2 IU
Carbohydrate	6 g	Folate	91 µg
Fiber	2 g	Vitamin B_6	0.4 mg
Sugar	3 g	Vitamin B_{12}	0.9 µg
Protein	13 g	Magnesium	27 mg

Garlicky Kale Frittata

This delicious dish is packed full of healthy ingredients, including kale, garlic, turmeric and coconut. Your fork can be a vehicle to good health or illness; this dish turns it into a powerful healing tool.

Tips

An equal amount of packed baby spinach leaves (no need to chop) can be used in place of the kale. Reduce the cooking time for the greens to 1 to 2 minutes.

Leftovers can be wrapped in individual portions and stored in an airtight container for up to 3 days. Enjoy cold or at room temperature, or reheat each portion in the microwave on High for 20 to 30 seconds.

Nutrients per serving	
Calories	261
Fat	16 g
Carbohydrate	15 g
Fiber	5 g
Sugar	1 g
Protein	18 g
Vitamin C	82 mg
Vitamin E	0 IU
Folate	141 µg
Vitamin B$_6$	5.0 mg
Vitamin B$_{12}$	3.9 µg
Magnesium	26 mg

- Preheat oven to 400°F (200°C)
- 8-inch (20 cm) square glass baking pan or pie plate, greased with coconut oil

2 tbsp	virgin coconut oil	30 mL
6	cloves garlic, thinly sliced	6
4 cups	packed chopped kale leaves	1 L
	Fine sea salt and freshly ground black pepper	
1	package (16 oz/500 g) extra-firm or firm tofu, drained	1
¼ cup	nutritional yeast	60 mL
¼ tsp	ground turmeric	1 mL
2 tbsp	coconut cream or well-stirred coconut milk (full-fat)	30 mL
1 tsp	Dijon mustard	5 mL

1. In a medium skillet, melt coconut oil over medium heat. Add garlic and cook, stirring, for 3 to 4 minutes or until golden. Add kale, increase heat to medium-high and cook, stirring, for 4 to 5 minutes or until kale is wilted. Season to taste with salt and pepper.

2. Meanwhile, in a medium bowl, mash tofu with a fork until it resembles ricotta cheese. Add nutritional yeast, ¾ tsp (3 mL) salt, turmeric, coconut cream and mustard, mixing until well blended. Add kale mixture, stirring until combined. Season to taste with pepper.

3. Transfer tofu mixture to prepared baking pan, pressing down firmly and smoothing top.

4. Bake in preheated oven for 20 to 25 minutes or until frittata is firm and golden brown. Let cool in pan for 3 minutes, then invert onto a plate. Serve warm.

Red Lentil Frittata

Phase 3

Transform your usual frittata into a microbiota-building meal. Your taste buds will enjoy the combination of Middle Eastern flavors combined with rich, tangy goat cheese.

Tips

To increase lentils' digestibility, soak them for 8 hours, rinse, then cook.

It is best to use filtered water to avoid ingestion of chlorine and other contaminants. Chlorine can be irritating to your gut and add to your toxic load.

Nutrients per serving

Calories	187
Fat	9 g
Carbohydrate	12 g
Fiber	3 g
Sugar	1 g
Protein	15 g
Vitamin C	32 mg
Vitamin E	2 IU
Folate	77 µg
Vitamin B$_6$	0.3 mg
Vitamin B$_{12}$	0.6 µg
Magnesium	25 mg

Makes 6 servings

- 9-inch (23 cm) glass baking dish, sprayed with nonstick cooking spray (preferably olive oil)

½ cup	dried red lentils, rinsed	125 mL
2 cups	water	500 mL
8	large eggs	12
1	clove garlic, minced	1
1½ tsp	ground cumin	7 mL
¾ tsp	fine sea salt	3 mL
¼ tsp	freshly cracked black pepper	1 mL
1 cup	chopped drained roasted red bell peppers	250 mL
½ cup	packed fresh cilantro leaves, chopped	125 mL
2 oz	soft goat cheese, crumbled	60 g

1. In a medium saucepan, combine lentils and water. Bring to a boil over medium-high heat. Reduce heat and simmer for about 22 minutes or until very tender but not mushy. Drain and let cool slightly.

2. Preheat oven to 375°F (190°C).

3. In a large bowl, whisk together eggs, garlic, cumin, salt and pepper. Stir in cooked lentils, roasted peppers, cilantro and cheese. Spread evenly in prepared baking dish.

4. Bake in preheated oven for 25 to 30 minutes or until golden brown, puffed and set at the center. Let cool on a wire rack for at least 10 minutes before cutting. Serve warm or let cool completely.

Juices, Ghees and Broths

Juices

Ghees

Broths

Spicy Carrot and Ginger Juice

Phase 1

Makes 1 serving

Juiced vegetables are a great concentrated source of vitamins, minerals and phytonutrients. A small glass of this potent juice can help to reduce inflammation and provide your cells with the nutrients they need to optimize your health and wellness. Juiced vegetables have the majority of the fiber removed, making them easy to digest.

- Juicer

2	carrots	2
1	1-inch (2.5 cm) piece gingerroot	1
1 cup	roughly chopped bok choy	250 mL

1. Using a juicer, process carrots, ginger and bok choy. Drink within 30 minutes.

Nutrients per serving

Calories	60	Vitamin C	25 mg
Fat	0 g	Vitamin E	1 IU
Carbohydrate	13 g	Folate	52 µg
Fiber	4 g	Vitamin B_6	0.3 mg
Sugar	6 g	Vitamin B_{12}	0.0 µg
Protein	2 g	Magnesium	23 mg

Purple Haze Juice

Phase 1

Makes 1 serving

This beautiful juice provides anti-inflammatory and detoxifying nutrients to expedite the healing process.

2	slices beet	2
1	carrot	1
$\frac{1}{2}$ cup	roughly chopped bok choy	125 mL
$\frac{1}{4}$ cup	roughly chopped purple cabbage	60 mL
	Squeeze of lemon juice	

1. Using a juicer, process beet slices, carrot, bok choy, cabbage and lemon juice. Drink within 30 minutes.

Nutrients per serving

Calories	51	Vitamin C	27 mg
Fat	0 g	Vitamin E	1 IU
Carbohydrate	11 g	Folate	67 µg
Fiber	3 g	Vitamin B_6	0.2 mg
Sugar	6 g	Vitamin B_{12}	0.0 µg
Protein	2 g	Magnesium	23 mg

Refreshing Fennel, Cucumber and Ginger Juice

| Phase 1 |

Refresh with this delicious, gut-calming juice packed with flavor and healing nutrients.

	Makes 1 serving	
½ cup	roughly chopped fennel bulb	125 mL
1	large (5- to 6-inch/12.5 to 15 cm) cucumber	1
1	1-inch (2.5 cm) piece gingerroot	1

1. Using a juicer, process fennel, cucumber and ginger. Drink within 30 minutes.

Nutrients per serving

Calories	49
Fat	1 g
Carbohydrate	10 g
Fiber	3 g
Sugar	4 g
Protein	2 g
Vitamin C	14 mg
Vitamin E	0 IU
Folate	51 µg
Vitamin B_6	0.2 mg
Vitamin B_{12}	0.0 µg
Magnesium	42 mg

Basic Ghee

Ghee is a traditional staple in Indian cooking and has been used in Ayurvedic medicine for thousands of years. It is made from butter, but during a simple cooking process, the casein, whey and lactose are removed, leaving behind only fat. This improves tolerance for some people who are sensitive to dairy foods.

Makes about 1½ cups (375 mL)

- Sieve lined with 4 to 5 layers of cheesecloth
- Glass jar

1 lb	unsalted butter	500 mL

1. Cut butter into 5 pieces and place in a medium saucepan. Heat over medium heat until melted. Reduce heat to low and cook, stirring slowly and constantly, for 25 minutes. The butter will foam and bubble, and some white curds will fall to the bottom of the pan. It will smell like popcorn and turn a golden color; be sure not to let it brown (remove from heat periodically to cool pan, if necessary). The mixture will almost stop bubbling and then foam again. When this happens, the ghee is ready and should now be a clear, golden yellow.

2. Immediately remove ghee from heat and let cool for 5 minutes. Meanwhile, skim off and discard the top foam layer.

3. Slowly pour ghee through the cheesecloth-lined sieve into a glass jar; discard solids. Store in the refrigerator for up to 6 months.

Nutrients per 1 tsp (5 mL)	
Calories	43
Fat	5 g
Carbohydrate	0 g
Fiber	0 g
Sugar	0 g
Protein	0 g
Vitamin C	0 mg
Vitamin E	0 IU
Folate	0 µg
Vitamin B$_6$	0.0 mg
Vitamin B$_{12}$	0.0 µg
Magnesium	0 mg

Garlic-Infused Ghee

Ghee has a high smoke point, so it is a great fat to use for cooking, as it will not be damaged by heat. We recommend consuming 1 to 3 tbsp (15 to 45 mL) of ghee daily, especially in the first 2 phases of the Endometriosis Diet Plan.

Makes about 1½ cups (375 mL)

- Sieve lined with 4 to 5 layers of cheesecloth
- Glass jar

1 lb	unsalted butter	500 mL
5	cloves garlic, cut into thin slivers	5

1. Cut butter into 5 pieces and place in a medium saucepan. Heat over medium heat until melted. Add garlic, reduce heat to low and cook, stirring slowly and constantly, for 25 minutes. The butter will foam and bubble, and some white curds will fall to the bottom of the pan. It will smell like popcorn and turn a golden color; be sure not to let it brown (remove from heat periodically to cool pan, if necessary). The mixture will almost stop bubbling and then foam again. When this happens, the ghee is ready and should now be a clear, golden yellow.

2. Immediately remove ghee from heat and let cool for 5 minutes. Meanwhile, skim off and discard the top foam layer.

3. Slowly pour ghee through the cheesecloth-lined sieve into a glass jar; discard solids. Store in the refrigerator for up to 6 months.

Nutrients per 1 tsp (5 mL)

Calories	44
Fat	5 g
Carbohydrate	0 g
Fiber	0 g
Sugar	0 g
Protein	0 g
Vitamin C	0 mg
Vitamin E	0 IU
Folate	0 µg
Vitamin B$_6$	0.0 mg
Vitamin B$_{12}$	0.0 µg
Magnesium	0 mg

Anti-Inflammatory Ghee

Ghee is rich in conjugated linoleic acid and several vitamins, including A, E and K2, which all help to improve your health. It is also a great source of butyric acid, which aids in digestion, decreases inflammation in your intestinal wall and supports your immune system.

Tip

Choose Ceylon cinnamon (also called real cinnamon), not cassia cinnamon. Cassia contains much higher amounts of a compound called coumarin, which in higher doses can contribute to liver damage. Ceylon cinnamon contains only trace amounts of coumarin.

Makes about 1 cup (250 mL)

1 cup	Basic Ghee (page 190)	250 mL
2 tsp	ground turmeric	10 mL
2 tsp	ground cinnamon (see tip)	10 mL
2 tsp	ground ginger	10 mL

1. In a small, heavy-bottomed saucepan, combine ghee, turmeric, cinnamon and ginger. Heat over medium heat, stirring constantly, until starting to sizzle. Continue cooking, stirring constantly, for 1 to 2 minutes to infuse the flavors. Remove from heat. Store in the refrigerator for up to 6 months.

Nutrients per 1 tsp (5 mL)

Calories	33
Fat	4 g
Carbohydrate	0 g
Fiber	0 g
Sugar	0 g
Protein	0 g
Vitamin C	0 mg
Vitamin E	0 IU
Folate	0 µg
Vitamin B_6	0.0 mg
Vitamin B_{12}	0.0 µg
Magnesium	0 mg

Basic Vegetable Stock

Vegetable stock can be a powerful detoxification tool in your healing toolbox. This stock makes enough for two average soup recipes. It can be made ahead and frozen. For convenience, cook it overnight in the slow cooker. If your slow cooker is not large enough to make a full batch, you can halve the recipe.

Tips

To freeze this stock and all others, transfer to airtight containers in small, measured portions (2 cups/500 mL or 4 cups/1 L are handy), leaving at least 1 inch (2.5 cm) headspace for expansion. Mason jars work great! Refrigerate until chilled, cover and freeze for up to 3 months. Thaw in refrigerator before using.

It is best to use filtered water to avoid ingestion of chlorine and other contaminants. Chlorine can be irritating to your gut and add to your toxic load.

Makes about 12 cups (3 L)

- Large slow cooker (about 5 quarts)

8	carrots, scrubbed and coarsely chopped	8
6	stalks celery, coarsely chopped	6
3	onions, coarsely chopped	3
3	cloves garlic, coarsely chopped	3
6	sprigs parsley	6
3	bay leaves	3
10	black peppercorns	10
¼ cup	dried alfalfa leaves (optional)	60 mL
1 tsp	dried thyme	5 mL
	Fine sea salt (optional)	
12 cups	water	3 L

1. In slow cooker stoneware, combine carrots, celery, onions, garlic, parsley, bay leaves, peppercorns, alfalfa leaves (if using), thyme, salt to taste (if using) and water. Cover and cook on Low for 8 hours or on High for 4 hours. Strain and discard solids. Cover and refrigerate for up to 5 days or freeze in an airtight container.

Nutrients per 1 cup (250 mL)			
Calories	29	Vitamin C	5 mg
Fat	0 g	Vitamin E	1 IU
Carbohydrate	7 g	Folate	19 µg
Fiber	2 g	Vitamin B$_6$	0.1 mg
Sugar	3 g	Vitamin B$_{12}$	0.0 µg
Protein	1 g	Magnesium	12 mg

Bone Marrow Broth

Phase 1

This traditional superfood has been around for thousands of years. Bone broths are teeming with healing nutrients. Some of their well-known benefits include improving joint health, healing a leaky gut, improving skin tone, texture and appearance, strengthening the immune system, boosting detoxification and supporting muscle repair. Bone broths are easy to make and are a must for optimizing your health.

Tips

Ask the butcher for beef marrow bones. They are usually quite inexpensive.

Portions of broth frozen in muffin cups are very handy for use in soups and other dishes; simply plop them in frozen. Each portion is about 2 tbsp (30 mL). For a warm cup of broth, add 1 to 2 cubes per 1 cup (500 mL) water and heat to desired temperature.

Makes 7 cups (1.75 L)

- Preheat oven to 450°F (230°C)
- Roasting pan or rimmed baking sheet
- Large slow cooker (minimum 6 quarts)
- Fine-mesh sieve
- Mason jars and/or silicone mini muffin pan

4 to 6	beef marrow bones (each about 3 to 4 inches/7.5 to 10 cm long)	4 to 6
14 cups	water	3.5 L
6	cloves garlic	6
1	onion, finely chopped	1
2 cups	chopped carrots (1/2-inch/1 cm pieces)	500 mL
2	bay leaves	2
1 to 2 tbsp	fresh rosemary leaves	15 to 30 mL
2 tbsp	apple cider vinegar	30 mL

1. Arrange bones in a single layer in pan. Bake in preheated oven for 40 minutes, turning the bones over halfway through.

2. Transfer bones to slow cooker. Add a little bit of the water to the roasting pan, scrape up any browned bits stuck to the bottom of the pan and pour into the slow cooker. Pour in the remaining water. Add garlic, onion, carrots, bay leaves, rosemary and vinegar. Cover and cook on Low for 48 hours, resetting the slow cooker as necessary.

3. Let cool for 30 minutes, then strain through a fine-mesh sieve and discard solids.

4. Store in jars in the refrigerator for up to 3 days and/or pour into muffin cups set on a baking sheet and freeze; once frozen, transfer to an airtight container and store in the freezer for up to 3 months.

Nutrients per 1 cup (250 mL)			
Calories	23	Vitamin C	4 mg
Fat	0 g	Vitamin E	0 IU
Carbohydrate	5 g	Folate	9 µg
Fiber	1 g	Vitamin B_6	0.1 mg
Sugar	2 g	Vitamin B_{12}	0.0 µg
Protein	1 g	Magnesium	11 mg

Lunches and Dinners

Homemade Chicken Soup

There is nothing like homemade chicken soup to make you feel better. This soup has the healing benefits of a bone broth with the added protein from chicken meat. The vegetables included in this soup have a low potential for aggravating your GI symptoms and provide essential nutrients for detoxification.

Tips

If you don't have fresh herbs on hand, you can use ¼ tsp (1 mL) each dried rosemary, oregano, thyme and sage.

It is best to use filtered water to avoid ingestion of chlorine and other contaminants. Chlorine can be irritating to your gut and add to your toxic load.

Store leftover soup in glass jars in the refrigerator for up to 4 days or in the freezer for up to 6 months.

Makes 4 servings

- Large slow cooker (minimum 6 quarts)

2	bone-in skin-on chicken breasts (about 1 lb/500 g total)	2
2	stalks celery, cut into ½-inch (1 cm) chunks	2
1 tsp	chopped fresh rosemary	5 mL
1 tsp	chopped fresh oregano	5 mL
1 tsp	chopped fresh thyme	5 mL
1 tsp	chopped fresh sage	5 mL
1 tbsp	apple cider vinegar	15 mL
2	carrots, cut into ¼-inch (0.5 cm) thick slices	2
1	small bok choy, diced	1

1. Place chicken in slow cooker and cover with about ½ inch (1 cm) of water. Add celery, rosemary, oregano, thyme, sage and vinegar. Cover and cook on Low for 6 to 8 hours or until an instant-read thermometer inserted in the thickest part of a chicken breast registers 165°F (74°C).

2. Remove chicken, leaving broth and vegetables in slow cooker. Let chicken cool slightly, then remove the skin and bones. Discard skin and small bones. Place chicken meat in an airtight container and refrigerate. Add larger bones back to slow cooker, cover and cook on Low for 18 hours, resetting the slow cooker as necessary.

3. Strain soup, discarding solids, and return liquid to slow cooker. Return chicken meat to soup and add carrots and bok choy. Cover and cook on Low for 1 to 2 hours or until chicken is heated through and carrots are soft.

Nutrients per serving

Calories	107	Vitamin C	11 mg
Fat	2 g	Vitamin E	1 IU
Carbohydrate	4 g	Folate	27 µg
Fiber	1 g	Vitamin B_6	0.4 mg
Sugar	2 g	Vitamin B_{12}	0.2 µg
Protein	17 g	Magnesium	26 mg

Carrot Bone Broth Soup

Phase 1

Makes 4 servings

You will feel the healing powers with each delicious spoonful of this soup. Enjoy it as a main dish or as a side.

Tips

Experiment with different spices. Ground Ceylon cinnamon and curry powder are a great addition.

For added flavor, chop the green parts of a few green onions and toss them in with the carrots.

• Blender, food processor or immersion blender

6 cups	Bone Marrow Broth (page 194)	1.5 L
4 cups	chopped carrots	1 L
1 tsp	finely grated or chopped gingerroot	5 mL
1 tsp	ground turmeric	5 mL
2 cups	Coconut Milk (page 168)	250 mL
1/2 tsp	fine sea salt	2 mL

1. In a large saucepan, bring broth to a boil over medium heat. Add carrots and boil for 10 minutes or until soft. Add ginger and turmeric; reduce heat and simmer for 5 minutes. Stir in coconut milk.

2. Working in batches, transfer soup to the blender and purée until smooth (or purée in the pan using an immersion blender). Return to pot (if needed) and reheat over medium heat until steaming.

Nutrients per serving	
Calories	153
Fat	6 g
Carbohydrate	24 g
Fiber	7 g
Sugar	10 g
Protein	3 g
Vitamin C	14 mg
Vitamin E	2 IU
Folate	41 µg
Vitamin B$_6$	0.4 mg
Vitamin B$_{12}$	0.0 µg
Magnesium	43 mg

Bone Marrow Soup

This delicious, filling soup is packed with nutrients to heal your body. It is easy to prepare and can be frozen for future meals. In phases 2 and 3, you can include both marrow and cartilage bones.

Tips

Ask the butcher for beef marrow bones. They are usually quite inexpensive.

If you don't have fresh herbs on hand, you can use ¼ tsp (1 mL) each dried rosemary, oregano, thyme and sage.

It is best to use filtered water to avoid ingestion of chlorine and other contaminants. Chlorine can be irritating to your gut and add to your toxic load.

Store leftover soup in glass jars in the refrigerator for up to 4 days or in the freezer for up to 6 months.

Makes 4 servings

- Large slow cooker (minimum 6 quarts)

4	beef marrow bones (each about 3 to 4 inches/7.5 to 10 cm long)	4
2	stalks celery, cut into ½-inch (1 cm) chunks	2
1 tsp	chopped fresh rosemary	5 mL
1 tsp	chopped fresh oregano	5 mL
1 tsp	chopped fresh thyme	5 mL
1 tsp	chopped fresh sage	5 mL
1 tbsp	apple cider vinegar	15 mL
1 lb	beef stewing meat, cut into 1-inch (2.5 cm) chunks	500 mL
2	carrots, cut into ¼-inch (0.5 cm) thick slices	2
1	small bok choy, diced	1

1. Place bones in slow cooker and cover with about 2 inches (5 cm) of water. Add celery, rosemary, oregano, thyme, sage and vinegar. Cover and cook on Low for 24 hours or until meat is tender and falling apart.

2. Strain soup, discarding solids, and return liquid to slow cooker. Add beef, carrots and bok choy. Cover and cook on Low for 6 to 10 hours or until beef is fall-apart tender.

Nutrients per serving

Calories	181		Vitamin C	11 mg
Fat	7 g		Vitamin E	1 IU
Carbohydrate	4 g		Folate	33 µg
Fiber	1 g		Vitamin B_6	0.9 mg
Sugar	2 g		Vitamin B_{12}	4.0 µg
Protein	24 g		Magnesium	37 mg

Anti-Inflammatory Baked Cod

Phase 1

This omega-3-rich, anti-inflammatory meal is almost effortless to prepare. Packed with healing power and flavor, it is sure to become a household favorite.

Tip

Natural salt contains over 50 minerals, which are all important for balancing blood pressure and other bodily functions. Table salt has been chemically stripped of all its natural minerals, except sodium and chloride, by the use of harsh chemicals. Table salt also contains additives that have been shown to be toxic to human health. We recommend using sea salt (look at the ingredients to ensure that the only ingredient is "sea salt").

Makes 4 servings

- Preheat oven to 400°F (200°C)
- 13- by 9-inch (33 by 23 cm) glass baking dish

4	pieces skinless cod fillet (each 4 oz/125 g)	4
1/4 cup	chopped fresh parsley	60 mL
2 tbsp	Garlic-Infused Ghee (page 191), melted	30 mL
2 tsp	ground turmeric	10 mL
1/2 tsp	fine sea salt	2 mL
1/2 tsp	freshly ground black pepper	2 mL
2	large carrots, cut into 1/2-inch (1 cm) thick circles	1
1	zucchini, cut into 1-inch (2.5 cm) thick circles	1
2	lemon wedges	2

1. Arrange cod in a single layer in baking dish and sprinkle with parsley. In a small bowl, combine ghee and turmeric; drizzle over fish. Sprinkle fish with salt and pepper. Arrange carrots and zucchini around fish.

2. Bake in preheated oven for 20 to 25 minutes or until fish is opaque and flakes easily when tested with a fork and vegetables are tender. Squeeze lemon juice over fish.

Nutrients per serving	
Calories	188
Fat	8 g
Carbohydrate	6 g
Fiber	2 g
Sugar	3 g
Protein	21 g
Vitamin C	19 mg
Vitamin E	2 IU
Folate	33 µg
Vitamin B$_6$	0.4 mg
Vitamin B$_{12}$	1.0 µg
Magnesium	54 mg

Baked Salmon

This entrée is an omega-3 power punch with almost zero preparation. Enjoy it with a side of greens and roasted root vegetables for a fast, delicious meal.

Tip

If you don't have fresh herbs on hand, you can use ¼ tsp (1 mL) each dried oregano and thyme.

Makes 4 servings

- Preheat oven to 350°F (180°C)
- Large glass baking dish

4	pieces skinless salmon fillet (each 4 oz/125 g)	4
3 tbsp	Garlic-Infused Ghee (page 191), melted	45 mL
1 tsp	chopped fresh oregano	5 mL
1 tsp	chopped fresh thyme	5 mL
½ tsp	fine sea salt	2 mL
½	lemon	½

1. Place salmon in baking dish. In a small bowl, combine ghee, oregano, thyme and salt; drizzle over fish.

2. Bake in preheated oven for 15 to 20 minutes or until fish is opaque and flakes easily when tested with a fork. Squeeze lemon juice over fish.

Nutrients per serving	
Calories	245
Fat	16 g
Carbohydrate	1 g
Fiber	0 g
Sugar	0 g
Protein	23 g
Vitamin C	5 mg
Vitamin E	1 IU
Folate	7 µg
Vitamin B_6	0.7 mg
Vitamin B_{12}	4.7 µg
Magnesium	32 mg

Easy Herbed Shrimp

Phase 1

This is an easy protein option to top a bed of cooked greens (or a salad in later phases, when you are able to tolerate raw vegetables). You also get the added bonus of the healing nutrients in the herbs and spices. Healthy eating never tasted so good!

Tip

If you don't have fresh herbs on hand, you can use ¼ tsp (1 mL) each dried rosemary, oregano, thyme and sage.

Makes 4 servings

2 tbsp	Garlic-Infused Ghee (page 191)	30 mL
1 tsp	chopped fresh rosemary	5 mL
1 tsp	chopped fresh oregano	5 mL
1 tsp	chopped fresh thyme	5 mL
1 tsp	chopped fresh sage	5 mL
1 tsp	ground turmeric	5 mL
1 lb	medium shrimp, peeled and deveined	500 g

1. In a medium saucepan, melt ghee over medium heat. Stir in rosemary, oregano, thyme, sage and turmeric. Add shrimp and cook, stirring, for 1 to 3 minutes or until shrimp are firm, pink and opaque.

Nutrients per serving	
Calories	148
Fat	8 g
Carbohydrate	2 g
Fiber	0 g
Sugar	0 g
Protein	16 g
Vitamin C	1 mg
Vitamin E	2 IU
Folate	22 µg
Vitamin B$_6$	0.2 mg
Vitamin B$_{12}$	1.3 µg
Magnesium	27 mg

Brined and Tender Lemon Roast Chicken

This recipe courtesy of dietitian Joanne Rankin.

This meal may be the most tender, flavorful chicken dish you have ever eaten! Brining is an effective way to add flavor and moisture to meats. The light salt solution helps to loosen the meat muscle fibers, making them more tender. The salt also helps the meat retain some water from the brine, again helping to tenderize. Any flavors in the brine will also infuse into the meat, adding flavor to the final product.

Nutrients per serving	
Calories	194
Fat	6 g
Carbohydrate	1 g
Fiber	0 g
Sugar	0 g
Protein	32 g
Vitamin C	7 mg
Vitamin E	1 IU
Folate	13 µg
Vitamin B$_6$	0.7 mg
Vitamin B$_{12}$	0.6 µg
Magnesium	42 mg

Makes 6 servings

- Roasting pan

1	whole roasting chicken (3 to 4 lbs/ 1.5 to 2 kg)	1
3 tbsp	kosher salt	45 mL
12 cups	water	3 L
1	lemon	1
2 tsp	olive oil	10 mL
½ tsp	fine sea salt	2 mL

1. Trim excess fat from chicken. Rinse inside and out under cold running water.

2. In a large pot, combine kosher salt and water, stirring to dissolve salt. Add chicken, breast side down, making sure it is fully submerged. Cover and refrigerate for at least 4 hours or for up to 8 hours.

3. About 30 minutes before cooking, drain brine from chicken and discard. Rinse chicken under running water and pat dry. Place on a clean plate and let stand at room temperature.

4. Place oven rack in center of oven, place empty roasting pan on rack and preheat oven to 425°F (220°C).

5. Meanwhile, place whole lemon in a small saucepan and add water to cover. Bring to a boil over high heat. Reduce heat and simmer for 5 minutes. Remove from heat and leave lemon in hot water until ready to use.

6. Rub chicken all over with oil and sprinkle with ½ tsp (2 mL) salt. Remove the lemon from the hot water, discarding water. Poke several holes in the lemon and insert it into the cavity of the chicken.

7. Carefully remove the hot roasting pan from the oven, place chicken, breast side up, in pan, and roast for 30 minutes. Reduce heat to 400°F (200°C). Roast chicken for 60 minutes or until skin is dark golden and crispy, drumsticks wiggle when touched and a meat thermometer inserted in the thickest part of a thigh registers 185°F (85°C). Transfer chicken to a cutting board, tent with foil and let rest for 10 to 15 minutes before carving.

Tips

Brining chicken in a mild salt solution produces delightfully tender meat. Do not brine the chicken for longer than 8 hours. Over-brining may adversely affect the texture of the cooked chicken.

Tenting the chicken with foil and letting it rest before carving allows the juices to redistribute throughout the meat, creating a much moister chicken.

8. Using kitchen tongs, remove lemon from the chicken. Cut lemon in half and squeeze juice over hot chicken pieces.

Variation

For added flavor, insert fresh or dried herbs, such as thyme, rosemary, savory or marjoram, into the cavity of the chicken along with the lemon.

Easy Baked Chicken Breasts over Arugula

Phase 1	Makes 2 servings

With only three ingredients, this is an easy, delicious meal. When you come home after a busy day at work, place it in the oven and relax while it cooks.

- Preheat oven to 350°F (180°C)
- 12-cup (3 L) casserole dish with lid

4 cups	arugula	1 L
2	boneless skinless chicken breasts (each 4 oz/125 g)	2
2 tbsp	Anti-Inflammatory Ghee (page 192)	30 mL

1. Arrange arugula in casserole dish and lay chicken on top. Crumble 1 tbsp (15 mL) ghee over each breast.

2. Cover and bake in preheated oven for 15 to 25 minutes or until an instant-read thermometer inserted in the thickest part of a chicken breast registers 165°F (74°C).

Nutrients per serving	
Calories	269
Fat	17 g
Carbohydrate	1 g
Fiber	1 g
Sugar	1 g
Protein	25 g
Vitamin C	7 mg
Vitamin E	1 IU
Folate	43 µg
Vitamin B_6	0.9 mg
Vitamin B_{12}	0.2 µg
Magnesium	48 mg

Chinese Chicken and Greens

Turn everyday chicken into a mouthwatering, anti-inflammatory feast for two, or double or triple the recipe to serve at your next dinner party. Your guests will think you slaved over this meal for hours. They don't need to know it took only minutes to prepare!

Makes 2 servings

4 tbsp	Garlic-Infused Ghee (page 191), divided	60 mL
2 tsp	grated gingerroot	10 mL
1 tsp	Chinese five-spice powder	5 mL
3 tbsp	coconut amino acids	45 mL
2	boneless skinless chicken breasts (each 4 oz/125 g)	2
4 cups	arugula	1 L
2 cups	finely chopped trimmed kale leaves	500 mL
1 cup	drained canned chopped bamboo shoots	250 mL
2 tbsp	water (if needed)	30 mL

1. In a medium skillet or wok, melt 2 tbsp (30 mL) ghee over medium heat. Stir in ginger, five-spice powder and coconut amino acids. Add chicken and cook, turning once, for about 10 minutes per side or until an instant-read thermometer inserted in the thickest part of a chicken breast registers 165°F (74°C). Transfer chicken to a bowl, cover with foil and set aside.

2. In the same skillet, melt the remaining ghee over medium heat. Add arugula, kale and bamboo shoots; cook, stirring, until all the greens are evenly covered with ghee. Reduce heat to low, cover and cook, stirring occasionally, for 10 minutes. If greens start to stick, stir in water.

3. Divide greens among plates and top with chicken.

Nutrients per serving

Calories	491
Fat	32 g
Carbohydrate	19 g
Fiber	3 g
Sugar	11 g
Protein	28 g
Vitamin C	89 mg
Vitamin E	1 IU
Folate	65 µg
Vitamin B_6	1.2 mg
Vitamin B_{12}	0.2 µg
Magnesium	75 mg

Turmeric Ginger Chicken Skewers

These are a mouthwatering anti-inflammatory twist on your regular chicken skewers. They make great appetizers or a fantastic meat entrée.

Tip

Natural salt contains over 50 minerals, which are all important for balancing blood pressure and other bodily functions. Table salt has been chemically stripped of all its natural minerals, except sodium and chloride, by the use of harsh chemicals. Table salt also contains additives that have been shown to be toxic to human health. We recommend using sea salt (look at the ingredients to ensure that the only ingredient is "sea salt").

Makes 4 servings

- Preheat oven to 350°F (180°C)
- Four 12-inch (30 cm) metal skewers
- Rimmed baking sheet

1 tbsp	finely grated gingerroot	15 mL
2 tsp	ground turmeric	10 mL
¼ tsp	fine sea salt	1 mL
¼ tsp	freshly ground black pepper	1 mL
1 lb	boneless skinless chicken breasts, cut into 1-inch (5 cm) cubes	500 g

1. In a large bowl, combine ginger, turmeric, salt and pepper. Add chicken and stir until evenly coated. Thread chicken onto skewers and arrange in a single layer on baking sheet.

2. Bake in preheated oven for 12 minutes, turning skewers over halfway through, until chicken is no longer pink inside.

Nutrients per serving	
Calories	134
Fat	3 g
Carbohydrate	1 g
Fiber	0 g
Sugar	0 g
Protein	24 g
Vitamin C	2 mg
Vitamin E	0 IU
Folate	5 µg
Vitamin B$_6$	0.9 mg
Vitamin B$_{12}$	0.2 µg
Magnesium	33 mg

Slow Cooker Chicken Wraps

Let your next dinner party meal virtually cook itself, or have a meal ready when you return home from a long day at work. This meal has the healing properties of bone broth, herbs and ghee, and is packed with nutrients to fuel your body.

Tips

If you don't have fresh herbs on hand, you can use ¼ tsp (1 mL) each dried rosemary, oregano, thyme and sage.

Make sure to choose a gluten-free chicken broth.

After step 1, you can save the broth for a healing snack. Pour it into a mason jar and store in the refrigerator for up to 3 days.

Nutrients per serving	
Calories	211
Fat	8 g
Carbohydrate	2 g
Fiber	0 g
Sugar	0 g
Protein	32 g
Vitamin C	4 mg
Vitamin E	1 IU
Folate	15 µg
Vitamin B$_6$	1.1 mg
Vitamin B$_{12}$	0.4 µg
Magnesium	41 mg

Makes 4 servings

- Large slow cooker (minimum 6 quarts)

4	bone-in skinless chicken breasts (each 6 oz/175 g)	4
1 tsp	chopped fresh rosemary	5 mL
1 tsp	chopped fresh oregano	5 mL
1 tsp	chopped fresh thyme	5 mL
1 tsp	chopped fresh sage	5 mL
½ tsp	fine sea salt	2 mL
½ tsp	freshly ground black pepper	2 mL
2 cups	ready-to-use reduced-sodium chicken broth (see tip)	500 mL
4	large collard green leaves	4
1 cup	water	250 mL
1 tbsp	Garlic-Infused Ghee (page 191), melted	15 mL

1. Rub chicken with rosemary, oregano, thyme, sage, salt and pepper. Add to slow cooker and pour in broth. Cover and cook on Low for 8 hours or on High for 4 hours, until chicken is falling off the bones.

2. Place collard green leaves in a large skillet and pour in water. Cover and cook over medium heat for about 10 minutes or until collard green leaves are flexible and tender. Drain leaves.

3. Spread ghee over collard green leaves. Place a chicken breast (bones removed) in the center of each leaf and wrap leaf around chicken.

Turkey Wraps

Enjoy these mouthwatering wraps on their own or, in later phases, dipped in one of the delicious dips provided in this book (pages 258 and 260–262). You can make the turkey ahead and have it on hand for a quick lunch or a no-hassle dinner.

Tips

Look for coconut wraps at reputable paleo bakeries, such as Julian Bakery. If coconut wraps are not available, substitute 2 large collard green leaves, prepared as in step 2 of Slow Cooker Chicken Wraps (page 206).

In phase 2, you can spread Zucchini Garlic Hummus (page 261) over the wrap before adding the turkey.

Nutrients per serving	
Calories	321
Fat	17 g
Carbohydrate	9 g
Fiber	1 g
Sugar	1 g
Protein	28 g
Vitamin C	9 mg
Vitamin E	0 IU
Folate	28 µg
Vitamin B$_6$	0.7 mg
Vitamin B$_{12}$	0.5 µg
Magnesium	48 mg

Makes 2 servings

- Preheat oven to 350°F (180°C)
- 12-cup (3 L) casserole dish with lid

2 cups	arugula	500 mL
1	small boneless turkey breast (8 oz/250 g)	1
2 tbsp	Anti-Inflammatory Ghee (page 192)	30 mL
2	6-inch (15 cm) coconut wraps	2

1. Arrange arugula in casserole dish and lay turkey on top. Crumble ghee over turkey.

2. Cover and bake in preheated oven for 50 to 60 minutes or until an instant-read thermometer inserted in the thickest part of the breast registers 165°F (74°C). Let turkey cool for 10 to 15 minutes, then cut into thin slices.

3. Arrange turkey slices and arugula in the center of the coconut wrap and wrap up like a burrito.

Anti-Inflammatory Meatballs

Phase 1

Craving meatballs without the gluten? Pair these anti-inflammatory balls of goodness with Spaghetti Squash Noodles (page 238). You'll never miss your traditional bread crumb meatballs!

Tip

Natural salt contains over 50 minerals, which are all important for balancing blood pressure and other bodily functions. Table salt has been chemically stripped of all its natural minerals, except sodium and chloride, by the use of harsh chemicals. Table salt also contains additives that have been shown to be toxic to human health. We recommend using sea salt (look at the ingredients to ensure that the only ingredient is "sea salt").

Nutrients per serving

Calories	159
Fat	6 g
Carbohydrate	1 g
Fiber	0 g
Sugar	0 g
Protein	24 g
Vitamin C	0 mg
Vitamin E	1 IU
Folate	6 µg
Vitamin B$_6$	0.5 mg
Vitamin B$_{12}$	2.5 µg
Magnesium	27 mg

Makes 4 servings

- Preheat oven to 350°F (180°C)
- Medium glass baking dish

1 lb	ground beef or bison	500 mL
1 tsp	finely chopped fresh basil	5 mL
1 tsp	ground turmeric	5 mL
1 tsp	freshly ground black pepper	5 mL
½ tsp	fine sea salt	2 mL

1. In a large bowl, combine beef, basil, turmeric, pepper and salt until thoroughly mixed. Form into 8 balls of equal size and place in baking dish, spacing them evenly.

2. Bake in preheated oven for 20 minutes or until meatballs are no longer pink inside.

Mediterranean-Style Mahi-Mahi

Phase 2

This dish is easy to prepare and tastes incredible! Get your daily dose of healthy fats in a mouthwatering meal.

Tips

It is difficult to be specific about the timing because of the configuration of the fish, but you should begin checking for doneness after 1 hour. Be aware it may take up to 1½ hours.

This recipe can be halved, but use a small slow cooker (1½ to 3 quarts) in that case.

Makes 4 servings

- Medium to large oval slow cooker (3½ to 5 quarts)

2 lbs	mahi-mahi steaks	1 kg
1 tsp	dried oregano	5 mL
1	lemon, thinly sliced	1
1	can (28 oz/796 mL) no-salt-added tomatoes, with juice, coarsely chopped	1
½ cup	dry white wine	125 mL
¼ cup	extra virgin olive oil, divided	60 mL
½ tsp	fine sea salt	2 mL
	Freshly ground black pepper	

Gremolata

½ cup	finely chopped fresh parsley	125 mL
3 tbsp	drained capers, minced	45 mL
2	whole anchovies, rinsed and finely chopped	2
	Freshly ground black pepper	
	Chopped black olives	

1. Place fish in slow cooker stoneware. Sprinkle with oregano and lay lemon slices evenly over top. In a bowl, combine tomatoes, wine, 2 tbsp (30 mL) oil, salt, and pepper to taste. Pour over fish. Cover and cook on High for 1 hour (see tip) or until fish flakes easily when pierced with a knife.

2. *Gremolata:* Meanwhile, in a bowl, combine parsley, capers, anchovies, the remaining oil, and pepper to taste. Mix well and set aside in refrigerator until fish is cooked.

3. To serve, transfer fish and tomato sauce to a warm platter. Spoon gremolata evenly over top and garnish with olives.

Nutrients per serving	
Calories	377
Fat	15 g
Carbohydrate	11 g
Fiber	3 g
Sugar	5 g
Protein	44 g
Vitamin C	30 mg
Vitamin E	5 IU
Folate	30 µg
Vitamin B$_6$	1.2 mg
Vitamin B$_{12}$	1.4 µg
Magnesium	92 mg

Grilled Salmon with Lemon Oregano Pesto

Makes 4 servings

This simple pesto sauce keeps the salmon extra-moist and adds a burst of fresh flavor. Oregano and garlic help to balance the bacteria in your gut and add a fantastic flavor to your salmon.

Tips

Double the quantity of the pesto ingredients. Use half to marinate the fish and refrigerate the other half to use as a quick baste when grilling chicken, pork or lamb. Pesto can be stored in an airtight container in the refrigerator for up to 2 days.

Broiler Method: Preheat broiler, with rack set 4 inches (10 cm) from heat. In step 3, arrange salmon on a broiler pan and broil for 5 minutes per side or until fish is opaque and flakes easily when tested with a fork.

Healing Help

To decrease your carcinogen exposure when barbecuing, keep the flame low to prevent it from touching the steak. In addition, clean your barbecue rack well before each use to reduce the buildup of carcinogens. Finally, marinate your meats for at least 5 minutes before cooking.

- Preheat greased barbecue grill to medium
- Food processor or mini chopper
- Shallow glass baking dish

1	clove garlic, chopped	1
½ cup	lightly packed fresh parsley sprigs	125 mL
2 tbsp	lightly packed fresh oregano (or 2 tsp/10 mL dried)	30 mL
2 tsp	grated lemon zest	10 mL
2 tbsp	freshly squeezed lemon juice	30 mL
4 tsp	olive oil	20 mL
¼ tsp	freshly ground black pepper	1 mL
4	skinless salmon fillets (each 4 oz/125 g)	4

1. In food processor, combine garlic, parsley, oregano, lemon zest and juice, oil and pepper; purée until very smooth.

2. Pat salmon dry with paper towels. Arrange in baking dish and coat both sides with pesto. Marinate at room temperature for 15 minutes, or cover and refrigerate for up to 1 hour.

3. Place salmon on preheated grill and cook for 5 to 7 minutes per side (depending on thickness) or until fish is opaque and flakes easily when tested with a fork.

Nutrients per serving			
Calories	209	Vitamin C	16 mg
Fat	12 g	Vitamin E	1 IU
Carbohydrate	2 g	Folate	42 µg
Fiber	0 g	Vitamin B_6	1.0 mg
Sugar	0 g	Vitamin B_{12}	3.6 µg
Protein	23 g	Magnesium	39 mg

Pan-Roasted Trout with Fresh Tomato Basil Sauce

This healthy meal requires very little preparation or cooking time. It's the perfect meal for a last-minute dinner party or after a long day of work.

Tip

Learn more about how to choose sustainable seafood by checking out these websites: Marine Stewardship Council (www.msc.org), Monterey Bay Aquarium Seafood Watch (www.seafoodwatch.org) or SeaChoice (www.seachoice. org).

Nutrients per serving

Calories	197
Fat	9 g
Carbohydrate	5 g
Fiber	1 g
Sugar	3 g
Protein	24 g
Vitamin C	16 mg
Vitamin E	2 IU
Folate	30 µg
Vitamin B$_6$	0.5 mg
Vitamin B$_{12}$	5.1 µg
Magnesium	47 mg

Makes 4 servings

Fresh Tomato Basil Sauce

2	large ripe red tomatoes, seeded and diced	2
1/2	clove garlic, minced	1/2
2 tbsp	minced green onion	30 mL
2 tbsp	chopped fresh basil	30 mL
1/8 tsp	fine sea salt	0.5 mL
	Freshly ground black pepper	
1 tbsp	balsamic vinegar	15 mL
1 tbsp	extra virgin olive oil	15 mL

Fish

1 tsp	extra virgin olive oil	5 mL
1 lb	trout fillets with skins	500 g

1. *Sauce:* Shortly before serving, in a bowl, combine tomatoes, garlic, green onion, basil, salt, pepper to taste, vinegar and oil.

2. *Fish:* Pat trout dry with paper towels. Brush a large nonstick skillet with oil and heat over medium-high heat. Place trout, skin side down, in skillet. Cook for 2 minutes, without turning. Reduce heat to medium-low, cover and cook for 3 to 5 minutes or until fish is opaque and flakes easily when tested with a fork (time depends on thickness of fish; increase time as needed).

3. Arrange fish on plates and top with sauce.

Variation

Substitute Mexico's famous pico de gallo (also called salsa fresca) for the fresh tomato basil sauce. The preparation is very similar; just use cilantro instead of basil, replace the vinegar with freshly squeezed lime juice, and add 1 minced jalapeño pepper.

Lemon Garlic Chicken

Phase 2

This tasty version of lemon garlic chicken is sure to delight your taste buds. The combination of herbs and spices helps to decrease inflammation and rebalance your microbiota.

Tips

Chicken can be marinated at room temperature for up to 30 minutes if you are short of time. Any longer, make sure it is refrigerated. Throw out the plastic bag used for marinating.

Can't find the cover that fits your casserole? Cover it with foil, dull side out. Trace around the rim with your fingers to be sure foil forms a tight seal.

Makes 4 servings

- 8-cup (2 L) covered casserole dish

1	clove garlic, minced	1
2 tbsp	freshly squeezed lemon juice	30 mL
1 tbsp	extra virgin olive oil	15 mL
1 tsp	dried thyme	5 mL
1/4 tsp	fine sea salt	1 mL
Pinch	ground nutmeg	Pinch
Pinch	paprika	Pinch
Pinch	freshly ground white pepper	Pinch
4	skinless boneless chicken breasts	4

1. In a resealable plastic freezer bag set in a bowl, combine garlic, lemon juice, olive oil, thyme, salt, nutmeg, paprika and white pepper. Add chicken breasts to marinade, seal bag and refrigerate for 1 hour.

2. Preheat oven to 375°F (190°C). Place chicken breasts with marinade in the casserole dish and cover tightly. Bake for 45 minutes or until juices run clear and meat thermometer registers 170°F (78°C).

Variation

Substitute an equal amount of oregano for the thyme. Or use 1 tbsp (15 mL) snipped fresh thyme or oregano.

Nutrients per serving	
Calories	170
Fat	7 g
Carbohydrate	1 g
Fiber	0 g
Sugar	0 g
Protein	25 g
Vitamin C	5 mg
Vitamin E	1 IU
Folate	7 µg
Vitamin B_6	0.9 mg
Vitamin B_{12}	0.2 µg
Magnesium	32 mg

Grilled Steak with Arugula and Parmesan

Phase 2

This meal is sure to be a hit at your next barbecue. Arugula is a great peppery counterpart to grilled steak, and is a good source of vitamins C, A and K, bioflavonoids, iron and potassium.

Tip

To decrease your carcinogen exposure when barbecuing, keep the flame low to prevent it from touching the steak. In addition, clean your barbecue rack well before each use to reduce the buildup of carcinogens. Finally, marinate your meats for at least 5 minutes before cooking. You can make extra dressing from this recipe to use as a marinade.

Makes 4 servings

- Preheat barbecue grill to medium-high

12 oz	boneless beef top loin (strip loin) or top sirloin steak, trimmed	375 g
	Nonstick cooking spray	
½ tsp	fine sea salt, divided	2 mL
½ tsp	freshly cracked black pepper, divided	2 mL
1 tbsp	extra virgin olive oil	15 mL
1 tsp	freshly squeezed lemon juice	5 mL
1 tsp	balsamic vinegar	5 mL
4 cups	packed arugula	1 L
¼ cup	shaved Parmesan cheese	60 mL

1. Pat steak dry with paper towels. Lightly spray with cooking spray and sprinkle with half the salt and half the pepper. Grill on preheated barbecue, turning once, for 5 to 6 minutes per side for medium-rare, or to desired doneness. Transfer to a cutting board and let rest for 5 minutes.

2. Meanwhile, in a small bowl, whisk together oil, lemon juice, vinegar and the remaining salt and pepper.

3. Divide arugula among four dinner plates. Thinly slice steak and arrange on top of arugula. Drizzle with dressing and scatter cheese over top.

Nutrients per serving	
Calories	167
Fat	8 g
Carbohydrate	1 g
Fiber	0 g
Sugar	1 g
Protein	21 g
Vitamin C	3 mg
Vitamin E	1 IU
Folate	31 µg
Vitamin B_6	0.6 mg
Vitamin B_{12}	0.9 µg
Magnesium	32 mg

Green Thai Curry with Spinach and Sweet Potatoes

This grain-, gluten- and meat-free variation of Thai green curry is sure to be a family favorite. It is packed with ingredients that help reduce inflammation and improve gut health.

Tips

Most Thai curry pastes are naturally gluten-free. Still, read the label before purchase to be certain.

If you can only find a 19-oz (540 mL) can of chickpeas, use about three-quarters of the can (about 1½ cups/375 mL drained).

Makes 4 servings

1 tbsp	virgin coconut oil	15 mL
1	large onion, thinly sliced	1
2 tbsp	Thai green curry paste	30 mL
2 lbs	sweet potatoes, peeled and cut into 1-inch (2.5 cm) chunks	1 kg
1½ cups	coconut water or water	375 mL
	Fine sea salt	
1	can (14 to 15 oz/398 to 425 mL) chickpeas, drained and rinsed	1
1	can (14 oz/398 mL) coconut milk (full-fat), well-stirred	1
8 cups	packed baby spinach (about 6 oz/175 g)	2 L
2 tbsp	freshly squeezed lime juice	30 mL
	Cayenne pepper	

1. In a large saucepan, melt coconut oil over low heat. Add onion, increase heat to medium-high and cook, stirring, for 6 to 8 minutes or until softened. Add curry paste and cook, stirring, for 30 seconds.

2. Stir in sweet potatoes, coconut water and 1 tsp (5 mL) salt; bring to a boil. Reduce heat and simmer, stirring occasionally, for 12 minutes.

3. Stir in chickpeas and coconut milk; reduce heat and simmer, stirring occasionally, for 3 to 7 minutes or until sweet potatoes are tender.

4. Stir in spinach and lime juice; simmer for 1 to 2 minutes or until spinach is wilted. Season to taste with salt and cayenne.

Nutrients per serving

Calories	296
Fat	13 g
Carbohydrate	42 g
Fiber	8 g
Sugar	7 g
Protein	6 g
Vitamin C	12 mg
Vitamin E	1 IU
Folate	58 µg
Vitamin B$_6$	0.5 mg
Vitamin B$_{12}$	0.0 µg
Magnesium	79 mg

Coconut Squash Pizza

Hankering for a great pizza without grains? Here's your recipe. Not only is this pizza crust delicious, but it also benefits the beneficial bacteria in your gut to reduce inflammation and improve your overall health.

Tips

An equal amount of pumpkin purée (not pie filling) or mashed cooked sweet potato can be used in place of the squash.

Add meat as a topping for more protein.

Makes one 10-inch (25 cm) crust

- Preheat oven to 400°F (200°C)
- Food processor
- Large pizza pan or baking sheet, greased with coconut oil

¾ cup	chickpea flour	175 mL
½ cup	coconut flour	125 mL
¼ cup	potato starch	60 mL
1 tbsp	gluten-free baking powder	15 mL
½ tsp	fine sea salt	2 mL
1 cup	canned butternut squash purée or thawed frozen winter squash purée	250 mL
1 tbsp	melted virgin coconut oil	15 mL

Suggested Toppings

Marinara sauce

Basil pesto

Hummus

Shredded or grated cheese

Parmesan cheese

Chopped, thinly sliced or coarsely shredded vegetables (zucchini, red onion, carrots, broccoli, cauliflower)

Leftover grilled or roasted vegetables, coarsely chopped

Pitted ripe or brine-cured black olives, sliced or chopped

1. In food processor, combine chickpea flour, coconut flour, potato starch, baking powder and salt. Pulse to combine. Add squash and coconut oil; pulse until a cohesive dough forms.

2. Press out dough on prepared pan, pressing to a 10-inch (25 cm) circle. Top with any of the suggested toppings.

3. Bake in preheated oven for 20 to 25 minutes or until crust is set and golden brown at the edges.

Nutrients per ¼ crust	
Calories	221
Fat	11 g
Carbohydrate	28 g
Fiber	4 g
Sugar	3 g
Protein	5 g
Vitamin C	8 mg
Vitamin E	1 IU
Folate	86 µg
Vitamin B$_6$	0.2 mg
Vitamin B$_{12}$	0.0 µg
Magnesium	51 mg

Stuffed Portobellos

Looking for a tasty alternative to your usual meat dish? Mushrooms are high in vitamin D and may also help with estrogen metabolism. A win-win for your health!

Tips

Extra-large portobello mushrooms work best in this dish to accommodate the volume of filling. If they are unavailable, use 8 regular portobello mushrooms in their place.

An equal amount of trimmed kale or Swiss chard can be used in place of the spinach.

If you do not like olives, omit them and increase the sun-dried tomatoes to 6 tbsp (90 mL).

Makes 4 servings

- Preheat oven to 500°F (260°C)
- Large rimmed baking sheet, lined with foil and greased with coconut oil

4	extra-large portobello mushrooms	4
2 tbsp	melted virgin coconut oil, divided	30 mL
2 tsp	balsamic vinegar	10 mL
2 tbsp	coconut flour	30 mL
1/2 cup	coconut water or water	125 mL
6 cups	packed baby spinach, roughly torn (about 6 oz/175 g)	1.5 L
2 tbsp	nutritional yeast	30 mL
3 tbsp	chopped drained oil-packed sun-dried tomatoes	45 mL
3 tbsp	chopped pitted brine-cured black olives (such as kalamata)	45 mL
	Fine sea salt and freshly cracked black pepper	

1. Remove stems from mushrooms. Chop stems and set aside. Using a spoon, gently scoop out black gills on underside of mushroom caps. Discard gills. Place mushroom caps, hollow side down, on prepared baking sheet. Brush 1 tbsp (15 mL) oil and the vinegar over tops of mushrooms. Bake in preheated oven for 5 to 7 minutes or until tender.

2. Meanwhile, in a small bowl, combine coconut flour and coconut water; let stand for 5 minutes.

3. In a large skillet, heat the remaining oil over low heat. Add spinach and mushroom stems, increase heat to medium-high and cook, stirring, for 1 to 2 minutes or until wilted. Add coconut flour mixture, nutritional yeast, sun-dried tomatoes and olives; cook, stirring, for 1 to 2 minutes to heat through and blend the flavors. Season to taste with salt and pepper.

4. Turn mushrooms over on baking sheet and fill caps with spinach mixture. Bake for 7 to 10 minutes or until filling is golden brown.

Nutrients per serving	
Calories	144
Fat	10 g
Carbohydrate	10 g
Fiber	4 g
Sugar	4 g
Protein	6 g
Vitamin C	19 mg
Vitamin E	2 IU
Folate	204 µg
Vitamin B$_6$	0.4 mg
Vitamin B$_{12}$	0.1 µg
Magnesium	66 mg

Black Bean Coconut Burgers

Black beans are a fantastic choice for vegan burgers, providing high amounts of protein, iron and fiber. These patties are delicious and incredibly nutritious!

Tips

If you can only find 19-oz (540 mL) cans of beans, you will need about 1½ cans (about 3 cups/750 mL drained).

The moisture content of canned beans can vary. If the patty mixture appears too wet, add a small amount of additional coconut flour; if too dry, add a small amount more coconut milk.

Nutrients per serving

Calories	322
Fat	14 g
Carbohydrate	37 g
Fiber	17 g
Sugar	1 g
Protein	14 g
Vitamin C	6 mg
Vitamin E	0 IU
Folate	130 µg
Vitamin B$_6$	0.2 mg
Vitamin B$_{12}$	0.0 µg
Magnesium	107 mg

Makes 4 servings

- Food processor

¼ cup	packed fresh cilantro leaves	60 mL
¼ cup	coconut flour	60 mL
3 tbsp	ground flax seeds (flaxseed meal)	45 mL
2 tsp	ground cumin	10 mL
1 tsp	dried oregano	5 mL
¼ tsp	cayenne pepper	1 mL
⅓ cup	well-stirred coconut milk (full-fat)	75 mL
2	cans (each 14 to 15 oz/ 398 to 425 mL) black beans, drained and rinsed, divided	2
1 tbsp	virgin coconut oil	15 mL

1. In food processor, combine cilantro, coconut flour, flax seeds, cumin, oregano, cayenne, coconut milk and half the beans; pulse until a chunky purée forms.

2. Transfer purée to a medium bowl and stir in the remaining beans. Form into four ¾-inch (2 cm) thick patties.

3. In a large skillet, melt coconut oil over low heat. Add patties, increase heat to medium and cook for 4 minutes. Turn patties over and cook for 3 to 5 minutes or until crispy on the outside and hot in the center.

Healing Help
For easier digestion, use ½ to ¾ cup (125 to 175 mL) dried black beans; soak them overnight, rinse and then cook them before use.

Black Cod with Fresh Herb Sauce

Get your daily dose of anti-inflammatory omega-3 fatty acids along with your healing herbs. Enjoy each bite, knowing you are healing your body.

Tips

An equal amount of chopped green onions (green parts only) may be used in place of the chives.

Use either Basic Vegetable Stock (page 193) or a gluten-free ready-to-use vegetable broth to prepare this soup.

Some black cod has been sustainably fished and others not. Learn more about how to choose sustainable seafood by checking out Marine Stewardship Council (www.msc.org), Monterey Bay Aquarium Seafood Watch (www.seafoodwatch.org) or SeaChoice (www.seachoice.org). If you cannot find sustainable black cod, you can use sea bass, halibut, cod or any other firm white fish fillets in its place.

Makes 4 servings

- Preheat broiler, with rack set 4 to 6 inches (10 to 15 cm) from the heat source
- Blender or food processor
- Broiler pan, sprayed with nonstick cooking spray (preferably olive oil)

½ cup	packed fresh basil leaves	125 mL
½ cup	packed fresh flat-leaf (Italian) parsley leaves	125 mL
3 tbsp	coarsely chopped fresh chives	45 mL
3 tbsp	vegetable stock (see tip)	45 mL
2 tbsp	freshly squeezed lemon juice	30 mL
5 tsp	extra virgin olive oil, divided	30 mL
4	skin-on black cod (sablefish) fillets (each about 5 oz/150 g and 1 inch/ 2.5 cm thick)	4
¼ tsp	fine sea salt	1 mL

1. In blender, combine basil, parsley, chives, stock, lemon juice and 3 tsp (15 mL) oil; purée until smooth. Set aside.

2. Place fish, skin side down, on prepared pan. Brush with the remaining oil and sprinkle with salt. Broil for 6 to 8 minutes or until fish is opaque and flakes easily when tested with a fork. Serve with sauce spooned over top.

Nutrients per serving

Calories	173	Vitamin C	17 mg
Fat	7 g	Vitamin E	3 IU
Carbohydrate	1 g	Folate	29 µg
Fiber	0 g	Vitamin B$_6$	0.4 mg
Sugar	0 g	Vitamin B$_{12}$	1.3 µg
Protein	26 g	Magnesium	54 mg

White Fish with Mediterranean Flavors

This recipe courtesy of Isla Horvath.

The Mediterranean diet is said to be one of the healthiest in the world. Dress your next fish dinner up with the healing ingredients of the region.

Tips

The cooking time will vary depending on the thickness of the fish. The general rule of thumb for fish is 10 minutes per inch (2.5 cm) of thickness.

Cod or any other firm white fish fillets may be used in place of the halibut. To learn more about how to choose sustainable seafood, see tip on page 218.

Nutrients per serving	
Calories	277
Fat	14 g
Carbohydrate	7 g
Fiber	2 g
Sugar	3 g
Protein	25 g
Vitamin C	7 mg
Vitamin E	3 IU
Folate	32 µg
Vitamin B$_6$	0.8 mg
Vitamin B$_{12}$	1.6 µg
Magnesium	40 mg

Makes 4 servings

2 tsp	dried basil	10 mL
1 tsp	dried oregano	5 mL
2 tbsp	olive oil, divided	30 mL
	Juice of 1 lemon	
4	skinless halibut steaks (about 1 lb/ 500 g total)	4
¾ cup	finely chopped onion	175 mL
2	cloves garlic, minced	2
¾ cup	chopped plum (Roma) tomatoes	175 mL
½ cup	sliced black olives	125 mL
½ cup	dry white wine	125 mL
½ cup	crumbled feta cheese	125 mL
	Lemon wedges	

1. In a medium shallow dish, combine basil, oregano, 1 tbsp (15 mL) oil and lemon juice. Add halibut, turning to coat both sides. Marinate at room temperature for 5 to 10 minutes.

2. Heat a large nonstick skillet over medium heat. Add halibut and fry for 3 to 4 minutes per side or until browned on both sides. Transfer to a plate and keep warm.

3. Wipe out skillet, add the remaining oil. Add onion and cook, stirring, for 3 to 4 minutes or until softened. Add garlic and cook, stirring, for 30 seconds. Add tomatoes, olives and wine; boil, stirring, until wine is slightly reduced. Return fish to skillet and spoon sauce over top; reduce heat and simmer for 1 to 2 minutes or until fish is opaque and flakes easily when tested with a fork.

4. Place each steak on a plate and drizzle sauce evenly over top. Sprinkle evenly with feta cheese and garnish with lemon wedges.

Variation

Use pimento-stuffed green olives instead of black olives.

Grilled Salmon with Mustard Maple Vinaigrette

With a nod to the Pacific Northwest, this super-quick mustard and maple glaze keeps the salmon fillets incredibly moist. A peppery bed of fresh watercress balances and brightens the dish.

Tips

Instead of buying aerosol cans of cooking spray, you can buy a pump oil sprayer and use any oil you like.

According to the Monterey Bay Aquarium Seafood Watch, some of the best choices for wild salmon are those caught in Alaska, British Columbia, California, Oregon and Washington. Compared with salmon caught in other regions, these options are abundant, well managed and caught in an environmentally friendly way.

To decrease your carcinogen exposure when barbecuing, keep the flame low to prevent it from touching the fillet. In addition, clean your barbecue rack well before each use to reduce the buildup of carcinogens. Finally, marinate your meats for at least 5 minutes before cooking. You can make extra dressing from this recipe to use as a marinade.

Makes 4 servings

- Preheat barbecue grill to medium-high

1 tbsp	apple cider vinegar	15 mL
1 tbsp	pure maple syrup	15 mL
1 tbsp	extra virgin olive oil	15 mL
2 tsp	whole-grain Dijon mustard	10 mL
4	skinless wild salmon fillets (each about 5 oz/150 g)	4
	Nonstick cooking spray (preferably olive oil)	
1/4 tsp	fine sea salt	1 mL
1/4 tsp	freshly cracked black pepper	1 mL
4 cups	packed watercress sprigs	1 L

1. In a small bowl or cup, whisk together vinegar, maple syrup, oil and mustard. Set aside.

2. Lightly spray both sides of fish with cooking spray, then sprinkle with salt and pepper. Grill on preheated barbecue, turning once, for 3 to 4 minutes per side or until fish is opaque and flakes easily when tested with a fork.

3. Divide watercress among four dinner plates. Top with salmon and drizzle fish and watercress with vinaigrette.

Nutrients per serving			
Calories	302	Vitamin C	15 mg
Fat	16 g	Vitamin E	2 IU
Carbohydrate	5 g	Folate	40 µg
Fiber	0 g	Vitamin B_6	1.2 mg
Sugar	3 g	Vitamin B_{12}	3.9 µg
Protein	33 g	Magnesium	55 mg

Swedish Salmon, Asparagus and Potato Omelet

This is a simplified version of laxpudding (salmon pudding), which is based on the traditional Swedish housewife's firm conviction that a good dinner provides an excellent basis for the next day's lunch. With a little salmon, some eggs and a few potatoes, you can go a long way.

Tip

Other varieties of waxy potatoes, such as purple potatoes, may be used in place of the red-skinned potatoes.

Nutrients per serving

Calories	257
Fat	9 g
Carbohydrate	14 g
Fiber	2 g
Sugar	3 g
Protein	30 g
Vitamin C	25 mg
Vitamin E	2 IU
Folate	56 µg
Vitamin B$_6$	0.4 mg
Vitamin B$_{12}$	5.5 µg
Magnesium	53 mg

Makes 6 servings

- Preheat broiler, with rack set 4 to 6 inches (10 to 15 cm) from the heat source
- Large ovenproof skillet

12 oz	red-skinned potatoes (3 to 4 medium), cut into ½-inch (1 cm) cubes	375 g
8 oz	asparagus, trimmed and cut into ½-inch (1 cm) pieces	250 g
6	large eggs, lightly beaten	6
3	large egg whites, lightly beaten	3
½ tsp	fine sea salt	2 mL
¼ tsp	freshly ground black pepper	1 mL
2 tsp	extra virgin olive oil	10 mL
1	small red bell pepper, chopped	1
1 cup	chopped onion	250 mL
1	can (15 oz/425 g) wild Alaskan salmon, drained and flaked (skin removed, if necessary)	1
3 tbsp	chopped fresh dill	45 mL

1. Place potatoes in a medium saucepan and cover with cold water. Bring to a boil over medium-high heat. Boil for about 7 minutes or until just tender. Add asparagus and cook for 30 seconds. Drain and set aside.

2. In a medium bowl, whisk together eggs, egg whites, salt and pepper. Set aside.

3. In ovenproof skillet, heat oil over medium-high heat. Add red pepper and onion; cook, stirring, for 6 to 8 minutes or until softened. Add potato mixture and cook, stirring, for 5 minutes. Add salmon and dill; cook, stirring, for 1 minute.

4. Pour in egg mixture, reduce heat to low and cook, stirring occasionally, for about 5 minutes or until eggs begin to set but are still wet on top. Cook, without stirring, for 5 minutes.

5. Place skillet under the preheated broiler and broil for 2 to 3 minutes or until golden and set at center. Let cool for at least 15 minutes before serving.

Mediterranean Quinoa-Stuffed Chicken Breasts

Phase 3

Dress up your chicken with the healing ingredients of the Mediterranean. Quinoa adds a great source of fiber to round off this healthy dish.

Tip

Make sure to use fine sea salt in the water you use to cook the quinoa. Conventional table salt contains chemicals and additives, whereas sea salt contains an abundance of naturally occurring trace minerals.

Makes 4 servings

- Large ovenproof skillet
- Toothpicks

¼ cup	white, red or black quinoa, rinsed	60 mL
2	cloves garlic, minced	2
2 tbsp	chopped fresh flat-leaf (Italian) parsley	30 mL
1 tsp	dried oregano	5 mL
3 tbsp	chopped drained oil-packed sun-dried tomatoes	45 mL
2 tbsp	chopped pitted brine-cured black olives (such as kalamata)	30 mL
2 tbsp	crumbled feta cheese	30 mL
2 tbsp	olive oil, divided	30 mL
	Fine sea salt and freshly cracked black pepper	
4	boneless skinless chicken breasts (each about 6 oz/175 g)	4

1. In a small saucepan of boiling salted water, cook quinoa for 9 minutes. Drain and rinse under cold water until cool. Transfer to a medium bowl and add garlic, parsley, oregano, tomatoes, olives, feta and half the oil, gently stirring to combine. Season to taste with salt and pepper.

2. Preheat oven to 400°F (200°C).

3. Place a chicken breast between two sheets of plastic wrap. Using a kitchen mallet or rolling pin, pound to ¼-inch (0.5 cm) thickness. Repeat with the remaining breasts.

4. Spread quinoa mixture over chicken breasts, dividing evenly. Starting at a long side, roll up like a jelly roll and secure with toothpicks. Sprinkle chicken with salt and pepper.

5. In ovenproof skillet, heat the remaining oil over medium-high heat. Add chicken and cook for 5 to 6 minutes or until browned on the bottom. Turn chicken over (browned side up). Place skillet in oven and bake for 4 to 6 minutes or until chicken is no longer pink inside.

Nutrients per serving	
Calories	324
Fat	14 g
Carbohydrate	9 g
Fiber	1 g
Sugar	0 g
Protein	39 g
Vitamin C	10 mg
Vitamin E	3 IU
Folate	33 µg
Vitamin B$_6$	1.4 mg
Vitamin B$_{12}$	0.4 µg
Magnesium	72 mg

Herbed Chicken and Pomegranate Salad

Phase 3

This stellar salad relies on varied tastes and textures — nutty quinoa, succulent roast chicken, aromatic fresh herbs, tart, crunchy pomegranate seeds and rich, slightly sweet pine nuts — to impress one and all.

Tip

To remove pomegranate seeds from the fruit, score the pomegranate around the circumference and place it in a large bowl of water. Break the pomegranate open underwater to free the white seed sacs. The seeds will sink to the bottom of the bowl, and the membrane will float to the top. Strain out the seeds and put them in a separate bowl. You can refrigerate or freeze any remaining seeds for another use.

Makes 4 servings

3 cups	cooked quinoa, cooled	750 mL
2 cups	shredded rotisserie, grilled or poached chicken breast	500 mL
1 cup	pomegranate seeds	250 mL
2 tsp	finely grated lime zest	10 mL
2 tbsp	freshly squeezed lime juice	30 mL
2 tbsp	extra virgin olive oil	30 mL
1 tbsp	liquid honey	15 mL
	Fine sea salt and freshly cracked black pepper	
¼ cup	packed fresh mint leaves, chopped	60 mL
¼ cup	packed fresh cilantro leaves, chopped	60 mL
⅓ cup	toasted pine nuts or sliced almonds	75 mL

1. In a large bowl, combine quinoa, chicken and pomegranate seeds.

2. In a small bowl, whisk together lime zest, lime juice, oil and honey. Add to quinoa mixture and gently toss to coat. Season to taste with salt and pepper. Cover and refrigerate for at least 30 minutes, until chilled, or for up to 4 hours.

3. Just before serving, add mint and cilantro, gently tossing to combine. Sprinkle with pine nuts.

Healing Help

For easier digestion, soak the quinoa overnight, rinse and then cook.

Nutrients per serving

Calories	419	Vitamin C	11 mg
Fat	13 g	Vitamin E	4 IU
Carbohydrate	48 g	Folate	89 µg
Fiber	7 g	Vitamin B_6	0.7 mg
Sugar	14 g	Vitamin B_{12}	0.2 µg
Protein	29 g	Magnesium	118 mg

Japanese Sesame Chicken Skewers

Phase 3

Makes 4 servings

A riff on a Japanese classic, this easy, healthy version of chicken teriyaki gets a boost of fresh flavor and bold red color from red peppers. A quick spell on the grill does more than just enhance the flavor of a bell pepper — it also releases the beta-carotene, a potent antioxidant, from the pepper's fiber cells

Tips

If desired, you can use coconut amino acids in place of the tamari.

To toast sesame seeds, place up to 3 tbsp (45 mL) seeds in a medium skillet set over medium heat. Cook, shaking the skillet, for 3 to 5 minutes or until seeds are golden brown and fragrant. Let cool completely before use.

- Six 10-inch (25 cm) metal skewers, or wooden skewers soaked in warm water for 30 minutes

1 tbsp	minced gingerroot	15 mL
1/4 cup	mirin or sherry	60 mL
1/4 cup	reduced-sodium tamari	60 mL
1 tsp	toasted sesame oil	5 mL
1 lb	boneless skinless chicken breasts, cut into 1-inch (2.5 cm) strips	500 g
1	large red bell pepper, cut into 1-inch (2.5 cm) pieces	1
2 tbsp	toasted sesame seeds (see tip)	30 mL

1. In a large bowl, whisk together ginger, mirin, tamari and sesame oil. Add chicken and toss to coat. Let stand for 15 minutes.

2. Meanwhile, preheat barbecue grill to medium-high.

3. Remove chicken from marinade, reserving marinade. Alternately thread chicken and red pepper onto skewers.

4. In a small saucepan, bring reserved marinade to a boil over medium-high heat. Boil until reduced by about half. Brush skewers with marinade.

5. Grill skewers for 3 to 5 minutes per side, brushing occasionally with marinade, until chicken is no longer pink inside. Serve sprinkled with sesame seeds.

Nutrients per serving			
Calories	221	Vitamin C	39 mg
Fat	6 g	Vitamin E	1 IU
Carbohydrate	12 g	Folate	26 µg
Fiber	1 g	Vitamin B_6	1.0 mg
Sugar	6 g	Vitamin B_{12}	0.2 µg
Protein	27 g	Magnesium	57 mg

Roasted Pork Tenderloin with Pear Slaw

This dish turns basic pork into a healing culinary masterpiece. Pears are a sweet complement to pork's rich, meaty flavor. Pears contain vitamin C, potassium, a good amount of fiber and antioxidants with anticancer and antibacterial properties.

Makes 4 servings

- Preheat oven to 400°F (200°C)
- Large ovenproof skillet

½ tsp	fine sea salt, divided	2 mL
½ tsp	freshly ground black pepper, divided	2 mL
2 tbsp	apple cider vinegar	30 mL
4 tsp	extra virgin olive oil, divided	20 mL
1 tbsp	liquid honey	15 mL
1 tsp	Dijon mustard	5 mL
1	firm-ripe Bosc pear, cut into very thin wedges	1
4 cups	thinly sliced napa cabbage	1 L
½ cup	thinly sliced green onions	125 mL
1 lb	pork tenderloin, trimmed	500 g

1. In a large bowl, whisk together half the salt, half the pepper, vinegar, half the oil, honey and mustard. Add pear, cabbage and green onions, gently tossing to combine. Set aside.

2. Sprinkle pork with the remaining salt and pepper. In ovenproof skillet, heat the remaining oil over medium-high heat. Add pork and cook, turning several times, for 3 to 4 minutes or until browned all over.

3. Transfer skillet to preheated oven and roast for 12 to 14 minutes or until an instant-read thermometer inserted in the thickest part of the tenderloin registers 145°F (63°C) for medium-rare, or until desired doneness. Let rest for at least 5 minutes before slicing. Serve with slaw.

Nutrients per serving	
Calories	240
Fat	9 g
Carbohydrate	16 g
Fiber	3 g
Sugar	10 g
Protein	25 g
Vitamin C	28 mg
Vitamin E	2 IU
Folate	11 µg
Vitamin B_6	0.9 mg
Vitamin B_{12}	0.6 µg
Magnesium	37 mg

Beef and Quinoa Soup

This hearty, rich soup is a meal in a bowl. Prepare it in the slow cooker (see variation) for a hot, nutritious meal ready to eat when you get home from a long day at work.

Tips

Make sure to choose a gluten-free beef broth.

Look for organic tomatoes in BPA-free cans.

Browning the beef in small batches before adding the broth results in a richer beef flavor.

This recipe can be halved or quartered.

This soup can be divided into 2-cup (500 mL) portions and frozen for up to 1 month. Reheat in the microwave on High for 5 to 7 minutes or until steaming.

Nutrients per serving

Calories	178
Fat	11 g
Carbohydrate	8 g
Fiber	1 g
Sugar	3 g
Protein	12 g
Vitamin C	7 mg
Vitamin E	1 IU
Folate	19 µg
Vitamin B$_6$	0.3 mg
Vitamin B$_{12}$	1.5 µg
Magnesium	26 mg

Makes 14 servings

2 tbsp	extra virgin olive oil (approx.)	30 mL
1½ lbs	stewing beef, cut into ¾-inch (2 cm) cubes	750 g
1	large onion, coarsely chopped	1
4 cups	ready-to-use beef broth (see tip)	1 L
3	carrots, coarsely chopped	3
2	stalks celery, coarsely chopped	2
¼ cup	quinoa, rinsed	60 mL
1	can (28 oz/796 mL) diced tomatoes, with juice	1
1 tbsp	snipped fresh thyme	15 mL
	Fine sea salt and freshly ground black pepper	

1. In a large saucepan, heat 1 tbsp (15 mL) oil over medium heat. Working in small batches, add beef and onion; cook, stirring, for 20 minutes or until beef is browned on all sides, adding oil as needed between batches. Transfer each batch to a plate lined with paper towels as completed. Drain off fat.

2. Add broth and scrape up any brown bits from bottom of pan. Return the beef mixture to the pan. Reduce heat to low and simmer for 35 minutes or until beef is tender.

3. Add carrots, celery and quinoa; simmer for 30 minutes or until vegetables are tender and quinoa is transparent and the tiny, spiral-like germ is separated.

4. Add tomatoes and thyme, increase heat to medium-high and heat until steaming. Season to taste with salt and pepper.

Variations

To make this recipe more alkaline, add more vegetables and greens, such as kale or collard greens.

After step 1, transfer beef mixture to the stoneware of a large slow cooker (minimum 5 quarts). Add broth, carrots, celery, tomatoes and thyme. Cover and cook on Low for 8 to 10 hours. Meanwhile, cook quinoa. Fifteen minutes before you're ready to serve, add the quinoa to the slow cooker.

Persian Ground Beef Kebabs

Phase 3

Makes 4 servings

These Persian-inspired kebabs make a delicious change of pace from the usual ground beef dishes. The combination of spices and herbs — vitamin C–packed cilantro and mint — is nothing short of addictive.

Tips

The kebabs can be broiled instead of grilled. Preheat broiler and place kebabs on a broiler tray sprayed with nonstick cooking spray. Broil for 6 to 10 minutes, turning once halfway through, until no longer pink inside.

To decrease your carcinogen exposure when barbecuing, keep the flame low to prevent it from touching the meat. In addition, clean your barbecue rack well before each use to reduce the buildup of carcinogens.

- Preheat barbecue grill to medium-high
- Eight 10-inch (25 cm) metal skewers, or wooden skewers soaked in warm water for 30 minutes

1 lb	extra-lean ground beef	500 g
1	large egg	1
⅔ cup	grated onion	150 mL
⅔ cup	packed fresh cilantro leaves, chopped	150 mL
⅓ cup	packed fresh mint leaves, chopped	75 mL
1 tsp	ground coriander	5 mL
½ tsp	ground ginger	2 mL
½ tsp	ground cinnamon (see tip, page 192)	2 mL
½ tsp	fine sea salt	2 mL
¼ tsp	freshly ground black pepper	1 mL

1. In a large bowl, gently combine beef, egg, onion, cilantro, mint, coriander, ginger, cinnamon, salt and pepper.

2. Divide meat mixture into 8 portions. Form each portion around a skewer, shaping the meat into a 6- by 1-inch (15 by 2.5 cm) cylinder around the skewer.

3. Grill kebabs on preheated barbecue, turning once or twice, for 6 to 10 minutes or until no longer pink inside.

Nutrients per serving	
Calories	189
Fat	7 g
Carbohydrate	4 g
Fiber	1 g
Sugar	1 g
Protein	26 g
Vitamin C	3 mg
Vitamin E	1 IU
Folate	19 µg
Vitamin B_6	0.5 mg
Vitamin B_{12}	2.7 µg
Magnesium	33 mg

Bison Stew with Kumquats

Bison seems to be the new meat of choice, and it's no wonder, as it is delicious, lean and has a healthier fatty acid profile than conventionally raised beef. All in all, it's a nutritious anti-inflammatory choice!

- Preheat oven to 300°F (150°C)

2¾ lbs	bison cubes, cut from the shoulder (each 2 oz/60 g)	1.375 kg
7 oz	pork belly (uncured)	210 g
5 oz	bison or veal fat (around the kidneys)	150 g
8	cloves garlic	8
1	bay leaf	1
2	whole cloves	2
3	dried orange peels	3
7 oz	kumquats	210 g
4 cups	red wine	1 L
	Fine sea salt and freshly ground black pepper	

1. Place bison, pork, bison fat, garlic, bay leaf, cloves, orange peels and kumquats in a stoneware casserole, an ovenproof stockpot or a Dutch oven with a recessed lid that has a small hole. Cover with red wine. Season with salt and pepper.

2. Place lid on pot, upside down, and fill with ½ cup (125 mL) water. Cook in preheated oven for 2 to 3 hours, making sure there is always water in the upside-down lid during the entire cooking process. Note that none of the ingredients are browned and no vegetables are added to the stew.

Variations

Instead of bison, use muskox, caribou, deer, moose, grass-fed beef or veal.

If kumquats are not in season, substitute black olives.

A pig's trotter can be added, if desired.

Nutrients per serving	
Calories	383
Fat	19 g
Carbohydrate	11 g
Fiber	2 g
Sugar	2 g
Protein	26 g
Vitamin C	15 mg
Vitamin E	0 IU
Folate	5 µg
Vitamin B_6	0.6 mg
Vitamin B_{12}	2.5 µg
Magnesium	44 mg

Side Dishes

Blended Vegetable Soup

This is a great side dish or main meal, especially if you have trouble digesting your foods. The blending virtually predigests the vegetables.

Tips

For the protein powder, we recommend using grass-fed hydrolyzed collagen powder or collagen peptides, which are easily digested. A reputable brand that is easy to find is Great Lakes collagen hydrolysate.

This soup is best served hot. If necessary after step 2, transfer it to a small saucepan and heat over medium heat until steaming.

Makes 2 servings

- Steamer basket
- Blender or food processor

2	green onions (green part only)	2
1	carrot, cut into 1-inch (2.5 cm) thick slices	1
1 cup	cubed rutabaga (1-inch/2.5 cm cubes)	250 mL
½ cup	broccoli florets	125 mL
½ cup	sliced zucchini (2-inch/5 cm thick slices)	125 mL
1	small (3- to 4-inch/7.5 to 10 cm) cucumber, peeled and seeded	1
¼ cup	protein powder (see tip)	60 mL

1. In a steamer basket placed over boiling water, steam green onions, carrot and rutabaga for 10 minutes. Add broccoli and zucchini; steam for 5 to 10 minutes or until vegetables are very tender.

2. Transfer all steamed vegetables to the blender and add cucumber. Blend on high for 1 minute. Add protein powder and blend on high for 1 to 2 minutes or until smooth and creamy (see tip).

Nutrients per serving	
Calories	123
Fat	1 g
Carbohydrate	13 g
Fiber	4 g
Sugar	7 g
Protein	19 g
Vitamin C	44 mg
Vitamin E	1 IU
Folate	54 µg
Vitamin B_6	0.2 mg
Vitamin B_{12}	0.0 µg
Magnesium	40 mg

Roasted Vegetables

These roasted veggies go great with almost anything. Enjoy the beautiful colors and natural sweetness of nature's root vegetables!

Tip

Cut up a large amount of root vegetables and store them in airtight containers in the fridge for later use; they'll stay fresh for about 3 to 4 days.

- Preheat oven to 350°F (180°C)
- 12-cup (3 L) casserole dish with lid

4	carrots, cut into $\frac{1}{2}$-inch (1 cm) thick slices	4
1	small red beet, cut into 1-inch (2.5 cm) cubes	1
2 cups	cubed butternut squash (1-inch/ 2.5 cm cubes)	500 mL
2 cups	cubed rutabaga (1-inch/2.5 cm cubes)	500 mL
2 tbsp	Basic Ghee (page 190)	30 mL

1. In casserole dish, combine carrots, beet, squash and rutabaga. Dot with ghee.

2. Cover and bake in preheated oven for 20 minutes. Remove lid and stir. Bake, uncovered, for 30 minutes or until all vegetables are fork-tender.

Nutrients per serving	
Calories	156
Fat	7 g
Carbohydrate	22 g
Fiber	5 g
Sugar	10 g
Protein	2 g
Vitamin C	37 mg
Vitamin E	2 IU
Folate	68 µg
Vitamin B_6	0.3 mg
Vitamin B_{12}	0.0 µg
Magnesium	52 mg

Sautéed Kale

Transform this superfood into a mouthwatering side dish your friends and family will beg for at meals. It's easy to make and chock-full of healing nutrients.

Tip

Natural salt contains over 50 minerals, which are all important for balancing blood pressure and other bodily functions. Table salt has been chemically stripped of all its natural minerals, except sodium and chloride, by the use of harsh chemicals. Table salt also contains additives that have been shown to be toxic to human health. We recommend using sea salt (look at the ingredients to ensure that the only ingredient is "sea salt").

Makes 2 servings

Amount	Ingredient	Metric
3 tbsp	Basic Ghee (page 190)	45 mL
¼ tsp	fine sea salt	1 mL
4 cups	trimmed kale leaves	1 L
2 tbsp	water (if needed)	30 mL
1 tsp	sesame seeds	5 mL

1. In a large skillet, melt ghee over medium heat. Stir in salt. Stir in kale until evenly coated with ghee. Reduce heat to low, cover and cook, stirring occasionally, for 10 minutes, until very tender. If kale starts to stick, stir in water.

2. Remove from heat and sprinkle with sesame seeds.

Nutrients per serving

Calories	271
Fat	23 g
Carbohydrate	14 g
Fiber	3 g
Sugar	0 g
Protein	5 g
Vitamin C	161 mg
Vitamin E	1 IU
Folate	40 µg
Vitamin B$_6$	0.4 mg
Vitamin B$_{12}$	0.0 µg
Magnesium	51 mg

Carrot Chips

Strengthen your eyesight and your immune system with this healthy alternative to french fries. These crunchy treats take just minutes to prepare! They make a great side for a burger or wrap.

Makes 2 servings

- Preheat oven to 350°F (180°C)
- Rimmed baking sheet

4	large carrots, cut into ¼-inch (0.5 cm) thick rounds	4
2 tbsp	virgin coconut oil	30 mL
	Fine sea salt	

1. Arrange carrots in a single layer on baking sheet. Dot or drizzle with coconut oil.

2. Bake in preheated oven for 5 minutes. Remove from oven and toss carrots with coconut oil until evenly coated. Sprinkle with salt. Return to oven and bake for 7 minutes or until tender inside and crisp outside.

Nutrients per serving	
Calories	176
Fat	14 g
Carbohydrate	14 g
Fiber	4 g
Sugar	7 g
Protein	1 g
Vitamin C	9 mg
Vitamin E	1 IU
Folate	27 µg
Vitamin B_6	0.2 mg
Vitamin B_{12}	0.0 µg
Magnesium	17 mg

Carrot Mash

A sweet treat to pair with any meat! Add to a protein-packed breakfast or as a colorful side at dinner.

Tip

Choose Ceylon cinnamon (also called real cinnamon), not cassia cinnamon. Cassia contains much higher amounts of a compound called coumarin, which in higher doses can contribute to liver damage. Ceylon cinnamon contains only trace amounts of coumarin.

Makes 4 servings

- Steamer basket
- Blender or food processor

4	large carrots, each cut into 4 pieces	4
1 tsp	ground cinnamon (see tip)	5 mL
½ tsp	fine sea salt	2 mL
1 tbsp	virgin coconut oil	15 mL

1. In a steamer set over boiling water, steam carrots for about 10 minutes or until soft.

2. Transfer carrots to the blender and add cinnamon, salt and coconut oil. Purée until smooth.

Nutrients per serving	
Calories	61
Fat	4 g
Carbohydrate	7 g
Fiber	2 g
Sugar	3 g
Protein	1 g
Vitamin C	4 mg
Vitamin E	1 IU
Folate	14 µg
Vitamin B_6	0.1 mg
Vitamin B_{12}	0.0 µg
Magnesium	9 mg

Rutabaga Mash

Say goodbye to boring old mashed potatoes and hello to a delicious new mash. Rutabagas have a hint of spiciness and a texture similar to carrots. Plus, they are rich in nutrients that enhance detoxification.

Tip

It is best to use filtered water to avoid ingestion of chlorine and other contaminants. Chlorine can be irritating to your gut and add to your toxic load.

Makes 2 servings

- High-power blender or food processor

2 cups	cubed rutabaga (1-inch/2.5 cm cubes)	500 mL
2 tbsp	Garlic-Infused Ghee (page 191)	30 mL
2	green onions (green part only), finely chopped	2
½ tsp	fine sea salt	2 mL

1. In a large pot of boiling water (see tip), boil rutabaga for 10 to 15 minutes or until fork-tender. Drain and set aside.

2. In a small saucepan, melt ghee over medium heat. Add green onions and cook, stirring, for 5 minutes.

3. In blender, combine rutabagas, ghee mixture and salt; blend on high for 1 to 2 minutes or until creamy.

Nutrients per serving	
Calories	182
Fat	14 g
Carbohydrate	12 g
Fiber	4 g
Sugar	8 g
Protein	2 g
Vitamin C	36 mg
Vitamin E	1 IU
Folate	33 µg
Vitamin B_6	0.1 mg
Vitamin B_{12}	0.0 µg
Magnesium	33 mg

Baked Acorn Squash

"Yum, yum!" is the typical response after sampling this side dish. It is so tasty, it can even be served as dessert, scooped right out of its natural bowl!

Tips

If you don't have a casserole dish with a lid, you can use a large glass baking dish and cover it with foil.

It is best to use filtered water to avoid ingestion of chlorine and other contaminants. Chlorine can be irritating to your gut and add to your toxic load.

Makes 4 servings

- Preheat oven to 350°F (180°C)
- 12-cup (3 L) deep casserole dish with lid (see tip)

1	acorn squash (3 to 4 lbs/1.5 to 2 kg), halved and seeded	1
4 tbsp	Anti-Inflammatory Ghee (page 192) or virgin coconut oil, divided	60 mL
10	drops liquid stevia extract, divided	10
	Fine sea salt	
	Ground Ceylon cinnamon (optional)	

1. Add ½ inch (1 cm) of water to casserole dish. Place squash halves, skin side down, in dish. Add 2 tbsp (30 mL) ghee and 5 drops stevia to the indentation in each squash and sprinkle with salt.

2. Cover and bake in preheated oven for 45 to 60 minutes or until squash is fork-tender. Sprinkle with cinnamon, if desired. Cut each half into 2 pieces to serve.

Nutrients per serving	
Calories	223
Fat	14 g
Carbohydrate	24 g
Fiber	10 g
Sugar	0 g
Protein	2 g
Vitamin C	25 mg
Vitamin E	1 IU
Folate	39 µg
Vitamin B$_6$	0.4 mg
Vitamin B$_{12}$	0.0 µg
Magnesium	73 mg

Cinnamon-Roasted Kabocha Squash and Carrots

Phase 1

This dish is so tasty you could almost serve it for dessert! It goes great with meats and fish.

Tips

Cut up a large amount of the vegetables and store them in airtight containers in the fridge for later use; they'll stay fresh for about 3 to 4 days.

Choose Ceylon cinnamon (also called real cinnamon), not cassia cinnamon. Cassia contains much higher amounts of a compound called coumarin, which in higher doses can contribute to liver damage. Ceylon cinnamon contains only trace amounts of coumarin.

Makes 2 servings

- Preheat oven to 350°F (180°C)
- Glass baking dish

1½ cups	chopped carrots (1-inch/ 2.5 cm pieces)	375 mL
½ cup	cubed kabocha squash (1-inch/ 2.5 cm cubes)	125 mL
3 tbsp	Anti-Inflammatory Ghee (page 192)	45 mL
1 tsp	ground cinnamon (see tip)	5 mL

1. Place carrots and squash in baking dish. Dot vegetables with ghee and sprinkle evenly with cinnamon.

2. Bake in preheated oven for 15 minutes. Stir vegetables to coat evenly with ghee. Bake for 30 minutes or until vegetables are fork-tender.

Nutrients per serving	
Calories	242
Fat	21 g
Carbohydrate	11 g
Fiber	4 g
Sugar	5 g
Protein	1 g
Vitamin C	11 mg
Vitamin E	2 IU
Folate	27 µg
Vitamin B$_6$	0.2 mg
Vitamin B$_{12}$	0.0 µg
Magnesium	17 mg

Spaghetti Squash Noodles

This is a great alternative to pasta, and is filling and easy to make. Spaghetti squash has a mild flavor that is easily enhanced by herbs and spices.

Tips

If you don't have a casserole dish with a lid, you can use a large glass baking dish and cover it with foil.

It is best to use filtered water to avoid ingestion of chlorine and other contaminants. Chlorine can be irritating to your gut and add to your toxic load.

Makes 6 servings

- Preheat oven to 350°F (180°C)
- 12-cup (3 L) deep casserole dish with lid (see tip)

1	spaghetti squash (5 to 7 lbs/2.5 to 3.5 kg), halved lengthwise and seeded	1
2 tsp	Garlic-Infused Ghee (page 191), melted	10 mL
1/2 tsp	fine sea salt	2 mL
1/2 tsp	freshly ground black pepper	2 mL

1. Add 1/2 inch (1 cm) of water (see tip) to casserole dish. Place squash halves, skin side down, in dish and brush squash flesh with ghee.

2. Cover and bake in preheated oven for 45 to 60 minutes or until squash is fork-tender. Let squash cool for 10 to 15 minutes, until cool enough to handle, then use a fork to gently scrape the flesh away from the skin in long, spaghetti-like strands. Season with salt and pepper.

Nutrients per serving	
Calories	132
Fat	4 g
Carbohydrate	26 g
Fiber	5 g
Sugar	10 g
Protein	2 g
Vitamin C	8 mg
Vitamin E	0 IU
Folate	45 µg
Vitamin B$_6$	0.4 mg
Vitamin B$_{12}$	0.0 µg
Magnesium	46 mg

Sautéed Bell Pepper and Eggplant

Phase 2

Makes 2 servings

This beautiful, tasty dish is sure to become a family favorite. It's perfect with fish and poultry.

Tip

Natural salt contains over 50 minerals, which are all important for balancing blood pressure and other bodily functions. Table salt has been chemically stripped of all its natural minerals, except sodium and chloride, by the use of harsh chemicals. Table salt also contains additives that have been shown to be toxic to human health. We recommend using sea salt (look at the ingredients to ensure that the only ingredient is "sea salt").

1	medium eggplant, cubed	1
¼ tsp	fine sea salt	1 mL
3 tbsp	Garlic-Infused Ghee (page 191)	45 mL
1	red bell pepper, sliced	1
1 tsp	ground cumin	5 mL
	Freshly ground black pepper	

1. In a large bowl, toss eggplant with salt. Let stand for 30 minutes, then pat dry with a paper towel.

2. In a large skillet, melt ghee over medium heat. Add eggplant, red pepper and cumin; cook, stirring, for 8 to 10 minutes or until tender. Season with pepper and serve hot.

Nutrients per serving	
Calories	284
Fat	22 g
Carbohydrate	20 g
Fiber	11 g
Sugar	9 g
Protein	4 g
Vitamin C	82 mg
Vitamin E	3 IU
Folate	88 µg
Vitamin B$_6$	0.4 mg
Vitamin B$_{12}$	0.0 µg
Magnesium	46 mg

Lemon Rosemary Glazed Parsnips

Parsnips are a tasty, high-fiber root vegetable. Dressed up with rosemary, coconut and lemon, they are sure to be a household favorite.

Tip

The rosemary can be replaced with 1 tbsp (15 mL) chopped tender-leaf herbs, such as cilantro, mint, basil or parsley.

1 cup	coconut water or water	250 mL
2 tbsp	virgin coconut oil	30 mL
1½ tbsp	coconut sugar or coconut nectar	22 mL
½ tsp	fine sea salt	2 mL
1¼ lbs	parsnips (about 8 medium), cut into ¼-inch (0.5 cm) thick slices	625 g
1½ tsp	minced fresh rosemary leaves	7 mL
1 tsp	freshly squeezed lemon juice	5 mL

1. In a large skillet, combine coconut water, coconut oil, coconut nectar and salt. Bring to a boil over medium-high heat, stirring occasionally. Add parsnips, reduce heat to medium, cover and boil gently for 10 to 12 minutes or until just tender. Using a slotted spoon, transfer parsnips to a dish.

2. Add rosemary to skillet, increase heat to medium-high and return cooking liquid to a boil. Boil, stirring occasionally, until reduced to a glaze (about 2 tbsp/30 mL). Return parsnips to the pan, reduce heat and simmer, stirring, until heated through and coated with glaze. Stir in lemon juice.

Variation

Substitute carrots for the parsnips, or use a combination.

Nutrients per serving	
Calories	131
Fat	5 g
Carbohydrate	22 g
Fiber	5 g
Sugar	9 g
Protein	1 g
Vitamin C	18 mg
Vitamin E	2 IU
Folate	65 µg
Vitamin B$_6$	0.1 mg
Vitamin B$_{12}$	0.0 µg
Magnesium	38 mg

Radish and Cucumber Salad

Phase 2

Radishes and cucumbers are highly detoxifying. They also taste great together, combined with the lemon, tarragon and chives in this dish.

2 tsp	minced fresh tarragon	10 mL
¼ tsp	fine sea salt	1 mL
2 tbsp	melted virgin coconut oil	30 mL
1 tbsp	freshly squeezed lemon juice	15 mL
1	large English cucumber, peeled and sliced	1
1 cup	thinly sliced (crosswise) red radishes	250 mL
3 tbsp	chopped fresh chives	45 mL

1. In a small bowl, whisk together tarragon, salt, coconut oil and lemon juice.

2. In a large bowl, combine cucumber, radishes and chives. Add dressing and gently toss to coat.

Tips

You can replace the fresh tarragon with 1 tsp (5 mL) dried.

A large field cucumber can be used in place of the English cucumber. Peel the cucumber, slice it in half lengthwise and scrape out the seeds with a spoon before slicing crosswise.

An equal amount of finely chopped green onions can be used in place of the chives.

Nutrients per serving	
Calories	74
Fat	7 g
Carbohydrate	3 g
Fiber	1 g
Sugar	2 g
Protein	1 g
Vitamin C	9 mg
Vitamin E	0 IU
Folate	20 µg
Vitamin B$_6$	0.1 mg
Vitamin B$_{12}$	0.0 µg
Magnesium	13 mg

Lentil-Stuffed Tomatoes

Makes 4 servings

- Preheat oven to 400°F (200°C)
- 6- or 12-cup muffin pan

4	firm tomatoes	4
1/4 cup	finely chopped celery	60 mL
1 tbsp	finely chopped onion	15 mL
1 tbsp	finely chopped green bell pepper	15 mL
1/2 tsp	curry powder	2 mL
1 cup	rinsed drained canned brown lentils	250 mL
1 tbsp	freshly grated Parmesan cheese	15 mL

1. Core tomatoes and cut a thin slice from the top of each. Scoop pulp and juice into a skillet and mash pulp. Place tomato shells cut side down on a paper towel to drain.

2. Add celery, onion, green pepper and curry powder to tomato pulp and juice. Cook, stirring, over medium heat for about 5 minutes or until vegetables are tender. Add lentils and cook, stirring, until mixture is thickened.

3. Spoon lentil mixture into tomato shells. Sprinkle with Parmesan. Place stuffed tomatoes in 4 muffin cups. Set muffin pan on a baking sheet.

4. Bake in preheated oven for 10 minutes or until heated through.

Healing Help
For easier digestion, use 1/2 cup (125 mL) dried brown lentils; soak them overnight, rinse and then cook them before adding them in step 2.

Nutrients per serving

Calories	81
Fat	1 g
Carbohydrate	14 g
Fiber	6 g
Sugar	5 g
Protein	6 g
Vitamin C	19 mg
Vitamin E	1 IU
Folate	22 µg
Vitamin B$_6$	0.1 mg
Vitamin B$_{12}$	0.0 µg
Magnesium	16 mg

Beet Soup with Lemongrass and Lime

This Thai-inspired soup, which is served cold, is elegant and refreshing. Its jewel-like appearance and intriguing flavors make it a perfect prelude to any meal.

Tips

Coconut oil's pleasantly nutty taste complements the Thai flavors in this soup. Moreover, in recent years, significant health benefits have been identified in this food.

Use either Basic Vegetable Stock (page 193) or a gluten-free ready-to-use vegetable broth to prepare this soup.

This recipe can be halved, but use a small slow cooker (1½ to 3½ quarts) in that case.

Makes 8 servings

- Medium to large slow cooker (3½ to 5 quarts)
- Food processor, blender or immersion blender

1 tbsp	olive oil or virgin coconut oil	15 mL
1	onion, chopped	1
4	cloves garlic, minced	4
2 tbsp	minced gingerroot	30 mL
2	stalks lemongrass, trimmed, smashed and cut in half crosswise	2
2 tsp	cracked black peppercorns	10 mL
6	beets, peeled and chopped (about 2½ lbs/1.25 kg)	6
6 cups	vegetable stock (see tip)	1.5 L
1	red bell pepper, finely chopped	1
1	long red chile pepper, seeded and minced (optional)	1
	Grated zest and juice of 1 lime	
	Fine sea salt (optional)	
	Coconut cream (optional)	
	Finely chopped fresh cilantro	

1. In a skillet, heat oil over medium heat. Add onion and cook, stirring, until softened, about 3 minutes. Add garlic, ginger, lemongrass and peppercorns and cook, stirring, for 1 minute. Transfer to slow cooker stoneware.

2. Add beets and stock. Cover and cook on Low for 6 to 8 hours or on High for 3 to 4 hours or until beets are tender. Add red pepper and chile pepper (if using). Cover and cook on High for 30 minutes or until peppers are tender. Remove lemongrass and discard.

3. Working in batches, purée soup in food processor. (You can also do this in the stoneware using an immersion blender.) Transfer to a large bowl. Stir in lime zest and juice. Season to taste with salt (if using). Chill thoroughly, preferably overnight.

4. When ready to serve, spoon into individual bowls, drizzle with coconut cream (if using) and garnish with cilantro.

Nutrients per serving	
Calories	79
Fat	2 g
Carbohydrate	15 g
Fiber	4 g
Sugar	7 g
Protein	2 g
Vitamin C	27 mg
Vitamin E	1 IU
Folate	92 µg
Vitamin B$_6$	0.2 mg
Vitamin B$_{12}$	0.0 µg
Magnesium	29 mg

Thai-Style Pumpkin Soup

This soup is both versatile and delicious. It has an exotic combination of flavors and works well as a prelude to a meal. If you prefer a more substantial soup, top each serving with cooked shrimp or scallops.

Tips

For best results, toast and grind cumin seeds yourself. Place in a dry skillet over medium heat and cook, stirring, until fragrant, about 3 minutes. Immediately transfer to a spice grinder or mortar and grind finely.

Use either Basic Vegetable Stock (page 193) or a gluten-free ready-to-use vegetable or chicken broth to prepare this soup.

Check the label to make sure your curry paste does not contain gluten.

Nutrients per serving	
Calories	126
Fat	8 g
Carbohydrate	14 g
Fiber	1 g
Sugar	4 g
Protein	2 g
Vitamin C	13 mg
Vitamin E	2 IU
Folate	28 µg
Vitamin B_6	0.1 mg
Vitamin B_{12}	0.0 µg
Magnesium	31 mg

Makes 8 servings

- Large slow cooker (about 5 quarts)
- Food processor, blender or immersion blender

1 tbsp	olive oil or virgin coconut oil	15 mL
2	onions, finely chopped	2
4	cloves garlic, minced	4
2 tbsp	minced gingerroot	30 mL
1 tsp	cracked black peppercorns	5 mL
2	stalks lemongrass, trimmed, smashed and cut in half crosswise	2
1 tbsp	ground cumin (see tip)	15 mL
6 cups	vegetable stock (see tip), divided	1.5 L
8 cups	cubed peeled pumpkin or other orange squash (2-inch/5 cm cubes)	2 L
1 cup	coconut milk	250 mL
1 tsp	Thai red curry paste	5 mL
	Finely grated zest and juice of 1 lime	
¼ cup	toasted pumpkin seeds (optional)	60 mL
	Cherry tomatoes, halved (optional)	
	Finely chopped cilantro	

1. In a skillet, heat oil over medium heat. Add onions and cook, stirring, until softened, about 3 minutes. Add garlic, ginger, peppercorns, lemongrass and cumin and cook, stirring, for 1 minute. Add 1 cup (250 mL) stock and stir well.

2. Transfer to slow cooker stoneware. Add pumpkin and the remaining stock. Cover and cook on Low for 6 hours or on High for 3 hours, until pumpkin is tender. Skim off 1 tbsp (15 mL) coconut milk. In a small bowl, combine with curry paste and blend well. Add to slow cooker along with the remaining coconut milk and lime zest and juice. Cover and cook on High until heated through, about 20 minutes. Discard lemongrass.

This soup can be partially prepared before it is cooked. Complete step 1. Cover and refrigerate overnight or for up to 2 days. When you're ready to cook, complete the recipe.

This recipe can be halved, but use a small slow cooker (2 to 3½ quarts) in that case.

3. Working in batches, purée soup in food processor. (You can also do this in the stoneware using an immersion blender.) Ladle into bowls, and garnish with pumpkin seeds (if using), tomatoes (if using) and cilantro.

Variation

For added protein, finish the soup with 2 to 3 oz (60 to 90 g) cooked wild shrimp, wild scallops, organic chicken or organic tempeh.

Garlic Soup

Phase 3	Makes 4 to 6 servings

Garlic is nature's antibiotic. This is a great soup to incorporate into your diet on a regular basis to help balance your gut health.

Tips

Sixteen cloves of garlic is about 2 large heads.

If you prefer a less peppery soup, halve the amount of black pepper or replace it with ¼ tsp (1 mL) freshly ground white pepper.

Make sure to choose a gluten-free chicken broth.

• Blender

2 tbsp	extra virgin olive oil or butter	30 mL
16	cloves garlic	16
1	white onion, chopped	1
½ tsp	freshly ground black pepper	2 mL
1	potato, peeled and diced	1
2 cups	ready-to-use chicken broth (see tip)	500 mL
2 cups	water	500 mL
1 tsp	fine sea salt	5 mL
¼ cup	chopped fresh parsley	60 mL

1. In a large saucepan, heat oil over medium heat. Add garlic, onion and pepper; cook, stirring often, until onion is soft and garlic is lightly browned, about 6 minutes. Add potato, broth, water and salt; bring to a boil. Cover, reduce heat to low and simmer until potatoes are soft, about 20 minutes.

2. Transfer to blender in batches and purée on high speed.

3. Return purée to saucepan and simmer until heated through. Stir in parsley. Ladle into bowls.

Nutrients per serving (1 of 6)			
Calories	95	Vitamin C	9 mg
Fat	5 g	Vitamin E	1 IU
Carbohydrate	10 g	Folate	9 µg
Fiber	1 g	Vitamin B_6	0.2 mg
Sugar	2 g	Vitamin B_{12}	0.0 µg
Protein	2 g	Magnesium	11 mg

Gingered Carrot and Coconut Soup

Here, fresh ginger adds gentle heat to a lush soup. Fresh mint and lime juice take the dish from good to grand.

Tips

When puréeing the soup in a food processor or blender, fill the bowl or jug no more than halfway full at a time.

Store the cooled soup in an airtight container in the refrigerator for up to 2 days or in the freezer for up to 6 months. Thaw overnight in the refrigerator or in the microwave using the Defrost function. Warm soup in a medium saucepan over medium-low heat.

Makes 6 servings

- Food processor, blender or immersion blender

1 tbsp	virgin coconut oil	15 mL
1 cup	chopped onion	250 mL
1 lb	carrots, chopped (about 4 cups/1 L)	500 g
1	1-inch (5 cm) piece gingerroot, chopped	1
1 tsp	fine sea salt	5 mL
3½ cups	coconut water	875 mL
1 cup	well-stirred coconut milk (full-fat)	250 mL
1 tbsp	coconut sugar	15 mL
1 tbsp	freshly squeezed lime juice	15 mL
¼ cup	minced fresh mint	60 mL

Suggested Accompaniments

Plain coconut yogurt

Lime wedges

Toasted unsweetened flaked coconut

1. In a large saucepan, melt coconut oil over low heat. Add onions and increase heat to medium-high; cook, stirring, for 5 to 6 minutes or until softened.

2. Stir in carrots, ginger, salt and coconut water; bring to a boil. Reduce heat and simmer, stirring occasionally, for 25 to 30 minutes or until carrots are very soft.

3. Working in batches, transfer soup to food processor (or use immersion blender in pan) and purée until smooth. Return soup to pan (if necessary) and whisk in coconut milk, sugar and lime juice. Warm over medium heat, stirring, for 1 minute.

4. Ladle soup into bowls and sprinkle with mint. Serve with any of the suggested accompaniments, as desired.

Nutrients per serving	
Calories	182
Fat	12 g
Carbohydrate	18 g
Fiber	5 g
Sugar	10 g
Protein	3 g
Vitamin C	12 mg
Vitamin E	1 IU
Folate	32 µg
Vitamin B$_6$	0.2 mg
Vitamin B$_{12}$	0.0 µg
Magnesium	63 mg

Gut-Building Blended Vegetable Soup

Take your gut healing to a new level with this tasty soup. The added gelatin aids in healing the gut, provides protein and gives this soup a smooth, consistent texture.

Tips

Adjust the amount of gelatin powder according to how thick you like your soup. Two tbsp (30 mL) will give it a creamy texture similar to a thin yogurt.

NOW Real Food is a reputable, easy-to-find brand of beef gelatin powder.

This soup is best served hot. If necessary after step 2, transfer it to a small saucepan and heat over medium heat until steaming.

Makes 2 servings

- Steamer basket
- Blender or food processor

1	carrot, cut into 1-inch (2.5 cm) thick slices	1
1	2-inch (5 cm) piece jicama (raw or steamed)	1
1 cup	cubed rutabaga (1-inch/2.5 cm cubes)	250 mL
½ cup	broccoli florets	125 mL
½ cup	sliced zucchini (2-inch/5 cm thick slices)	
2	green onions (green and white parts)	2
1	small (4-inch/10 cm) cucumber, peeled and seeded	1
2 tbsp	beef gelatin powder (see tips)	30 mL

1. In a steamer basket placed over boiling water, steam carrot, jicama (if you prefer cooked) and rutabaga for 10 minutes. Add broccoli and zucchini; steam for 5 to 10 minutes or until vegetables are very tender.

2. Transfer all steamed vegetables to the blender and add green onions, cucumber and jicama (if using raw). Blend on high for 1 minute. Add gelatin powder and blend on high for 1 to 2 minutes or until smooth and creamy (see tip).

Nutrients per serving	
Calories	197
Fat	1 g
Carbohydrate	40 g
Fiber	20 g
Sugar	12 g
Protein	10 g
Vitamin C	108 mg
Vitamin E	3 IU
Folate	83 µg
Vitamin B_6	0.3 mg
Vitamin B_{12}	0.0 µg
Magnesium	71 mg

Mexican Jicama Slaw

Jicama is a refreshing vegetable that tastes like a blend of apple, celery and potato. It feeds the beneficial bacteria in your gut, lowering inflammation and improving your overall health. In this salad, it is mixed with cumin and chili powder for an authentic Mexican experience.

Tips

To peel the jicama, use a sharp chef's knife to cut a small slice from each end, exposing the flesh. Starting from the top, in a downward motion, cut away the dark brown skin around the flesh and discard.

Use a mandoline to slice the jicama approximately ¼ inch (0.5 cm) thick. Then stack the slices on a cutting board and, using a sharp chef's knife, cut into thin, even strips.

Makes 2 servings

- Food processor

¼ cup	extra virgin olive oil	60 mL
3 tbsp	freshly squeezed lime juice	45 mL
1 tsp	chili powder	5 mL
½ tsp	ground cumin	2 mL
¼ tsp	fine sea salt	1 mL
2 cups	finely sliced peeled jicama	500 mL

1. In food processor, process olive oil, lime juice, chili powder, cumin and salt. Transfer to a bowl.

2. Add jicama to dressing and toss until well coated. Cover and set aside for 10 minutes or until softened. Serve immediately or cover and refrigerate for up to 2 days.

Nutrients per serving			
Calories	296	Vitamin C	31 mg
Fat	27 g	Vitamin E	8 IU
Carbohydrate	13 g	Folate	17 µg
Fiber	7 g	Vitamin B$_6$	0.1 mg
Sugar	3 g	Vitamin B$_{12}$	0.0 µg
Protein	1 g	Magnesium	20 mg

Crunchy, Colorful Thai Cabbage Slaw

Phase 3

This fresh, crunchy slaw has just the right balance of sweet and tart. Leftovers are terrific tucked into sandwiches the next day. Ginger and cayenne are strong anti-inflammatories, and apple cider vinegar, cabbage, onions and cilantro are potent detoxifiers.

Tip

An equal amount of thickly sliced or shredded green or purple cabbage can be used in place of the napa cabbage.

Makes 6 servings

1 tbsp	grated gingerroot	15 mL
1/4 tsp	cayenne pepper	1 mL
1/4 tsp	fine sea salt	1 mL
3 tbsp	apple cider vinegar	45 mL
2 tbsp	melted virgin coconut oil	30 mL
1 tbsp	coconut nectar or coconut sugar	15 mL
6 cups	sliced napa cabbage (about 1 small head)	1.5 L
1 cup	shredded carrots	250 mL
1 cup	thinly sliced green onions	250 mL
1/4 cup	packed fresh basil leaves, chopped	60 mL
1/4 cup	packed fresh cilantro or mint leaves, chopped	60 mL

1. In a small bowl, whisk together ginger, cayenne, salt, vinegar, coconut oil and coconut nectar.

2. In a large bowl, combine cabbage, carrots, green onions, basil and cilantro. Add dressing and gently toss to coat. Cover and refrigerate for at least 30 minutes, until chilled, or for up to 2 hours.

Nutrients per serving

Calories	437
Fat	29 g
Carbohydrate	45 g
Fiber	14 g
Sugar	23 g
Protein	10 g
Vitamin C	102 mg
Vitamin E	2 IU
Folate	330 µg
Vitamin B$_6$	1.0 mg
Vitamin B$_{12}$	0.0 µg
Magnesium	88 mg

Fast and Easy Greek Salad

This recipe courtesy of dietitian Jane Bellman.

Here's a simple salad that's an old favorite. It's especially good when tomatoes are in season.

Tip

If desired, substitute 1 tbsp (15 mL) chopped fresh basil for the dried.

2 cups	diced tomatoes	500 mL
2 cups	diced cucumbers	500 mL
1 cup	cubed feta cheese (about 8 oz/250 g)	250 mL
½ cup	thinly sliced onions	125 mL
¼ cup	sliced black olives (optional)	60 mL
2 tbsp	white wine vinegar	30 mL
2 tbsp	olive oil	30 mL
½ tsp	minced garlic	2 mL
½ tsp	dried basil	2 mL
½ tsp	dried oregano	2 mL
	Freshly ground black pepper	

1. In a large bowl, combine tomatoes, cucumbers, cheese, onions and olives (if using). Set aside.

2. In a small bowl or measuring cup, whisk together vinegar, oil, garlic, basil, oregano, and pepper to taste. Add to tomato mixture; toss gently to combine. Chill before serving.

Nutrients per serving	
Calories	192
Fat	15 g
Carbohydrate	8 g
Fiber	2 g
Sugar	5 g
Protein	7 g
Vitamin C	15 mg
Vitamin E	2 IU
Folate	37 µg
Vitamin B_6	0.3 mg
Vitamin B_{12}	0.6 µg
Magnesium	27 mg

Pan-Braised Brussels Sprouts

Phase 3

Brussels sprouts, with their delicate, nutty flavor, take on a pleasant sweetness in this easy-to-prepare recipe that can be doubled to serve a crowd. Like other vegetables in the cabbage family, they are fantastic for detoxifying the body.

Tips

Make sure to choose a gluten-free chicken broth.

Serve Brussels sprouts when they are tender-crisp and bright green in color. Be sure not to overcook them.

Makes 4 to 6 servings

1½ lbs	Brussels sprouts, trimmed and halved	750 g
2 tbsp	ready-to-use chicken broth (see tip)	30 mL
2 tbsp	red wine vinegar	30 mL
1½ tsp	granulated sugar	7 mL
1 tbsp	butter	15 mL
2	cloves garlic, finely chopped	2
	Fine sea salt and freshly ground black pepper	

1. In a saucepan of boiling salted water, blanch Brussels sprouts for 3 minutes or until bright green and crisp; drain well. (If preparing sprouts ahead, chill in ice water. Drain well and wrap in a clean, dry kitchen towel to absorb moisture. Place in an airtight container and refrigerate for up to a day.)

2. In a glass measuring cup, stir together broth, vinegar and sugar.

3. In a wok or large nonstick skillet, melt butter over medium-high heat and heat until foamy. Cook garlic, stirring, for 30 seconds or until fragrant. Add sprouts and cook, stirring, for 3 minutes or until lightly browned.

4. Add stock mixture. Reduce heat to medium and cook, stirring often, for about 4 minutes or until sprouts are barely tender. Season to taste with salt and pepper.

Nutrients per serving (1 of 6)	
Calories	73
Fat	2 g
Carbohydrate	12 g
Fiber	4 g
Sugar	4 g
Protein	4 g
Vitamin C	97 mg
Vitamin E	2 IU
Folate	69 µg
Vitamin B$_6$	0.3 mg
Vitamin B$_{12}$	0.0 µg
Magnesium	27 mg

Sugar Snap Peas in Ginger Butter

Here's a quick stir-fry with ginger and shallots that nicely complements the sweetness of emerald-green sugar snap peas.

Tip

Snow peas can be prepared in the same way, but reduce the cooking time to 1 minute or until bright green and crisp.

Makes 4 servings

1½ lbs	sugar snap peas	750 g
1 tbsp	butter	15 mL
¼ cup	minced shallots	60 mL
2 tsp	minced gingerroot	10 mL
	Fine sea salt and freshly ground black pepper	

1. Remove strings from both sides of sugar snap peas. In a large nonstick skillet, melt butter over medium heat. When hot and foamy, cook shallots and ginger, stirring, for 2 minutes.

2. Add peas and cook, stirring often, for 4 minutes or until just tender. Season to taste with salt and pepper.

Nutrients per serving	
Calories	171
Fat	4 g
Carbohydrate	26 g
Fiber	9 g
Sugar	10 g
Protein	10 g
Vitamin C	69 mg
Vitamin E	1 IU
Folate	114 µg
Vitamin B$_6$	0.3 mg
Vitamin B$_{12}$	0.0 µg
Magnesium	59 mg

Roasted Butternut Squash with Onion and Sage

Roasting brings out the best in winter squash. Most supermarkets now offer convenient packages of peeled, cubed ready-to-cook butternut squash in the produce department, making this fall dish a breeze to whip together.

Tip

Nonstick cooking sprays are sold in aerosol cans and pump sprays at supermarkets. We suggest buying a spray pump mister, available at specialty kitchen shops. This non-aerosol dispenser can be filled with any kind of oil.

- Preheat oven to 375°F (190°C)
- 11- by 7-inch (28 by 18 cm) glass baking dish, sprayed with nonstick cooking spray

4 cups	cubed butternut squash about 1 lb/500 g, (cut into ¾-inch/2 cm cubes)	1 L
1	small onion, cut into thin wedges	1
1 tbsp	finely chopped fresh sage	15 mL
⅛ tsp	fine sea salt	0.5 mL
	Freshly ground black pepper	
2 tsp	extra virgin olive oil	10 mL

1. In baking dish, combine squash, onion, sage, salt, and pepper to taste. Drizzle with oil and toss to coat. Spread out in an even layer.

2. Roast in preheated oven for 30 to 35 minutes, stirring occasionally, until squash is just tender when pierced with a fork.

Variation

Roasted Butternut Squash with Sweet Spices: Replace the sage with ¼ tsp (1 mL) each ground cinnamon and ground cumin.

Nutrients per serving	
Calories	91
Fat	2 g
Carbohydrate	18 g
Fiber	3 g
Sugar	4 g
Protein	2 g
Vitamin C	31 mg
Vitamin E	4 IU
Folate	41 µg
Vitamin B$_6$	0.2 mg
Vitamin B$_{12}$	0.0 µg
Magnesium	50 mg

Baked Sweet Potato Fries

Baked fries are a terrific alternative to the deep-fried variety, and when they're made with sweet potatoes, you get added vitamins and fiber — and they taste great, too!

Tip

Sweet potatoes are sometimes incorrectly labeled "yams." True yams are larger than sweet potatoes and have fewer nutrients. Be sure to pick up sweet potatoes with orange-colored flesh.

Makes 4 servings

- Preheat oven to 400°F (200°C)
- Large baking sheet, lined with parchment paper

1	large sweet potato (about 1 lb/500 g)	1
1 tbsp	olive oil, divided	15 mL
¼ tsp	fine sea salt	1 mL
	Freshly ground black pepper	

1. Peel sweet potato and rinse. Cut in half crosswise, then cut lengthwise into sticks about ½ inch (1 cm) square. Place on prepared baking sheet. Drizzle with oil and sprinkle with salt and pepper. Spread out in a single layer, leaving space between each fry.

2. Bake for about 30 minutes, flipping sweet potatoes halfway through, until browned and tender.

Nutrients per serving	
Calories	127
Fat	3 g
Carbohydrate	23 g
Fiber	3 g
Sugar	5 g
Protein	2 g
Vitamin C	3 mg
Vitamin E	1 IU
Folate	13 µg
Vitamin B_6	0.2 mg
Vitamin B_{12}	0.0 µg
Magnesium	28 mg

Veggie Kabobs

Phase 3

In summer and early fall, when fresh vegetables are in season, this dish is a standby. The kabobs are equally delicious served hot or at room temperature.

Tips

The longer the marinating time, the deeper the flavors.

Any leftover veggies from these kabobs make a perfect beginning for tasty salads.

For convenience, cook the vegetables in a nonstick grill basket, being aware that some may cook more quickly than others.

Nutrients per serving (1 of 8)

Calories	99
Fat	7 g
Carbohydrate	8 g
Fiber	2 g
Sugar	5 g
Protein	2 g
Vitamin C	58 mg
Vitamin E	3 IU
Folate	43 µg
Vitamin B$_6$	0.3 mg
Vitamin B$_{12}$	0.0 µg
Magnesium	22 mg

Makes 6 to 8 servings

- Preheat grill or broiler
- 16 bamboo or metal skewers

⅓ cup	freshly squeezed lemon juice	75 mL
¼ cup	olive oil	60 mL
1	clove garlic, minced (about 1 tsp/5 mL)	1
2 tsp	dried oregano (or 2 tbsp/30 mL finely chopped fresh)	10 mL
	Fine sea salt and freshly ground black pepper	
2	bell peppers (any color), cut into 1-inch (2.5 cm) strips	2
2	small zucchini, cut into 1-inch (2.5 cm) thick slices	2
2 cups	grape tomatoes or cherry tomatoes (about 16)	500 mL
2 cups	whole button mushrooms (about 16)	500 mL
1	large onion, cut into 8 wedges and halved crosswise, separated into single layers	1
1	yellow summer squash (such as golden zucchini) cut into 1-inch (2.5 cm) cubes	1

1. In a large bowl or resealable plastic bag, combine lemon juice, olive oil, garlic, oregano, and salt and pepper to taste. Add peppers, zucchini, tomatoes, mushrooms, onion and squash and stir to evenly coat. Marinate at room temperature for 15 to 20 minutes or in the refrigerator for up to 12 hours.

2. Thread vegetables onto skewers, alternating to form an attractive pattern and leaving a bit of space between the pieces to allow air to circulate.

3. Grill or broil, turning and basting often with the remaining marinade, for 8 to 10 minutes or until vegetables are browned on all sides and tender. While cooking, rotate location of the skewers on the grill or broiler to ensure even cooking.

Variation

The vegetables (unskewered) can also be spread in a single layer on two greased rimmed baking sheets and baked in a preheated 400°F (200°C) oven for 30 to 35 minutes. Turn the vegetables and rotate the pans after 20 minutes.

Coconut Flax Tortillas

Phase 3

With a rustic texture reminiscent of corn tortillas, these flax and coconut tortillas make a great bread alternative for quick and easy sandwich roll-ups. They are a fantastic source of fiber, increasing estrogen elimination and improving your gut health.

Tip

Stack the cooled tortillas between sheets of waxed paper and store, wrapped in foil or plastic wrap, in the refrigerator for up to 3 days. Alternatively, wrap them in plastic wrap, then foil, completely enclosing them, and freeze for up to 3 months. Let thaw at room temperature for 4 to 6 hours before serving.

Makes eight 6-inch (15 cm) tortillas

- Parchment paper or waxed paper

1¼ cups	ground flax seeds (flaxseed meal), divided	300 mL
6 tbsp	coconut water or water	90 mL
2 tbsp	coconut flour	30 mL
1 tsp	fine sea salt	5 mL
	Melted virgin coconut oil	

1. In a small bowl, combine ¼ cup (60 mL) flax seeds and coconut water until blended. Let stand for 5 minutes or until thickened.

2. In a large bowl, whisk together the remaining flax seeds, coconut flour and salt. Add the coconut water mixture, stirring until blended (mixture will be very thick). Turn out onto a flat surface and knead until dough is no longer sticky.

3. Divide dough into 8 equal pieces and roll each piece into a ball. Roll each ball out between two sheets of parchment paper into a 6-inch (15 cm) round.

4. Heat a medium skillet (preferably cast iron) over medium-high heat until hot, then lightly brush with coconut oil. Place one round in skillet and cook for 30 to 40 seconds or until edges begin to brown. Flip over and cook for 30 to 40 seconds or until tortilla appears dry. Transfer to a wire rack. Repeat with the remaining rounds, lightly brushing the pan with oil each time and adjusting heat as necessary to prevent burning.

Variations

Spiced Coconut Flax Tortillas: Add 1 tsp (5 mL) ground cumin, curry powder, chili powder, smoked paprika, garlic powder or onion powder with the coconut flour.

Herbed Coconut Flax Tortillas: Add 1 tsp (5 mL) dried herbs (crumbled rosemary, rubbed sage, basil, Italian seasoning, oregano) or 1 to 2 tbsp (15 to 30 mL) chopped fresh herbs (flat-leaf parsley, cilantro, basil) with the coconut flour.

Nutrients per tortilla	
Calories	104
Fat	8 g
Carbohydrate	6 g
Fiber	5 g
Sugar	1 g
Protein	3 g
Vitamin C	0 mg
Vitamin E	0 IU
Folate	16 µg
Vitamin B$_6$	0.1 mg
Vitamin B$_{12}$	0.0 µg
Magnesium	73 mg

Snacks, Dips, Sauces and Dressings

Olive Oil Dipping Sauce

Phase 1

This dipping sauce takes only minutes to make but packs a powerful flavor punch! Use it as a dressing, for dipping wraps or as a sauce on steamed vegetables.

Tip

This dipping sauce can be stored in an airtight container (small mason jars work well) in the refrigerator for up to 3 days.

Makes 4 servings

¼ cup	extra virgin olive oil	60 mL
1 tbsp	apple cider vinegar	15 mL
¼ tsp	finely chopped fresh thyme	1 mL
¼ tsp	finely chopped fresh basil	1 mL
¼ tsp	finely chopped fresh oregano	1 mL
⅛ tsp	fine sea salt	0.5 mL
	Freshly ground black pepper	

1. In a small glass jar with a lid, combine oil, vinegar, thyme, basil, oregano, salt and pepper. Seal jar and shake vigorously.

Nutrients per serving	
Calories	120
Fat	14 g
Carbohydrate	0 g
Fiber	0 g
Sugar	0 g
Protein	0 g
Vitamin C	0 mg
Vitamin E	3 IU
Folate	0 µg
Vitamin B$_6$	0.0 mg
Vitamin B$_{12}$	0.0 µg
Magnesium	0 mg

Salty Almonds with Thyme

Imagine — a snack as delicious as these almonds that is also an excellent source of vitamin E, a valuable antioxidant vitamin. Since numerous studies confirm that taking vitamin E in supplements has little benefit and may be harmful in some circumstances, obtaining this nutrient from food makes an enormous amount of sense. Feel free to truly enjoy every satisfying bite.

Tip

Sea salt is available in most supermarkets. It is much sweeter than table salt and is essential for this recipe, as table salt would impart an unpleasant acrid taste to the nuts.

Nutrients per 12 almonds	
Calories	119
Fat	11 g
Carbohydrate	4 g
Fiber	2 g
Sugar	1 g
Protein	4 g
Vitamin C	1 mg
Vitamin E	7 IU
Folate	9 µg
Vitamin B_6	0.0 mg
Vitamin B_{12}	0.0 µg
Magnesium	48 mg

Makes about 2 cups (500 mL)

- Small slow cooker (maximum $3\frac{1}{2}$ quarts)

2 cups	unblanched almonds	500 mL
$\frac{1}{2}$ tsp	freshly ground white pepper	2 mL
1 tbsp	fine sea salt (or to taste)	15 mL
2 tbsp	extra virgin olive oil	30 mL
2 tbsp	fresh thyme leaves	30 mL

1. In slow cooker stoneware, combine almonds and white pepper. Cover and cook on High for $1\frac{1}{2}$ hours, stirring every 30 minutes, until nuts are nicely toasted.

2. In a bowl, combine salt, olive oil and thyme. Add to hot almonds in stoneware and stir thoroughly to combine. Spoon mixture into a small serving bowl and serve hot or let cool.

Anti-Inflammatory Cucumber Dip

Phase 2

Makes 4 servings

This tasty dip also makes a great sandwich spread. It may become your new mayo alternative!

Tips

In place of the sprouted almonds, you can use raw almonds, soaked overnight and rinsed.

This dip can be stored in an airtight container (small mason jars work well) in the refrigerator for up to 3 days.

• Blender or food processor

2	small (4-inch/10 cm) cucumbers, peeled, seeded and cut into chunks	2
1	clove garlic, peeled	1
¼ cup	sprouted almonds	60 mL
1 tsp	ground turmeric	5 mL
⅛ tsp	fine sea salt (or to taste)	0.5 mL
2 tsp	extra virgin olive oil	10 mL

1. In blender, combine cucumbers, garlic, almonds, turmeric, salt and oil; blend until creamy.

Nutrients per serving

Calories	84	Sugar	1 g	Folate	16 µg
Fat	7 g	Protein	2 g	Vitamin B_6	0.1 mg
Carbohydrate	4 g	Vitamin C	3 mg	Vitamin B_{12}	0.0 µg
Fiber	2 g	Vitamin E	4 IU	Magnesium	35 mg

Goat's Milk Yogurt Dip

Phase 2

Makes 4 servings

This fantastic dip doesn't just taste amazing, it is also full of healthy bacteria to make your intestines happy. Try it as a sandwich spread, too.

1 cup	Homemade Goat's Milk Yogurt (page 175)	250 mL
1 tsp	Dijon mustard	5 mL
½ tsp	dried dillweed	2 mL
⅛ tsp	fine sea salt	0.5 mL

1. In a small bowl, combine yogurt, mustard, dill and salt.

Nutrients per serving

Calories	44	Sugar	3 g	Folate	1 µg
Fat	3 g	Protein	2 g	Vitamin B_6	0.0 mg
Carbohydrate	3 g	Vitamin C	1 mg	Vitamin B_{12}	0.0 µg
Fiber	0 g	Vitamin E	0 IU	Magnesium	9 mg

Zucchini Garlic Hummus

Say goodbye to boring old chickpea hummus and hello to this delicious low-carb alternative. It's a good source of calcium.

Tip

Hummus can be stored in an airtight container (small mason jars work well) in the refrigerator for up to 3 days.

Makes 4 servings

- Food processor or blender

1	large zucchini, cut into chunks	1
1	clove garlic, peeled	1
¼ cup	tahini	60 mL
2 tbsp	freshly squeezed lemon juice	30 mL
1 tbsp	extra virgin olive oil	15 mL
½ tsp	fine sea salt	2 mL

1. In food processor, combine zucchini, garlic, tahini, lemon juice, oil and salt; process until smooth.

Nutrients per serving

Calories	135
Fat	12 g
Carbohydrate	7 g
Fiber	1 g
Sugar	2 g
Protein	4 g
Vitamin C	18 mg
Vitamin E	1 IU
Folate	36 µg
Vitamin B$_6$	0.2 mg
Vitamin B$_{12}$	0.0 µg
Magnesium	29 mg

Lentil Tapenade

Phase 2

This yummy tapenade builds up the beneficial bacteria in your gut and helps decrease inflammation. Serve it with allowable raw vegetables or 2 to 3 gluten-free crackers.

Tips

Cooked dried lentils (which don't require presoaking) are so much better, both in flavor and texture, than mushy canned lentils, which are also very high in sodium.

Always rinse brined foods, such as olives and capers, to remove excess salt.

The spread can be stored in an airtight container in the refrigerator for up to 5 days.

Makes about 1¼ cups (300 mL)

• Food processor

3 cups	water	750 mL
½ cup	dried brown or green lentils, rinsed	125 mL
1	small bay leaf	1
1	clove garlic, coarsely chopped	1
⅓ cup	pitted kalamata olives, rinsed and coarsely chopped (about 12)	75 mL
1 tbsp	extra virgin olive oil	15 mL
¼ tsp	freshly ground black pepper	1 mL
¼ cup	chopped fresh parsley	60 mL
1 tsp	grated lemon zest	5 mL

1. In a medium saucepan, bring water to a boil over high heat. Add lentils and bay leaf. Reduce heat to medium-low, cover and simmer for 25 to 30 minutes or until lentils are tender. Drain and let cool to room temperature. Discard bay leaf.

2. In food processor, combine lentils, garlic, olives, olive oil and pepper; process until smooth. Add parsley and lemon zest; pulse until combined.

3. Transfer to a serving bowl, cover and refrigerate for 2 hours, until chilled, before serving.

Nutrients per ¼ cup (60 mL)	
Calories	103
Fat	4 g
Carbohydrate	13 g
Fiber	3 g
Sugar	0 g
Protein	5 g
Vitamin C	5 mg
Vitamin E	1 IU
Folate	44 µg
Vitamin B$_6$	0.1 mg
Vitamin B$_{12}$	0.0 µg
Magnesium	18 mg

Spicy Tamari Almonds

Phase 3

Serve these tasty tidbits as pre-dinner nibbles, with a glass of cold white wine, or enjoy them as a gluten-free snack. Nuts contain resistant starch, which is a fantastic food for the beneficial bacteria in your gut. Moreover, in the digestive process, resistant starch produces a substance that helps your body to absorb minerals, such as magnesium.

Tip

For a holiday gift, make up a batch or two and package in pretty jars. If well sealed, the nuts will keep for 10 days.

Makes about 2 cups (500 mL)

- Small slow cooker (2 to 3½ quarts)

2 cups	whole almonds	500 mL
¼ tsp	cayenne pepper	1 mL
2 tbsp	reduced-sodium tamari sauce or coconut amino acids	30 mL
1 tbsp	extra virgin olive oil	15 mL
	Fine sea salt	

1. In slow cooker stoneware, combine almonds and cayenne. Place a clean tea towel folded in half (so you will have 2 layers) over top of stoneware to absorb moisture. Cover and cook on High for 45 minutes.

2. In a small bowl, combine tamari and olive oil. Add to hot almonds and stir thoroughly to combine. Replace tea towel. Cover and cook on High for 1½ hours, until nuts are hot and fragrant, stirring every 30 minutes and replacing towel each time. Sprinkle with salt to taste. Store in an airtight container.

Nutrients per 12 almonds	
Calories	112
Fat	10 g
Carbohydrate	4 g
Fiber	2 g
Sugar	1 g
Protein	4 g
Vitamin C	0 mg
Vitamin E	7 IU
Folate	9 µg
Vitamin B_6	0.0 mg
Vitamin B_{12}	0.0 µg
Magnesium	48 mg

Spicy Cashews

Phase 3

Only slightly nippy and with just a hint of cinnamon, these cashews are a tasty anti-inflammatory treat any time of the year. Like all nuts, cashews are a source of healthy fats. They are also high in nutrients, including copper, magnesium, manganese, vitamin K and phosphorus.

Tips

Check your chili powder to make sure it doesn't contain gluten.

For a holiday gift, make up a batch or two and package in pretty jars. If well sealed, the nuts will keep for 10 days.

Nutrients per 12 cashews

Calories	213
Fat	18 g
Carbohydrate	11 g
Fiber	1 g
Sugar	2 g
Protein	5 g
Vitamin C	0 mg
Vitamin E	1 IU
Folate	24 µg
Vitamin B_6	0.1 mg
Vitamin B_{12}	0.0 µg
Magnesium	90 mg

Makes about 2 cups (500 mL)

- Small slow cooker (maximum $3\frac{1}{2}$ quarts)

2 cups	raw cashews	500 mL
1 tsp	chili powder	5 mL
$\frac{1}{2}$ tsp	cayenne pepper	2 mL
$\frac{1}{4}$ tsp	ground cinnamon (see tip, page 237)	1 mL
2 tsp	fine sea salt	10 mL
1 tbsp	extra virgin olive oil	15 mL

1. In slow cooker stoneware, combine cashews, chili powder, cayenne and cinnamon. Stir to combine thoroughly. Cover and cook on High for $1\frac{1}{2}$ hours, stirring every 30 minutes, until nuts are nicely toasted.

2. In a small bowl, combine sea salt and olive oil. Add to nuts in slow cooker and stir to thoroughly combine. Transfer mixture to a serving bowl and serve hot or let cool.

Artichoke and White Bean Spread

The flavor combinations in this spread — onion, garlic, cannellini beans, artichokes, Parmesan and parsley — are simple, elegant and synergistically delicious. Serve on gluten-free crackers or as a dip for vegetables.

Tips

For this quantity of beans, soak, cook and drain 1 cup (250 mL) dried cannellini beans or drain and rinse 1 can (14 to 19 oz/398 to 540 mL) cannellini beans.

If you prefer, use frozen artichokes, thawed, to make this recipe. You will need 6 artichoke hearts.

Nutrients per ¼ cup (60 mL)

Calories	113
Fat	6 g
Carbohydrate	12 g
Fiber	5 g
Sugar	1 g
Protein	5 g
Vitamin C	7 mg
Vitamin E	1 IU
Folate	73 µg
Vitamin B$_6$	0.1 mg
Vitamin B$_{12}$	0.1 µg
Magnesium	30 mg

Makes about 3 cups (750 mL)

- Small slow cooker (about 2 quarts)
- Food processor

½	red onion, finely chopped	½
2	cloves garlic, minced	2
¼ cup	extra virgin olive oil, divided	60 mL
2 cups	drained cooked cannellini (white kidney) beans	500 mL
1	can (14 oz/398 mL) artichoke hearts, drained and coarsely chopped	1
½ cup	freshly grated Parmesan cheese or vegan alternative	125 mL
1 tsp	sweet paprika	5 mL
½ tsp	fine sea salt	2 mL
¼ tsp	freshly ground black pepper	1 mL
½ cup	finely chopped fresh parsley	125 mL

1. In slow cooker stoneware, combine onion, garlic and 2 tbsp (30 mL) oil. Place a clean tea towel folded in half (so you will have two layers) over top of stoneware to absorb moisture. Cover and cook on High for 30 minutes or until onions are softened.

2. Meanwhile, in food processor, in batches, if necessary, pulse beans and artichokes until desired consistency is achieved. After onions have softened, add bean mixture to stoneware along with Parmesan, paprika, salt, pepper and the remaining oil. Replace tea towel. Cover and cook on Low for 4 hours or on High for 2 hours, until hot and bubbly. Add parsley and stir well.

Basic Pesto

Pesto is the perfect condiment atop meat, pizza, vegetables, crackers and so much more! This one is bursting with flavor and packs a healing punch.

Tip

The pesto can be stored in an airtight container in the refrigerator for up to 3 days or frozen for up to 6 months.

Makes about 2 cups (500 mL)

• Blender or food processor

3	cloves garlic	3
4 cups	fresh basil leaves (about 3 large bunches)	1 L
1/3 cup	pine nuts	75 mL
1/4 cup	freshly grated Parmesan cheese	60 mL
1 tsp	coarse kosher salt	5 mL
1/2 cup	extra virgin olive oil	125 mL
1 tsp	freshly squeezed lemon juice	5 mL

1. In blender, combine garlic, basil, pine nuts, cheese, salt, oil and lemon juice; blend until smooth.

Nutrients per 1 tbsp (15 mL)

Calories	42
Fat	4 g
Carbohydrate	0 g
Fiber	0 g
Sugar	0 g
Protein	1 g
Vitamin C	1 mg
Vitamin E	1 IU
Folate	4 µg
Vitamin B_6	0.0 mg
Vitamin B_{12}	0.0 µg
Magnesium	7 mg

Parsley Pesto Sauce

Phase 3	Makes about ⅔ cup (150 mL)

This twist on pesto is delicious and nutritious. Parsley is a fantastic source of potassium and a potent detoxifier.

Tip
Use either Basic Vegetable Stock (page 193) or a gluten-free ready-to-use vegetable broth to prepare this soup.

- Food processor

2	large cloves garlic	2
1 cup	fresh parsley leaves, tightly packed	250 mL
⅓ cup	fresh basil leaves, tightly packed	75 mL
1 tbsp	extra virgin olive oil	15 mL
¼ cup	freshly grated Parmesan cheese	60 mL
¼ cup	vegetable stock (see tip)	60 mL

1. In food processor, with the motor running, drop garlic through the tube and process until chopped. Add basil, parsley, oil and Parmesan cheese. Process until well mixed. With a rubber spatula, scrape the sides once or twice. Add stock, process until well blended.

Nutrients per 2 tbsp (30 mL)

Calories	49	Sugar	0 g	Folate	21 µg
Fat	4 g	Protein	2 g	Vitamin B_6	0.0 mg
Carbohydrate	2 g	Vitamin C	17 mg	Vitamin B_{12}	0.1 µg
Fiber	1 g	Vitamin E	1 IU	Magnesium	10 mg

Artichoke Salsa

Phase 3	Makes about 1½ cups (375 mL)

The beneficial bacteria in your gut love artichokes, and feeding them foods they love helps to decrease inflammation and improve your overall health. Serve this easy salsa with grilled steaks, lamb, fish or chicken.

- Food processor

1	small clove garlic	1
1	jar (6 oz/170 mL) marinated artichoke hearts, drained	1
⅓ cup	pine nuts	75 mL
	Juice of ½ large lemon	

1. In food processor, combine garlic, artichokes, pine nuts and lemon juice; process until finely chopped.

Nutrients per ¼ cup (60 mL)

Calories	71	Sugar	0 g	Folate	3 µg
Fat	7 g	Protein	1 g	Vitamin B_6	0.0 mg
Carbohydrate	3 g	Vitamin C	0 mg	Vitamin B_{12}	0.0 µg
Fiber	1 g	Vitamin E	1 IU	Magnesium	19 mg

Green Goddess Salad Dressing

Attractive, colorful, contrasting flecks of green — this is the dressing everyone requests. In addition to dressing salads, use it as a dip with cut-up vegetables, as a marinade for baked chicken or fish, or drizzled over cooked vegetables.

Tips

This recipe can be halved or doubled, depending on the amount you require.

For the best color, be sure to use fresh parsley.

• Food processor

1	small clove garlic	1
1	green onion	1
1/4 cup	fresh parsley	60 mL
1 1/2 tsp	dried tarragon or 1 to 2 tbsp (15 to 30 mL) snipped fresh	7 mL
1/2 cup	gluten-free sour cream	125 mL
1/2 cup	plain yogurt	125 mL
1 tbsp	freshly squeezed lemon juice	15 mL

1. In food processor, combine garlic, green onion, parsley, tarragon, sour cream, yogurt and lemon juice. Process until smooth. Cover and refrigerate for a minimum of 2 hours to allow flavors to develop and blend. Refrigerate for up to 2 weeks.

Nutrients per 1 tbsp (15 mL)	
Calories	21
Fat	1 g
Carbohydrate	1 g
Fiber	0 g
Sugar	1 g
Protein	1 g
Vitamin C	1 mg
Vitamin E	0 IU
Folate	1 µg
Vitamin B$_6$	0.0 mg
Vitamin B$_{12}$	0.0 µg
Magnesium	2 mg

Contributing Authors

Johanna Burkhard
500 Best Comfort Food Recipes
Recipes from this book are found on pages 251 and 252.

Johanna Burkhard and Barbara Allan
The Diabetes Prevention & Management Cookbook
Recipes from this book are found on pages 210, 211, 253 and 262.

Andrew Chase and Nicole Young
The Blender Bible
A recipe from this book is found on page 245 (bottom).

Danielle Cook
Recipes by this author, developed for this book, are found on pages 168–75, 177, 179–82, 188–92, 194, 196–201, 203 (bottom), 203–8, 230–39, 247, 258 and 260–61.

Dietitians of Canada
Cook!
Recipes from this book are found on pages 202 and 219.

Dietitians of Canada
Cook Great Food
A recipe from this book is found on page 250.

Maxine Effenson-Chuck and Beth Gurney
125 Best Vegan Recipes
A recipe from this book is found on page 255.

Judith Finlayson
The Healthy Slow Cooker, Second Edition
Recipes from this book are found on pages 193, 209, 243, 244, 259 and 263–65.

Jean-Paul Grappe
The Complete Wild Game Cookbook
A recipe from this book is found on page 228.

Dr. Nikolas R. Hedberg and Danielle Cook
The Complete Thyroid Health & Diet Guide
Recipes from this book are found on pages 178 and 266.

Douglas McNish
Eat Raw, Eat Well
A recipe from this book is found on page 183.

Douglas McNish
Raw, Quick & Delicious!
A recipe from this book is found on page 248.

Camilla V. Saulsbury
5 Easy Steps to Healthy Cooking
Recipes from this book are found on pages 184, 186, 213, 218, 220, 221, 224, 225 and 227.

Camilla V. Saulsbury
500 Best Quinoa Recipes
Recipes from this book are found on pages 222 and 223.

Camilla V. Saulsbury
Complete Coconut Cookbook
Recipes from this book are found on pages 176, 185, 214–17, 240, 241, 246, 249 and 256.

Andrew Schloss with Ken Bookman
2500 Recipes
A recipe from this book is found on page 267 (bottom).

Donna Washburn & Heather Butt
250 Gluten-Free Favorites
A recipe from this book is found on page 226.

Donna Washburn & Heather Butt
Easy Everyday Gluten-Free Cooking
Recipes from this book are found on pages 212, 267 (top) and 268.

Sharon Zeiler, ed.
250 Essential Diabetes Recipes
Recipes from this book are found on pages 242 and 254.

References

Chapter 1

[1] Vercellini P, Vigano P, Somigliana E, et al. Endometriosis: pathogenesis and treatment. Nat Rev Endocrinol, 2014 May; 10 (5): 261–75.

[2] Simoens S, Hummelshoj L, Dunselman G, et al. Endometriosis cost assessment (the EndoCost study): A cost-of-illness study protocol. Gynecol Obstet Invest, 2011; 71 (3): 170–76.

[3] Nnoaham KE, Hummelshoj L, Webster P, et al. Impact of endometriosis on quality of life and work productivity: A multicenter study across ten countries. Fertil Steril, 2011; 96 (2): 366–73.

[4] Noble LS, Simpson ER, Johns A, et al. Aromatase expression in endometriosis. J Clin Endocrinol Metab, 1996 Jan; 81 (1): 174–79; Clayton RD, Hawe JA, Love JC, et al. Recurrent pain after hysterectomy and bilateral salpingo-oophorectomy for endometriosis: Evaluation of laparoscopic excision of residual endometriosis. Br J Obstet Gynaecol, 1999 Jul; (106) 7: 740–44; Haas D, Chvatal R, Reichert B, et al. Endometriosis: A premenopausal disease? Age pattern in 42,079 patients with endometriosis. Arch Gynecol Obstet, 2012 Sep; 286 (3): 667–70; Redwine DB. Endometriosis persisting after castration: Clinical characteristics and results of surgical management. Obstet Gynecol, 1994 Mar; 83 (3): 405–13; Zeitoun KM, Bulun SE. Aromatase: A key molecule in the pathophysiology of endometriosis and a therapeutic target. Fertil Steril, 1999 Dec; 72 (6): 961–69.

[5] Chung MK, Chung RR, Gordon D, et al. The evil twins of chronic pelvic pain syndrome: Endometriosis and interstitial cystitis. JSLS, 2000 Oct–Dec; 6 (4): 311–14.

Chapter 3

[1] Muyldermans M, Cornillie FJ, et al. CA125 and endometriosis. Hum Reprod Update, 1995 Mar; 1 (2): 173–87.

[2] Koninckx PR, Muyldermans M, Meuleman C, et al. CA 125 in the management of endometriosis. Eur J Obstet Gynecol Reprod Biol, 1993 Apr; 49 (1–2): 109–13.

[3] Al-Jefout M, Dezarnaulds G, Cooper M, et al. Diagnosis of endometriosis by detection of nerve fibres in an endometrial biopsy: A double blind study. Hum Reprod, 2009 Dec; 24 (12): 3019–24.

[4] Saba L, Sulcis R, Melis GB, et al. Endometriosis: The role of magnetic resonance imaging. Acta Radiol, 2015 Mar; 56 (3): 355–67; Jung SI, Kim YJ, Jeon HJ, et al. Deep infiltrating endometriosis: CT imaging evaluation. J Comput Assist Tomogr, 2010 May–Jun; 34 (3): 338–42.

Chapter 4

[1] Simpson JL, Bischoff FZ, Kamat A, et al. Genetics of endometriosis. Obstet Gynecol Clin North Am, 2003 Mar; 30 (1): 21–40; Dunn E, Taylor R, Wieser F. Advances in the genetics of endometriosis. Genome Med, 2010 Oct; 2 (10): 1–6.

[2] Malinak LR, Buttram VC, Elias S, et al. Heritable aspects of endometriosis. II. Clinical characteristics of familial endometriosis. Am J Obstet Gynecol, 1980 Jun; 137 (3): 332–37; Lamb K, Hoffmann RG, Nichols TR. Family trait analysis: A case-control study of 43 women with endometriosis and their best friends. Am J Obstet Gynecol, 1986 Mar; 154 (3): 596–601; Moen MH, Magnus P. The familial risk of endometriosis. Acta Obstet Gynecol Scand, 1993 Oct; 72 (7): 560–64; Moen MH. Endometriosis in monozygotic twins. Acta Obstet Gynecol Scand, 1994 Jan; 73 (1): 59–62.

[3] Bischoff FZ, Simpson JL. Genetics of endometriosis. Global Library of Women's Medicine. Available at: https://www.glowm.com/section_view/heading/Genetics%2520of%2520Endometriosis/item/36 2; Arvanitis D, Koumantakis G, Goumenou A, et al. CYP1A1, CYP19, and GSTM1 polymorphisms increase the risk of endometriosis. Fertil Steril, 2003 Mar; 79 (1): 702–709.

[4] Xu X, Ding J, Rana N, et al. Association between COMT gene polymorphism and endometriosis-associated pain: An interim analysis. Fertil Steril, 2007; 88 (Suppl 1): S213.

[5] Xu X, Ding J, Rana N, et al. Association between COMT gene polymorphism and endometriosis-associated pain: An interim analysis. Fertil Steril, 2007; 88 (Suppl 1): S213.

[6] Guo SW. Epigenetics and endometriosis. Mol Hum Reprod, 2009 Oct; 15 (10): 587–607.

[7] Dyson MT, Roqueiro D, Monsivais D, et al. Genome-wide DNA methylation analysis predicts an epigenetic switch for GATA factor expression in endometriosis. PLoS Genet, 2014 Mar; 10 (3): e1004158.

[8] Guo SW. Epigenetics and endometriosis. Mol Hum Reprod, 2009 Oct; 15 (10): 587–607.

[9] Ahn S, Monsanto S, Miller C, et al. Pathophysiology and Immune Dysfunction in Endometriosis. Biomed Res Int, 2015 Jul; Article ID 795976: 1–12.

[10] Ballweg ML. Big picture of endometriosis helps provide guidance on approach to teens: comparative historical data show endo starting younger, is more severe. J Pediatr Adolesc Gynecol, 2003 Jun; 16 (3 Suppl): S21–26; Koninckx PR. The pathophysiology of endometriosis: Pollution and dioxin. Gynecol Obstet Investig, 1999; 47(Suppl 1): 47–50.

11 Ballweg ML. Big picture of endometriosis helps provide guidance on approach to teens: comparative historical data show endo starting younger, is more severe. J Pediatr Adolesc Gynecol, 2003 Jun; 16 (3 Suppl): S21–26.

12 Birnbaum LS, Cummings AM. Dioxins and endometriosis: A plausible hypothesis. Environ Health Perspect, 2002 Jan; 110 (1): 1–21.

13 Dioxins and furans: the most toxic chemicals known to science. Energy Justice Network. Available at: http://www.ejnet.org/dioxin/.

14 U.S. Environmental Protection Agency. Risk Characterization of Dioxin and Related Compounds: Dioxin Reassessment. Washington, DC: US Environmental Protection Agency, 1994.

15 U.S. Food and Drug Administration. Tampons and asbestos, dioxin, & toxic shock syndrome. Available at: http://www.fda.gov/MedicalDevices/Safety/AlertsandNotices/PatientAlerts/ucm070003.htm.

16 Mrema EJ, Rubino FM, Brambilla G, et al. Persistent organochlorinated pesticides and mechanisms of their toxicity. Toxicology, 2013 May; 307: 74–88.

17 Rier SE, Martin DC, Bowman RE, et al. Immunoresonsiveness in endometriosis: Implications of estrogenic toxicants. Environ Health Perspect, 1995 Oct; 103 (Suppl 7): 151–56; Bruner-Tran K, Ding T, Osteen K. Dioxin and endometrial progesterone resistance. Semin Reprod Med, 2010 Jan; 28 (1): 59–68.

18 Bailey MT, Coe CL. Endometriosis is associated with altered profile of intestinal microflora in female rhesus monkeys. Hum Reprod, 2002 Jul; 17 (7): 1704–1708; Bulun SE, Zeitoun KM, Kilic G. Expression of dioxin-related transactivating factors and target genes in human eutopic endometrial and endometriotic tissues. Am J Obstet Gynecol, 2000 Apr; 182 (4): 767–75; Herington JL, Bruner-Tran KL, Lucas JA, et al. Immune interactions in endometriosis. Expert Rev Clin Immunol, 2011 Sep; 7 (5): 611–26.

19 Schecter A, Colacino J, Haffner D, et al. Perfluorinated compounds, polychlorinated biphenyls, and organochlorine pesticide contamination in composite food samples from Dallas, Texas, USA. Environ Health Perspect, 2010 Jun; 118 (6): 796–802.

20 Rier S, Foster WG. Environmental dioxins and endometriosis. Toxicol Sci, 2002 Dec; 70 (2): 161–70; Bruner-Tran KL, Yeaman GR, Crispens MA, et al. Dioxin may promote inflammation-related development of endometriosis. Fertil Steril, 2008 May; 89(5 Suppl): 1287–98; Porpora MG, Medda E, Abballe A, et al. Endometriosis and organochlorinated environmental pollutants: a case-control study on Italian women of reproductive age. Environ Health Perspect, 2009 Jul; 117 (7): 1070–75.

21 Buck Louis GM, Peterson CM, Chen Z, et al. Bisphenol A and phthalates and endometriosis: The endometriosis: natural history, diagnosis and outcomes study. Fertil Steril, 2013 Jul; 100 (1): 162–169.e2.

22 Quesda I, Fuentes E, Viso-León MC, et al. Low doses of the endocrine disruptor bisphenol-A and the native hormone 17beta-estradiol rapidly activate transcription factor CREB. FASEB J, 2002 Oct; 16 (12): 1671–73.

23 Upson K, De Roos A, Thompson M, et al. Organochlorine pesticides and risk of endometriosis: findings from a population-based case-control study. Environ Health Perspect, 2013 Nov–Dec; 121 (11–12): 1319–24.

24 Harada T. Dysmenorrhea and endometriosis in young women. Yonago Acta Med, 2013 Dec; 56 (4): 81–84.

25 DeLeon FD, Vijayakumar R, Brown M, et al. Peritoneal fluid volume, estrogen, progesterone, prostaglandin, and epidermal growth factor concentrations in patients with and without endometriosis. Obstet Gynecol, 1986 Aug; 68 (2): 189–94.

26 Wu MH, Shoji Y, Chuang PC, et al. Endometriosis: Disease pathophysiology and the role of prostaglandins. Expert Rev Mol Med, 2007 Jan; 9 (2): 1–20.

27 Nobel LS, Takayama K, Zeitoun KM, et al. Prostaglandin E2 stimulates aromatase expression in endometriosis-derived stromal cells. J Clin Endocrinol Metab, 1997 Feb; 82 (2): 600–606.

28 Van Langendonckt A, Casanas-Roux F, Donnez J. Oxidative stress and peritoneal endometriosis. Fertil Steril, 2002 May; 77 (5): 861–70.

29 Esposito K, et al. Inflammatory cytokine concentrations are acutely increased by hyperglycemia in humans: Role of oxidative stress. Circulation, 2002, Oct: 106 (16); 2067–72.

30 Van Langendonckt A, Casanas-Roux F, Donnez J. Oxidative stress and peritoneal endometriosis. Fertil Steril, 2002 May; 77 (5): 861–70.

31 Hidden in Plain Sight. SugarScience. Available at: http://www.sugarscience.org/hidden-in-plain-sight/#.VyJSymMXJtl.

32 Hidden in Plain Sight. SugarScience. Available at: http://www.sugarscience.org/hidden-in-plain-sight/#.VyJSymMXJtl.

33 Lenoir M, Serre F, Cantin L, et al. Intense Sweetness Surpasses Cocaine Reward. PLoS ONE, 2007 Aug; 2 (8): e698.

34 Wang GJ, Volkow ND, Thanos PK, et al. Similarity between obesity and drug addiction as assessed by neurofunctional imaging: A concept review. J Addict Dis, 2004; 23 (3): 39–53.

35 Frank GK, Oberndorfer TA, Simmons AN, et al. Sucrose activates human taste pathways differently than artificial sweetener. Neuroimage, 2008 Feb; 39 (4): 1559–69.

36 Ahn S, Monsanto S, Miller C, et al. Pathophysiology and Immune Dysfunction in Endometriosis. Biomed Res Int, 2015 Jul; Article ID 795976: 1–12; Herington J, Bruner-Tran K, Lucas J, et al. Immune interactions in endometriosis. Expert Rev Clin Immunol, 2011 Sep; 7 (5): 611–26.

37 Lagana A, Sturlese E, Retto G, et al. Interplay between misplaced mullerian-derived stem cells and peritoneal immune dysregulation in the pathogenesis of endometriosis. Obstet Gynecol Int, 2013. Article ID 52704.

38 Herington J, Bruner-Tran K, Lucas J, et al. Immune interactions in endometriosis. Expert Rev Clin Immunol, 2011 Sep; 7 (5): 611–26.

39 Lagana A, Sturlese E, Retto G, et al. Interplay between misplaced mullerian-derived stem cells and peritoneal immune dysregulation in the pathogenesis of endo-metriosis. Obstet Gynecol Int, 2013. Article ID 52704.

40 Herington J, Bruner-Tran K, Lucas J, et al. Immune interactions in endometriosis. Expert Rev Clin Immunol, 2011 Sep; 7 (5): 611–26.

41 Berbic M, Hey-Cunningham A, Ng C, et al. The role of Foxp3 + regulatory T-cells in endometriosis: A potential controlling mechanism for a complex, chronic immunological condition. Hum. Reprod, 2010 Apr, 25 (4): 900–907; Slabe N, Meden-Vrtovec H, Verdenik I, et al. Cytotoxic T-Cells in Peripheral Blood in Women with Endometriosis. Geburtshilfe Frauenheilkd, 2013 Oct; 73 (10):1042–48.

42 Bailey MT, Coe CL. Endometriosis is associated with altered profile of intestinal microflora in female rhesus monkeys. Hum Reprod, 2002 Jul; 17 (7): 1704–1708.

43 Miniello VL, Colasanto A, Cristofori F, et al. Gut microbiota biomodulators, when the stork comes by the scalpel. Clin Chim Acta, 2015 Dec; 451 (Pt A): 88–96.

44 Jandhyala SM, Talukdar R, Subramanyam C, et al. Role of the normal gut microbiota. World J Gastroenterol, 2015 Aug; 21 (29): 8787–803. doi:10.3748/wjg.v21.i29.8787

45 Goldin BR, Gorbach SL. The effect of milk and lacto-bacillus feeding on human intestinal bacterial enzyme activity. Am J Clin Nutr, 1984 May; 39 (5): 756–61.

46 Samsel A, Seneff S. Glyphosate's suppression of cytochrome P450 enzymes and amino acid biosynthesis by the gut microbiome: Pathways to modern diseases. Entropy, 2013; 15 (4): 1416–63.

47 Samsel A, Seneff S. Glyphosate's suppression of cytochrome P450 enzymes and amino acid biosynthesis by the gut microbiome: Pathways to modern diseases. Entropy, 2013; 15 (4): 1416–63.

48 Mathias JR, Franklin R, Quast DC, et al. Relation of endometriosis and neuromuscular disease of the gastrointestinal tract: New insights. Fertil Steril, 1998 Jul; 70 (1): 81–88.

49 Gur T, Worly B, Bailey M. Stress and the commensal microbiota: Importance in parturition and infant neurodevelopment. Front Psychiatry, 2015 Feb; 6 (5).

50 Wacklin P, Mäkivuokko H, Alakulppi N, et al. Secretor Genotype (FUT2 gene) is strongly associated with the composition of Bifidobacteria in the human intestine. PLoS ONE, 2011; 6 (5) :e20113.

51 Bergstrom A, et al. Establishment of intestinal microbiota during early life: a longitudinal, explorative study of a large cohort of Danish infants. Appl Environ Microbiol, 2014 May; 80 (9): 2889–900.

52 Vangay, P, Ward T, Gerber J, et al. Antibiotics, pediatric dysbiosis, and disease. Cell Host Microbe, 2015 May; 17 (5): 553–64.

53 Filler K, Lyon D, Bennett J, et al. Association of mitochondrial dysfunction and fatigue: A review of the literature. BBA Clin, 2014 Jun; 1: 12–23.

54 Cho S, Lee YM, Choi YS, et al. Mitochondrial DNA polymorphisms are associated with susceptibility to endometriosis. DNA Cell Biol, 2012 Mar; 31 (3): 317–22.

55 Xing X, Wang L, Ren Y, et al. Differences in mitochondrial proteins in the eutopic endometrium of patients with adenomyosis and endometriosis identified using surface-enhanced laser absorption/ionization time-of-flight mass spectrometry. J Int Med Res, 2010 May–Jun: (38) 3: 987–93; Xu B, Guo N, Zhang X, et al. Oocyte quality is decreased in women with minimal or mild endometriosis. Sci Rep, 2015 May; Article ID 107798.

56 Kang YJ, Bang B-R, Han KH, et al. Regulation of NKT cell-mediated immune responses to tumours and liver inflammation by mitochondrial PGAM5-Drp1 signalling. Nat Commun, 2015 Sep; (6): 8371; Walker M, Volpi S, Sims K, et al. Powering the immune system: Mitochondria in immune function and deficiency. J Immunol Res, 2014; Article ID 164309.

57 Segura, G. Ketogenic diet — a connection between mitochondria and diet. August 9, 2013. Available at: http://www.drmyhill.co.uk/wiki/Ketogenic_diet_-_a_connection_between_mitochondria_and_diet#References.

58 Menshikova EV, Ritov VB, Fairfull L, et al. Effects of Exercise on Mitochondrial Content and Function in Aging Human Skeletal Muscle. J Gerontol A Biol Sci Med Sci, 2006 Jun; 61 (6): 534–40.

59 Hardie DG. AMP-activated protein kinase: A key system mediating metabolic responses to exercise. Med Sci Sports Exerc, 2004 Jan; 36 (1): 28–34.

60 Bulun SE, Zeitoun KM, Takayama K, et al. Estrogen bio-synthesis in endometriosis: Molecular basis and clinical relevance. J Mol Endocrinol, 2000 Aug; 25 (1): 35–42.

61 Hall D. Nutritional influences on estrogen metabolism. Applied Nutritional Science Reports. Advanced Nutrition Publications, Inc: 2001.

62 Hall D. Nutritional influences on estrogen metabolism. Applied Nutritional Science Reports. Advanced Nutrition Publications, Inc: 2001.

63 Bianco B, Barbosa C, Christofolini D. Polymmorphisms in the CYP2C19 and HSD17B1 genes associated to estrogen metabolism in women with endometriosis. Fertil Steril, 2013; 100 (3): S363.

64 Xu X, Ding J, Rana N, et al. Association between COMT gene polymorphism and endometriosis-associated pain: An interim analysis. Fertil Steril, 2007; 88 (Suppl 1): S21.

65 Hall D. Nutritional influences on estrogen metabolism. Applied Nutritional Science Reports. Advanced Nutrition Publications, Inc: 2001.

66 Segerstrom S, Miller G. Psychological stress and the human immune system: a meta-analytic study of 30 years of inquiry. Psychol Bull, 2004 Jul; 130 (4): 601-30.

67 Cohen S, Janicki-Deverts D, Doyle WJ, et al. Chronic stress, glucocorticoid receptor resistance, inflammation, and disease risk. Proc Natl Acad Sci USA, 2012 Apr; 109 (16): 5995-99.

68 Lloyd C, Smith J, Weinger K. Stress and diabetes: A review of the links. Diabetes Spectrum, 2005 Apr; 18 (2): 121-27.

69 Whirledge S, Cidlowski J. Glucocorticoid, stress, and fertility. Minerva Endocrinol, 2010 Jun; 35 (2): 109-25.

70 Bhatia V, Tandon RK. Stress and the gastrointestinal tract. J Gastroenterol Hepatol, 2005 Mar; 20 (3): 332-39.

71 Bharwani A, Mian M, Foster J, et al. Structural and functional consequences of chronic psychosocial stress on the microbiome and host. Psychoneuroendocrinology, 2016 Jan; 63: 217-27.

72 Cuevas m, Flores I, Thompson JK, et al. Stress exacerbates endometriosis manifestations and inflammatory parameters in an animal model. Reprod Sci, 2012 Aug; 19 (8): 851-62; Leyendecker G, Wildt L, Mall G, et al. The pathophysiology of endometriosis and adenomyosis: Tissue injury and repair. Arch Gynecol Obstet, 2009 Oct; 280 (4): 529-38; Wieser F, Vitonis A, Rich-Edwards J, et al. Abuse in childhood and risk of endometriosis. Fertil Steril, 2012 Sep; 98 (3): S218.

73 Felitti V, Anda RF, Nordenberg D, et al. Relationship of childhood abuse and household dysfunction to many of the leading causes of death in adults. Am J Prev Med, 1998 May; 14 (4): 245-58.

74 Nugent C, Black L. Sleep duration, quality of sleep, and use of sleep medication by sex and family type, 2013-2014. NCHS Data Brief, 2016 Jan; 230: 1-8.

75 Hirshkowitz M, Whiton K, Albert SM. National Sleep Foundation's sleep time duration recommendations: Methodology and results summary. Sleep Health, 2015 Mar; 1 (1): 40-43.

76 Nugent C, Black L. Sleep duration, quality of sleep, and use of sleep medication by sex and family type, 2013-2014. NCHS Data Brief, 2016 Jan; 230: 1-8.

77 Nunes FR, Ferreira JM, Bahamondes L. Pain threshold and sleep quality in women with endometriosis. Eur J Pain, 2015 Jan; 19 (1): 15-20.

78 Irwin MR, Olmstead R, Carrillo C, et al. Sleep loss exacerbates fatigue, depression, and pain in rheumatoid arthritis. Sleep, 2012 Apr; 35 (4): 537-43; McBeth J, Lacey R, Wilkie R. Predictors of new-onset pain in older adults: Results from a population-based prospective cohort study in the UK. Arthritis Rheumatol, 2014 Mar; 66 (3): 757-67.

79 National Sleep Foundation. Sleep-Wake Cycle: Its Physiology and Impact on Health. 2006. Available at: https://sleepfoundation.org/sites/default/files/SleepWakeCycle.pdf.

80 Waknine Y. Wake Time Influences Circadian Clock More Than Bed Time, Medscape, 2005 Jun 28. Available at: http://www.medscape.com/viewarticle/507491.

81 Parazzini F, Vigano P, Candiani M, et al. Diet and endometriosis risk: A literature review. Reprod BioMed Online, 2013; 26 (4): 323-36.

82 Bulun SE, Zeitoun KM, Takayama K, et al. Estrogen biosynthesis in endometriosis: Molecular basis and clinical relevance. J Mol Endocrinol, 2000 Aug; 25 (1): 35-42.

83 Mozaffarian D, Pischon T, Hankinson SE, et al. Dietary intake of trans fatty acids and systemic inflammation in women. Am J Clin Nutr, 2004 Apr; 79 (4): 606-12; Simopoulos AP. The importance of the ratio of omega-6/omega-3 essential fatty acids. Biomed Pharmacother, 2002 Oct; 56 (8): 365-79.

84 Hall D. Nutritional influences on estrogen metabolism. Applied Nutritional Science Reports. Advanced Nutrition Publications, Inc: 2001.

85 Hall D. Nutritional influences on estrogen metabolism. Applied Nutritional Science Reports. Advanced Nutrition Publications, Inc: 2001.

86 Olefsky JM, Glass CK. Macrophages, inflammation, and insulin resistance. Annu Rev Physiol, 2010; 72: 219-46; Orhan B, Hardy D, Carr B, et al. Inflammatory status influences aromatase and steroid receptor expression in endometriosis. Endocrinology, 2008 Mar; 149 (3): 1190-1204.

87 Parazzini F, Vigano P, Candiani M, et al. Diet and endometriosis risk: A literature review. Reprod BioMed Online, 2013; 26 (4): 323-36.

88 Handa Y, Fujita H, Honma S, et al. Estrogen concentrations in beef and human hormone-dependent cancers. Ann Oncol, 2009 Sep; 20 (9): 1610–11.

89 Handa Y, Fujita H, Watanabe Y, et al. Does dietary estrogen intake from meat relate to the incidence of hormone-dependent cancers? J Clin Oncol, 2010 May; 28 (15): 1553.

90 Evans JM. An integrative approach to fibroids, endometriosis, and breast cancer prevention. Integr Med, 2008 Oct–Nov; 7 (5): 28–31.

91 Parazzini F, Vigano P, Candiani M, et al. Diet and endometriosis risk: A literature review. Reprod BioMed Online, 2013; 26 (4): 323–36.

92 Evans JM. An integrative approach to fibroids, endometriosis, and breast cancer prevention. Integr Med, 2008 Oct–Nov; 7 (5): 28–31.

93 Marziali M, Venza M, Lazzaro S, et al. Gluten-free diet: A new strategy for management of painful endometriosis related symptoms? Minerva Chir, 2012 Dec; 67 (6): 499–504.

94 Parazzini F, Vigano P, Candiani M, et al. Diet and endometriosis risk: A literature review. Reprod BioMed Online, 2013; 26 (4): 323–36.

95 Parazzini F, Vigano P, Candiani M, et al. Diet and endometriosis risk: A literature review. Reprod BioMed Online, 2013; 26 (4): 323–36.

96 Parazzini F, Vigano P, Candiani M, et al. Diet and endometriosis risk: A literature review. Reprod BioMed Online, 2013; 26 (4): 323–36.

97 Guo SW. Epigenetics and endometriosis. Mol Hum Reprod, 2009 Oct; 15 (10): 587–607.

98 Mier-Cabrera J, Aburto-Soto T, Burrola-Mendez S, et al. Women with endometriosis improved their peripheral antioxidant markers after the application of a high antioxidant diet. Reprod Biol Endocrinol, 2009 May; 7 (54).

99 Porpora MG, Medda E, Abballe A, et al. Endometriosis and organochlorinated environmental pollutants: A case-control study on Italian women of reproductive age. Environ Health Perspect, 2009 Jul; 117 (7): 1070–75.

100 Milanski M, Degasperi G, Coope A, et al. Saturated fatty acids produce an inflammatory response predominantly through the activation of TLR4 signaling in hypothalamus: Implications for the pathogenesis of obesity. J Neurosci, 2009 Jan; 29 (2): 359–70.

Chapter 5

1 Haas D, Chvatal R, Reichert B, et al. Endometriosis: A premenopausal disease? Age pattern in 42,079 patients with endometriosis. Arch Gynecol Obstet, 2012 Sep; 286 (3): 667–70.

2 Food and Drug Administration. Mirena (fact sheet). Available at: http://www.accessdata.fda.gov/drugsatfda_docs/label/2009/021225s027lbl.pdf.

3 Fulop I, Rucz A, Szakonyi T, et al. Evaluation of the Efficacy of Different Operative Techniques in the Treatment of Peritoneal Endometriosis. P-265, 12th World Congress on Endometriosis, Apr 30–May 3, 2014, Sao Palo, Brazil.

4 Pain and Quality of Life Survey. Commissioned by the UK Endometriosis All-Party Parliamentary Group and presented at the 9th World Congress on Endometriosis. Maastricht, Netherlands, 2005.

5 Abbott J, Hawe J, Hunter D, et al. Laparoscopic excision of endometriosis: A randomized placebo-controlled trial. Fertil Steril, 2004 Oct; 82 (4): 878–84.

Chapter 6

1 Genuis SJ, Birkholz D, Rodushkin I, et al. Blood, urine, and sweat (BUS) study: Monitoring and elimination of bioaccumulated toxic elements. Arch Environ Contam Toxicol, 2011 Aug; 61 (2): 344–57.

2 Genuis SJ, Beesoon S, Lobo RA, et al. Human elimination of phthalate compounds: Blood, urine, and sweat (BUS) study. ScientificWorldJournal, 2012; 2012: 615068; Genuis SJ, Beesoon S, Birkholz D, et al. Human excretion of bisphenol A: Blood, urine, and sweat (BUS) study. J Environ Public Health, 2012; 2012: 185731.

3 Genuis SJ, Birkholz D, Rodushkin I, et al. Blood, urine, and sweat (BUS) study: Monitoring and elimination of bioaccumulated toxic elements. Arch Environ Contam Toxicol, 2011 Aug; 61 (2): 344–57.

4 Rier SE, Yeaman GR. Immune aspects of endometriosis: A relevance of the uterine mucosal immune system. Semin Reprod Endocrinol, 1997: 15 (3): 209-20.

5 Ahn S, Monsanto S, Miller C, et al. Pathophysiology and Immune Disfunction in Endometriosis. Biomed Res Int, 2015: Article ID 795976.

6 Schmulson M, Chang L. The treatment of functional abdominal bloating and distension. Aliment Pharmacol Ther, 2011 May; 33 (10): 1071–86.

7 Crinnion W. Components of practical clinical detox programs — sauna as a therapeutic tool. Altern Ther Health Med, 2007 Mar–Apr; 13 (2): S154–56.

8 Sen CK. Glutathione homeostasis in response to exercise training and nutritional supplements. Mol Cell Biochem, 1999 Jun; 196 (1–2): 31–42.

9 Ngo C, Chereau C, Nicco C, et al. Reactive oxygen species controls endometriosis progression. Am J Pathol, 2009 Jul; 175 (1): 225–34.

10 Li M, Chen K, Mo Z. Use of qigong therapy in the detoxification of heroin addicts. Altern Ther Health Med, 2002 Jan–Feb; 8 (1): 50–4.

Chapter 7

[1] Church D, Yount G, Brooks A. The Effect of Emotional Freedom Techniques on Stress Biochemistry: A Randomized Controlled Trial. J Nerv Ment Dis. 2012 Oct; 200 (10): 891–96.

[2] Ritter M, Low K. Effects of dance movement therapy: A meta-analysis. Arts in Psychotherapy, 1996; 23 (3): 249–60.

[3] Koch S, Bräuninger I. International Dance/Movement Therapy Research: Theory, Methods, and Empirical Findings. American Journal of Dance Therapy, 2005 Mar; 27 (1): 37–46.

Chapter 9

[1] Kohl HW, Craig CL, Lambert EV et al. The pandemic of physical inactivity: Global action for public health. Lancet, 2012 Jul; 380 (9838): 294–305.

[2] Young DR, Reynolds K, Sidell M, et al. Effects of physical activity and sedentary time on the risk of heart failure. Circ Heart Fail, 2014 Jan; 7: 21–27.

[3] Wilmot EG, Edwardson CL, Achana FA, et al. Sedentary time in adults and the association with diabetes, cardiovascular disease and death: Systematic review and meta-analysis. Diabetologia, 2012 Nov; 55 (11): 2895–2905.

[4] Balkau B, Mhamdi L, Oppert JM, et al. Physical activity and insulin sensitivity: The RISC study. Diabetes, 2008 Oct; 57 (10): 2613–18.

[5] Lew H, Quintanilha A. Effects of endurance training and exercise on tissue antioxidataive capacity and acetaminophen detoxification. Eur J Drug Metab Pharmacokinet, 1991 Jan–Mar; 16 (1): 59–68.

[6] Sen K. Glutathione homeostasis in response to exercise training and nutritional supplements. Mol Cell Biochem, 1999 Jun; 196 (1–2): 31–32.

[7] Ngo C, Chereau C, Nicco C, et al. Reactive oxygen species controls endometriosis progression. Am J Pathol, 2009 Jul; 175 (1): 225–34.

[8] Smith A, Phipps W, Thomas W, et al. The effects of aerobic exercise on estrogen metabolism in healthy premenopausal women. Cancer Epidemiol Biomarkers Prev, 2013 May; 22 (5): 756–64.

[9] Brinton LA, Gridley G, Persson I, et al. Cancer risk after a hospital discharge diagnosis of endometriosis. Am J Obstet Gynecol, 1997 Mar; 176 (3): 572–29; Melin A, Sparén P, Persson I, et al. Endometriosis and the risk of cancer with special emphasis on ovarian cancer. Hum Reprod, 2006 May; 21 (5): 1237–42; Yoshikawa H, Jimbo H, Okada S, et al. Prevalence of endometriosis in ovarian cancer. Gynecol Obstet Invest, 2000; 50 (Suppl 1): 11–17; DeLigdisch L, Pénault-Llorca F, Schlosshauer P, et al. Stage I ovarian carcinoma: Different clinical pathologic patterns. Fertil Steril, 2007 Oct; 88 (4): 906–10.

[10] Ennour-Idrissi K, Maunsell E, Diorio C. Effect of physical activity on sex hormones in women: A systematic review and meta-analysis of randomized controlled trials. Breast Cancer Res, 2015 Nov; 17 (1): 139.

[11] Vaziri F, Hoseini A, Kamali F, et al. Comparing the effects of aerobic and stretching exercises on the intensity of primary dysmenorrhea in the students of universities of bushehr. J Family Reprod Health, 2015 Mar; 9 (1): 23–28.

[12] La Gerche A, Burns AT, Mooney DJ, et al. Exercise-induced right ventricular dysfunction and structural remodeling in endurance athletes. Eur Heart J, 2012 Apr; 33 (8): 998–1006.

[13] Ober C, Sinatra S, Zucker M. Earthing: The most important health discovery ever? Laguna Beach, CA: Basic Health Publications, 2014.

Chapter 10

[1] Mann D. Negative ions create positive vibes. WebMD, 2002 May 6. Available at: http://www.webmd.com/balance/features/negative-ions-create-positive-vibe.

[2] Goldstein N, Arshavskaya TV. Is atmospheric superoxide vitally necessary? Accelerated death of animals in a quasi-neutral electric atmosphere. Z Naturforsch C, 1997 May–Jun; 52 (5–6): 396–404; Livanova LM, Levshina IP, Nozdracheva LV, et al. The protective action of negative air ions in acute stress in rats with different typological behavioral characteristics. Zh Vyssh Nerv Deiat Im I P Pavlova 1998 May–Jun; 48 (3): 554–57; Goel N, Etwaroo GR. Bright light, negative air ions and auditory stimuli produce rapid mood changes in a student population: A placebo-controlled study. Psychol Med, 2006 Sep; 36 (9): 1253–63; Thayer RE. Biopsychology of Mood and Arousal. New York: Oxford University Press, 1989; Chevalier, G, Sinatra, ST, Oschman, J. et al. Earthing (Grounding) the Human Body Reduces Blood Viscosity — a Major Factor in Cardiovascular Disease. J Altern Complement Medicine, 2013 Feb; 19 (2): 102–110; Oschman JL. Can electrons act as antioxidants? A review and commentary. J Altern Complement Med, 2007 Nov; 13: 955–67: Chevalier G, Sinatra ST, Oschman JL, et al. Earthing: Health implications of reconnecting the human body to the earth's surface electrons. J Environ Public Health, 2012: Article ID 291541.

Chapter 11

1 Therapeutic Research staff. Milk Thistle. Therapeutic Research 2016. Available at: https://naturalmedicines.therapeuticresearch.com/databases/food,-herbs-supplements/professional.aspx?productid=138# dosing. Last updated on 1/12/2016. Accessed 5/25/16.

2 Ngo C, Chereau C, Nicco C, et al. Reactive oxygen species controls endometriosis progression. Am J Pathol, 2009 Jul; 175 (1): 225–34; Radomska-Lesniewska D, Skopinski P. N-acetylcysteine as an anti-oxidant and anti-inflammatory drug and some of its clinical applications. Centr Eur J Immunol, 2012; 37 (1): 57–66.

3 Fulghesu A, Ciampelli M, Muzj G, et al. N-acetyl-cysteine treatment improves insulin sensitivity in women with polycystic ovary syndrome. Fertil Steril, 2002 Jun; 77 (6): 1128–35; Radomska-Lesniewska D, Skopinski P. N-acetylcysteine as an anti-oxidant and anti-inflammatory drug and some of its clinical applications. Centr Eur J Immunol, 2012; 37 (1): 57–66.

4 Schwertner A, Conceicao dos Santos C, Costa G, et al. Efficacy of melatonin in the treatment of placebo endometriosis: A phase II, randomized, double-blind, placebo controlled trial. Pain, 2013 Jun; 154 (6): 874–81.

5 No authors listed. Alpha-lipoic acid. Monograph. Altern Med Rev, 2006 Sept; 11 (3): 232–37.

6 Taguchi A, Wada-Hiraike O, Kawana K, et al. Resveratrol suppresses inflammatory responses in endometrial stromal cells derived from endometriosis: A possible role of the sirtuin 1 pathway. J Obstet Gynaecol Res, 2014 Mar; 40 (3): 770–78; Maia H Jr, Haddad C, Pinheiro N, et al. Advantages of the association of resveratrol with oral contraceptives for management of endometriosis-related pain. Int J Womens Health, 2012; 4: 543–49.

7 Kohama T, Herai K, Inoue M. Effect of French maritime pine bark extract on endometriosis as compared to leuprorelin acetate. J Reprod Med, 2007 Aug; 52 (8): 703–708; Suzuki N, Uebaba K, Kohama T, et al. French maritime pine bark extract significantly lowers the requirement for analgesic medication in dysmenorrhea. A multicenter, randomized, double-blind, placebo-controlled study. J Reprod Med, 2008 May; 53 (5): 338–46; Kohama T, Suzuki N, Ohno S, et al. Analgesic efficacy of French maritime pine bark extract in dysmenorrhea: An open clinical trial. J Reprod Med, 2004 Oct; 49 (10): 828–32.

8 Zhang Y, Cao H, Yu Z, et al. Curcumin inhibits endometriosis endometrial cells by reducing estradiol production. Iran J Reprod Med, 2013 May; 11 (5): 415–22; Swarnakar S, Paul S. Curcumin arrests endometriosis by downregulation of matrix metalloproteinase-9 activity. Indian J Biochem Biophys, 2009 Feb; 46 (1): 59–65.

9 Chandran B, Goel A. A randomized, pilot study to assess the efficacy and safety of curcumin in patients with active rheumatoid arthritis. Phytother Res, 2012 Nov; 26 (11): 1719–25; Ganjali S, Sahebkar A, Mahdipour E, et al. Investigation of the Effects of Curcumin on Serum Cytokines in Obese Individuals: A Randomized Controlled Trial. ScientificWorldJournal, 2014 Feb; Article ID 898361.

10 Safayhi H, Sailer ER, Ammon HP. Mechanism of 5-lipoxygenase inhibition by acetyl-11-keto-beta-boswellic acid. Mol Pharmacol, 1995 Jun; 47 (6): 1212–16.

11 Gupta PK, Samarakoon SMS, Chandola HM, et al. Clinical evaluation of Boswellia serrata (Shallaki) resin in the management of Sandhivata (osteoarthritis. Ayu, 2011 Oct; 32 (4): 478–82; Sengupta K, Alluri KV, Satish AR, et al. A double blind, randomized, placebo controlled study of the efficacy and safety of 5-Loxin® for treatment of osteoarthritis of the knee. Arthritis Res Ther, 2008; 10 (4): R85; Knaus U, Wagner H. Effects of boswellic acid of Boswellia serrata and other triterpenic acids on the complement system. Phytomedicine, 1996 May; 3 (1): 77–81.

12 Zhao RH, Liu Y, Tan Y, et al. Chinese medicine improves postoperative quality of life in endometriosis patients: a randomized controlled trial. Chin J Integr Med, 2013 Jan; 19 (1): 15–21: Herington JL, Glore DR, Lucas JA, et al. Dietary fish oil supplementation inhibits formation of endometriosis-associated adhesions in a chimeric mouse model. Fertil Steril, 2013 Feb; 99 (2): 543–50.

13 Calder P. Omega-3 polyunsaturated fatty acids and inflammatory processes: nutrition or pharmacology? Br J Clin Pharmacol, 2013 Mar; 75 (3): 645–62.

14 Zhang Q, Xinhua X, Ming L, et al. Berberine moderates glucose metabolism through the GnRH-GLP-1 and MARK pathway in the intestine. BMC Complement Altern Med, 2014 Jun; 14: 188; Li Y, Ma H, Zhang Y, et al. Effect of berberine on insulin resistance in women with polycystic ovary syndrome: Study protocol for a randomized multicenter controlled trial. Trials, 2013 Jul; 14 (226): 1–5.

15 Zhang Y, Li X, Zhang Q, et al. Berberine hydrochloride prevents postsurgery intestinal adhesion and inflammation in rats. J Pharmacol Exp Ther, 2014 Jun; 349 (3): 417–26.

16 Zhao L, Ma Z, Zhu J, et al. Characterization of polysaccharide from astragalus radix as the macrophage stimulator. Cell Immunol, 2011: 271 (2); 329–34; Abuelsaad A. Supplementation with astragalus polysaccharides alters aeromonas-induced tissue-specific cellular immune response. Microb Pathog, 2014 Jan; 66: 48–56.

17 Cho H, Kim Y, Lim E. Effects of Astragalus membranaceus on surgically induced endometriosis in rats. J Oriental Obstet Gynecol, 2007 Jan; 20 (2); 43–59.

18 Natural Medicines Database. Astragalus. Available at: https://naturalmedicines.therapeuticresearch.com/databases/food,-herbs-supplements/professional.aspx?productid=963#scientificName.

19 Groom S, Johns T, Oldfield P. The potency of immunomodulatory herbs may be primarily dependent upon macrophage activation. J Med Food, 2007 Mar; 10 (1): 73–79.

20 Nogueira Neto N, Coelho T, Agular G, et al. Experimental endometriosis reduction in rats treated with Uncaria tomentosa (cat's claw) extract. Eur J Obstet Gynecol Reprod Biol, 2011 Feb; 154 (2); 205–208.

21 Nogueira Neto N, Cavalcante F, Carvalho et al. Contraceptive effect of Uncaria tomentosa (cat's claw) in rats with experimental endometriosis. Acta Cir Bras, 2011; 26 (Suppl 2): 15-19.

22 Natural Medicines Database. Cat's Claw. Available at: https://naturalmedicines.therapeuticresearch.com/databases/food,-herbs-supplements/professional.aspx?productid=395#peopleUseThisFor.

23 Lull C, Wichers HJ, Savelkoul HFJ. Antiinflammatory and immunomodulating properties of fungal metabolites. Mediators Inflamm, 2005 Jun; 2005 (2): 63–80.

24 Wachtel-Galor S, Yuen J, Buswell JA, et al. Ganoderma lucidum (Lingzhi or Reishi: A medicinal mushroom. In: Benzie IFF, Wachtel-Galor S, eds. Herbal Medicine: Biomolecular and Clinical Aspects, 2nd edition. Boca Raton, FL: CRC Press/Taylor & Francis; 2011. Available at: http://www.ncbi.nlm.nih.gov/books/NBK92757/.

25 Chang CJ, Lin CS, Lu, CC et al. Ganoderma lucidum reduces obesity in mice by modulating the composition of the gut microbiota. Nat Commun, 2015; 6: Article ID 7489.

26 Wachtel-Galor S, Yuen J, Buswell JA, et al. Ganoderma lucidum (Lingzhi or Reishi: A medicinal mushroom. In: Benzie IFF, Wachtel-Galor S, eds. Herbal Medicine: Biomolecular and Clinical Aspects, 2nd edition. Boca Raton, FL: CRC Press/Taylor & Francis; 2011. Available at: http://www.ncbi.nlm.nih.gov/books/NBK92757/.

27 Soo T. Effective dosage of extract of Ganoderma lucidum in the treatment of various ailments. In Royse, ed. Mushroom Biology and Mushroom Products. University Park, PA: Penn State University, 1996.

28 Natural Medicines Database. Reishi. Available at: https://naturalmedicines.therapeuticresearch.com/databases/food,-herbs-supplements/professional.aspx?productid=905#dosing.

29 O'Mahony, McCarthy, J, Kelly P, et al. Lactobacillus and bifidobacterium in irritable bowel syndrome: Symptom responses and relationship to cytokine profiles. Gastroenterology, 2005 Mar; 128 (3): 541–51.

30 Iwai W, Abe Y, Iijima K, et al. Gastric hypochlorhydria is associated with an exacerbation of dyspeptic symptoms in female patients. J Gastroenterol, 2013 Feb; 48 (2): 214–21.

31 Rosch W, Vinson B, Sassin I. A randomized clinical trial comparing the efficacy of a herbal preparation of STW 5 with the prokinetic drug ciasapride in patients with dysmotility type of functional dyspepsia. Z Gastroenterol, 2002 Jun; 40 (6): 4401–4408.

32 Ianiro G, Pecere S, Giorgio V, et al. Digestive enzyme supplementation in gastrointestinal diseases. Curr Drug Metab, 2016; 17 (2): 187–93.

33 Mahmood A, FitzGerald AJ, Marchbank T, et al. Zinc carnosine, a health food supplement that stabilises small bowel integrity and stimulates gut repair processes. Gut, 2007 Feb; 56 (2): 168–75.

34 Canani RB, Costanzo MD, Leone L, et al. Potential beneficial effects of butyrate in intestinal and extraintestinal diseases. World J Gastroenterol, 2011 Mar; 17 (12): 1519–28.

35 Furusawa Y, Obata Y, Fukuda S, et al. Commensal microbe-derived butyrate induces the differentiation of colonic regulatory T cells. Nature. 2014 Feb; 13; 506 (7487): 446–50.

36 Rao R, Samak G. Role of glutamine in protection of intestinal epithelial tight junctions. J Epithel Biol Pharmacol, 2012 Jan; 5 (Suppl 1-M7): 47–54.

37 Therapeutic Research staff. Glutamine. Therapeutic Research 2016. Available at: https://naturalmedicines.therapeuticresearch.com/databases/food,-herbs-supplements/professional.aspx?productid=878#dosing.

38 O'Mahony, McCarthy, J, Kelly P, et al. Lactobacillus and bifidobacterium in irritable bowel syndrome: Symptom responses and relationship to cytokine profiles. Gastroenterology, 2005 Mar; 128 (3): 541–51.

39 Filler K, Lyon D, Bennett J, et al. Association of mitochondrial dysfunction and fatigue: A review of the literature. BBA Clin, 2014, Jun; 1: 12–23.

40 Mizuno K, Tanaka M, Nozaki S et al. Antifatigue effects of coenzyme Q10 during physical fatigue. Nutrition, 2008 Apr; 24 (4): 293–99; Cordero J, Alocer Gomez E, de Miguel M, et al. Can coenzyme q10 improve clinical and molecular parameters in fibromyalgia? Antioxid Redox Signal, 2013 Oct; 19 (12): 1356–61.

41 Natural Medicines Database. Astragalus. Available at: https://naturalmedicines.therapeuticresearch.com/databases/food,-herbs-supplements/professional.aspx?productid=998#dosing.

42 Liu J. The effects and mechanisms of mitochondrial nutrient alpha-lipoic acid on improving age-associated mitochondrial and cognitive dysfunction: an overview. Neurochem Res, 2008 Jan; 33 (1): 194–203.

[43] Hermann, R, Niebch, G. Enantioselective pharmacokinetics and bioavailability of different racemic alpha lipoic acid formulations in healthy volunteers. Eur J Pharm Sci, 1996; 4: 167–74.

[44] Khabbazi T, Mahdavi R, Safa J, et al. Effects of alpha-lipoic acid supplementation on inflammation, oxidative stress, and serum lipid profile levels in patients with end-stage renal disease on hemodialysis . J Ren Nutr, 2012 Mar; 22 (2): 244–50.

[45] Ferretta A, Gaballo A, Tanzarella P, et al. Effect of resveratrol on mitochondrial function: Implications in parkin-associated familiar Parkinson's disease. Biochem Biophys Acta, 2014 Jul; 1842 (7): 902–15.

[46] Taguchi A, Wada-Hiraike O, Kawana K, et al. Resveratrol suppresses inflammatory responses in endometrial stromal cells derived from endometriosis: A possible role of the sirtuin 1 pathway. J Obstet Gynaecol Res, 2014 Mar; 40 (3): 770–78; Maia H Jr, Haddad C, Pinheiro N, et al. Advantages of the association of resveratrol with oral contraceptives for management of endometriosis-related pain. Int J Womens Health, 2012; 4: 543–49.

[47] Maia H Jr, Haddad C, Pinheiro N, et al. Advantages of the association of resveratrol with oral contraceptives for management of endometriosis-related pain. Int J Womens Health, 2012; 4: 543–49.

[48] Roemheld-Hamm B. Chasteberry. Am Fam Physicia, 2005 Sep; 72 (5): 821–24.

[49] Aksoy AN, Gozukara I, Kabil Kocur S. Evaulation of the efficacy of Fructus agni casti in women with severe primary dysmenorrhea: A prospective comparative Doppler study. J Obstet Gynaecol Res, 2014 Mar; 40 (3): 84.

[50] Dalessandri KM, Firestone GL, Fitch MD, et al. Pilot study: Effect of 3,3'-diindolylmethane supplements on urinary hormone metabolites in postmenopausal women with a history of early-stage breast cancer. Nutr Cancer 2004; 50 (2), 161–67.

[51] Rajoria S, Suriano R, Parmar PS, et al. 3,3'-diindolylmethane modulates estrogen metabolism in patients with thyroid proliferation disease: A pilot study. Thyroid. 2011 Mar; 21 (3): 299–304; Dalessandri KM, Firestone GL, Fitch MD, et al. Pilot study: Effect of 3,3'-diindolylmethane supplements on urinary hormone metabolites in postmenopausal women with a history of early-stage breast cancer. Nutr Cancer 2004; 50 (2), 161–67 (used Bio-Response DIM).

[52] O'Mahony, McCarthy, J, Kelly P, et al. Lactobacillus and bifidobacterium in irritable bowel syndrome: Symptom responses and relationship to cytokine profiles. Gastroenterology, 2005 Mar; 128 (3): 541–51.

[53] Taguchi A, Wada-Hiraike O, Kawana K, et al. Resveratrol suppresses inflammatory responses in endometrial stromal cells derived from endometriosis: A possible role of the sirtuin 1 pathway. J Obstet Gynaecol Res, 2014 Mar; 40 (3): 770–78; Maia H Jr, Haddad C, Pinheiro N, et al. Advantages of the association of resveratrol with oral contraceptives for management of endometriosis-related pain. Int J Womens Health, 2012; 4: 543–49.

[54] Kohama T, Herai K, Inoue M. Effect of French maritime pine bark extract on endometriosis as compared to leuprorelin acetate. J Reprod Med, 2007 Aug; 52 (8): 703–708; Suzuki N, Uebaba K, Kohama T, et al. French maritime pine bark extract significantly lowers the requirement for analgesic medication in dysmenorrhea. A multicenter, randomized, double-blind, placebo-controlled study. J Reprod Med, 2008 May; 53 (5): 338–46; Kohama T, Suzuki N, Ohno S, et al. Analgesic efficacy of French maritime pine bark extract in dysmenorrhea: An open clinical trial. J Reprod Med, 2004 Oct; 49 (10): 828–32.

[55] No authors listed. Calcium-D-glucarate. Altern Med Rev, 2002 Aug; 7 (4): 336–39.

[56] Walaszek Z, Hanuasek M, Sherman U, et al. Antiproliferative effect of dietary glucarate on the Sprague-Dawley rat mammary gland. Cancer Lett, 1990 Jan; 49 (1): 51–57.

[57] Stough C, Scholey A, Lloyd J, et al. The effect of 90 day administration of a high dose vitamin B-complex on work stress. Hum Psychopharmacol, 2011 Oct; 26 (7): 470–76.

[58] American Chemical Society. Scientists say vitamin c may alleviate the body's response to stress. ScienceDaily. 1999 August 23. Available at: www.sciencedaily.com/releases/1999/08/990823072615.htm.

[59] Peters EM, Anderson R, Nieman DC, et al. Vitamin C supplementation attenuates the increases in circulating cortisol, adrenaline, and anti-inflammatory polypeptides following ultramarathon running. Int J Sports Med, 2001 Oct; 22 (7): 537–43.

[60] Brody S, Preut R, Schommer K, et al. A randomized controlled trial of high dose ascorbic acid for reduction of blood pressure, cortisol, and subjective responses to psychological stress. Psychopharmacol (Berl), 2002 Jan; 159 (3): 319–24.

[61] National Institutes of Health. Magnesium. Fact Sheet. Available at: http://dietary-supplements.info.nih.gov/factsheets/magnesium.asp.

[62] Sartori SB, Whittle, N, Hetzenauer A, et al. Magnesium deficiency induces anxiety and HPA axis dysregulation: Modulation by therapeutic drug treatment. Neuropharmacology, 2012 Jan; 62 (1): 304–12.

[63] Sribanditmonogkol V, Neal J, Patrick T, et al. Effect of perceived stress on cytokine production in healthy college students. West J of Nurs Res, 2015 Apr; 37 (4): 481–93.

64 Delarue J, Matzinger O, Binnert C, et al. Fish oil prevents the adrenal activation elicited by mental stress in healthy men. Diabetes Metab, 2003 Jun; 29 (3): 289–95.

65 Hellhammer J, Vogt D, Franz N, et al. A soy-based phosphatidylserine/phosphatidic acid complex (PAS) normalizes the stress reactivity of hypothalamus-pituitary-adrenal-axis in chronically stressed male subjects: a randomized, placebo-controlled study. Lipids Health Dis, 2014 Jul; 13: 121.

66 Cooper R, Morré DJ, Morré DM. Medicinal benefits of green tea: Part 1. Review of noncancer health benefits. J Altern Complement Med, 2005 Jun; 11 (3): 521–28.

67 Yamada T, Terashima T, Okubo T, et al. Effects of theanine, r-glutamylethylamide, on neurotransmitter release and its relationship with glutamic acid neurotransmission. Nutr Neurosci, 2005 Aug; 8 (4): 219–26.

68 Lu K, Gray MA, Oliver C, et al. The acute effects of L-theanine in comparison with alprazolam on anticipatory anxiety in humans. Hum Psychopharmacol. 2004 Oct; 19 (7): 457–65.

69 Kennedy DO, Little W, Scholey AB. Attenuation of laboratory-induced stress in humans after acute administration of Melissa officinalis (lemon balm). Psychosom Med, 2004 Jul–Aug; 66 (4): 607–13.

70 Bhattacharya SK, Bhattacharya A, Sairam K, et al. Anxiolytic-antidepressant activity of Withania somnifera glycowithanolides: An experimental study. Phytomedicine, 2000 Dec; 7 (6): 463–69.

71 Jain S, Shukla SD, Sharma K, et al. Neuroprotective effects of Withania somnifera Dunn. in hippocampal sub-regions of female albino rat. Phytother Res, 2001 Sep; 15 (6): 544–48.

72 Chandrasekhar K, Kapoor J, Anishetty S. A prospective, randomized double-blind, placebo-controlled study of safety and efficacy of a high-concentration full-spectrum extract of ashwagandha root in reducing stress and anxiety in adults. Indian J Psychol Med, 2012 Jul; 34 (3): 255–62.

73 Saratikov AS, Krasnov EA. Rhodiola rosea is a valuable medicinal plant (Golden root). Tomsk, Russia: Tomsk State University Press, 1987.

74 Ulbricht C, Chao W, Tanguay-Colucci S, et al. Rhodiola (Rhodiola spp.): An evidence-based systematic review by the natural standard research collaboration. Altern Complement Ther, 2011 May; 17 (2): 110–19.

75 Darbinyan V, Kteyan A, Panossian A, et al. Rhodiola rosea in stress induced fatigue—a double blind cross-over study of a standardized extract SHR-5 with a repeated low-dose regimen on the mental performance of healthy physicians during night duty. Phytomedicine, 2000 Oct; 7 (5): 365–71.

76 Shevtsov VA, Zholus BI, Shervarly VI, et al. A randomized trial of two different doses of a SHR-5 Rhodiola rosea extract versus placebo and control of capacity for mental work. Phytomedicine, 2003 Mar; 10 (2–3): 95–105.

77 National Institutes of Health. Magnesium. Fact Sheet. Available at: http://dietary-supplements.info.nih.gov/factsheets/magnesium.asp.

78 Sartori SB, Whittle, N, Hetzenauer A, et al. Magnesium deficiency induces anxiety and HPA axis dysregulation: Modulation by therapeutic drug treatment. Neuropharmacology, 2012 Jan; 62 (1): 304–12.

79 Paul S, Bhattacharya P, Das Mahapatra P, et al. Melatonin protects against endometriosis via regulation of matrix metalloproteinase-3 and an apoptatic pathway. J Pineal Res, 2010 Sep; 49 (2): 156–68.

80 Therapeutic Research staff. L-theainine. Therapeutic Research 2016. Available at: https://naturalmedicines.therapeuticresearch.com/databases/food,-herbs-supplements/professional.aspx?productid=1053#dosing.

81 Therapeutic Research staff. Hops. Therapeutic Research 2016. Available at: https://naturalmedicines.therapeuticresearch.com/databases/food,-herbs-supplements/professional.aspx?productid=856#dosing.

82 Mirabi P, Dolatian M, Mojab F, et al. Effects of valerian on the severity and systemic manifestations of dysmenorrhea. Int J Gynaecol Obstet, 2011 Dec; 115 (3): 285–88.

83 Therapeutic Research staff. Valerian. Therapeutic Research 2016. Available at: https://naturalmedicines.therapeuticresearch.com/databases/food,-herbs-supplements/professional.aspx?productid=870#dosing.

84 Therapeutic Research staff. Lemon Balm. Therapeutic Research 2016. Available at: https://naturalmedicines.therapeuticresearch.com/databases/food,-herbs-supplements/professional.aspx?productid=437#dosing.

85 Mirabi P, Dolatian M, Mojab F, et al. Effects of valerian on the severity and systemic manifestations of dysmenorrhea. Int J Gynaecol Obstet, 2011 Dec; 115 (3): 285–88.

86 Jonader M, Bastide J, Bastide P, et al. Enzyme inhibiting activites in vitro and in vivo angiopropective activity of Viburnum opulus L. Pharm Acta Helv, 1989; 64: 94–96.

Index

Library and Archives Canada Cataloguing in Publication

Cook, Andrew S. (Gynecologic surgeon), author
The endometriosis health & diet program : get your life back / Dr. Andrew S. Cook, MD, FACOG,
Danielle Cook, MS, RD, CDE.

Includes index.
ISBN 978-0-7788-0562-5 (softcover)

1. Endometriosis — Popular works. 2. Endometriosis — Diet therapy. 3. Endometriosis — Diet therapy
— Recipes. 4. Cookbooks. I. Cook, Danielle, 1975-, author II. Title. III. Title: Endometriosis health and
diet program.

RG483.E53C66 2017   618.1   C2017-900072-1